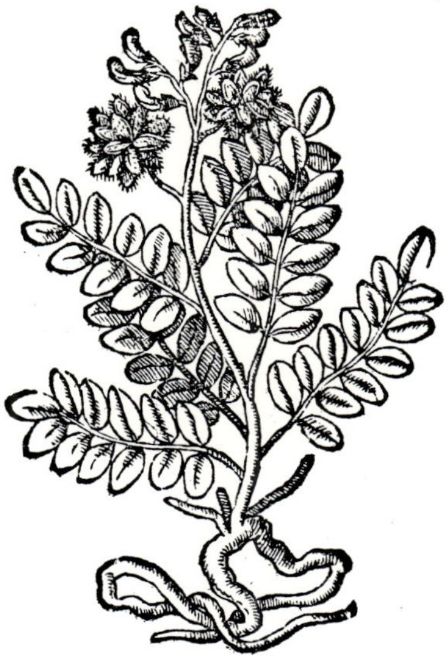

Healing Plants

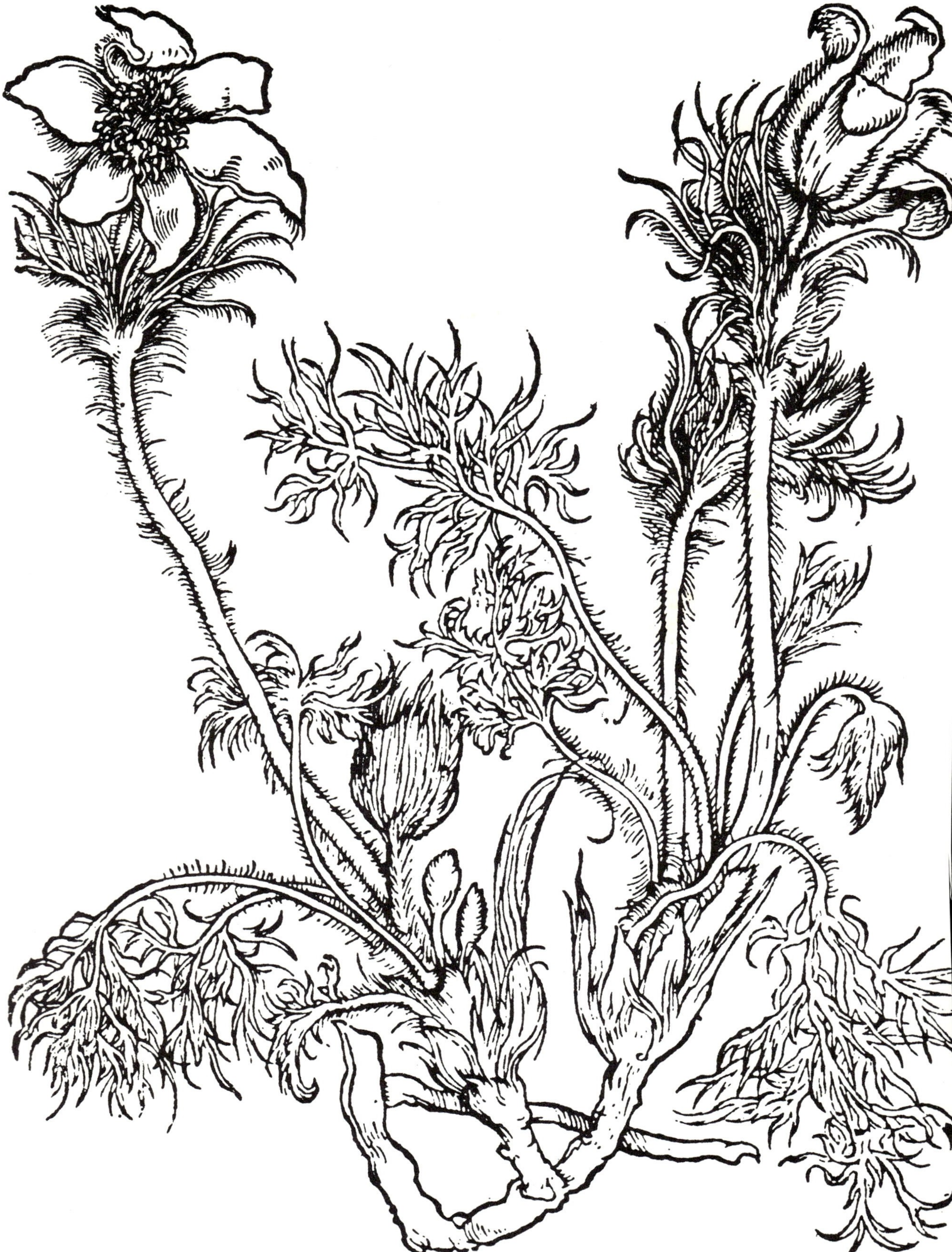

HEALING PLANTS

A MODERN HERBAL

EDITED BY

WILLIAM A.R. THOMSON, M.D.

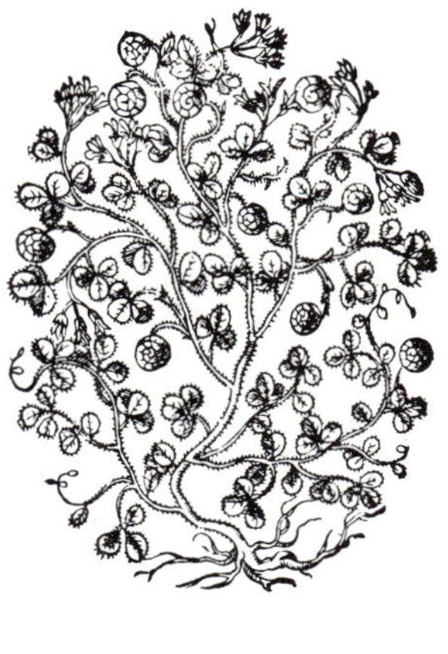

CAUTION

This book is not intended for prescribing medicines nor for curing afflictions. Its purpose is not to replace the services of a physician but rather to serve as a reference source on medicinal plants. We emphasize that the use of any of the information in this book for purposes of self-treatment without consulting a physician can be dangerous.

First published in the United Kingdom by
MACMILLAN LONDON LIMITED
London and Basingstoke
Associated companies in Delhi, Dublin, Hong Kong, Johannesburg, Lagos, Melbourne, New York, Singapore & Tokyo

Originally published in the USA by McGraw-Hill under the title
MEDICINES FROM THE EARTH
A Guide to Healing Plants
A McGraw-Hill Co-Publication

British Library Cataloguing in Publication Data
Healing plants.
1. Botany, Medical
I. Thomson, William Archibald Robson
581.6'34 QK99

ISBN 0-333-25604-2

Original Concept and Design by
EMIL M. BÜHRER

Translator:
R.E.K. MEUSS

Printed by:
IMPRIMERIES REUNIES, LAUSANNE, SWITZERLAND

Bound by:
MAURICE BUSENHART, LAUSANNE, SWITZERLAND

Composition by:
EDV+FILMSATZ AG, THUN, SWITZERLAND

Photolithography by:
FOTO-LITHO HEGO AG, LITTAU, SWITZERLAND

Printed in Switzerland

HEALING PLANTS

CONTENTS

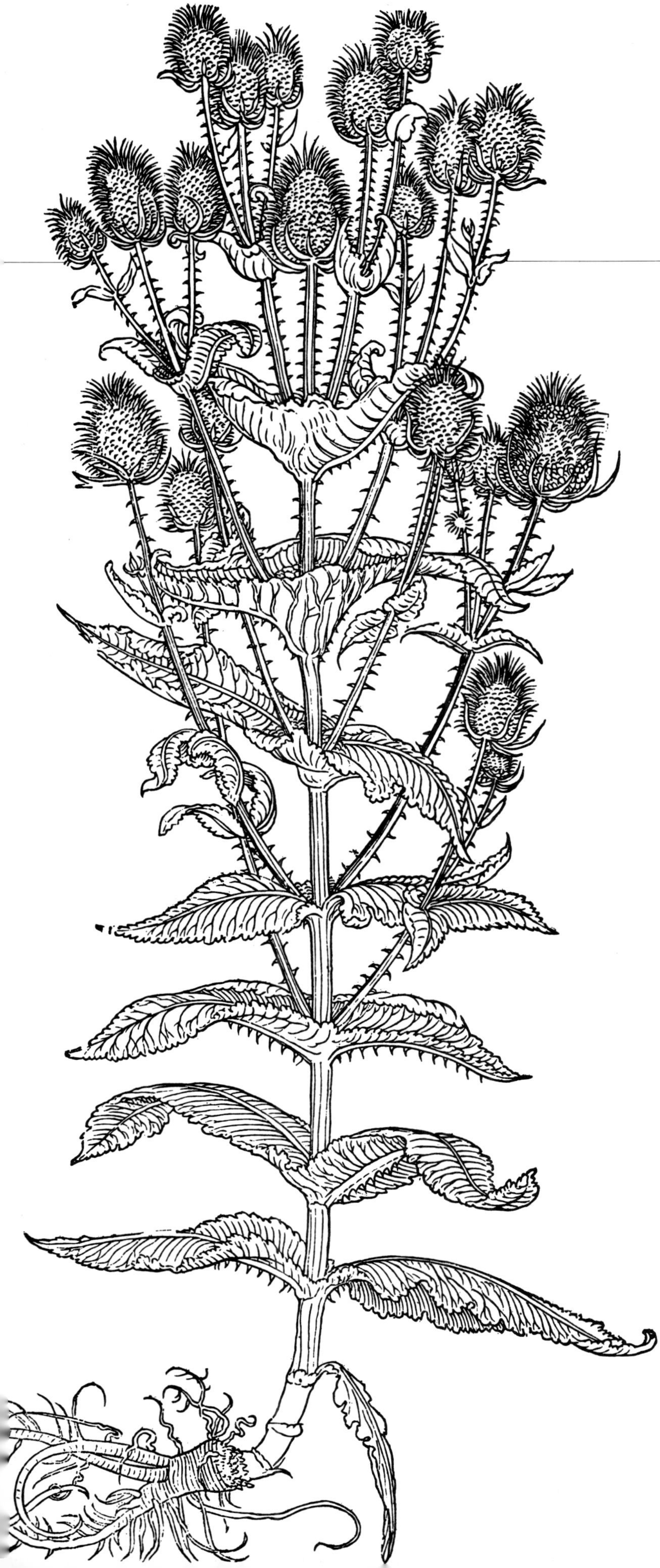

CONTRIBUTORS AND CONSULTANTS

General Editor

William A.R. Thomson, M.D.

Contributors

Richard Evans Schultes

Professor of Natural Sciences,
Harvard University;
Curator of Economic Botany,
Harvard Botanical Museum

Urte Knefeli

Specialist in Phytotherapy

Eugen Bossard

Druggist and Botanist
Pharmacological Journalist

Bruno Vonarburg

Phytotherapist

Consultants

Willem F. Daems

Lecturer,
Würzburg University, Germany,
and Ecole Suisse de Droguerie,
Neuchatel

Elias Landolt

Professor at the
Geobotanical Institute (Rübel Foundation),
Eidgenössische Technische Hochschule,
Zurich

Traugott Steger

Specialist in
Homeopathy and Phytotherapy

HOW TO USE THIS BOOK

This guide to healing plants can be considered two books in one: as both a botanical and a medical reference. It can be approached from either direction.

TO FIND INFORMATION ABOUT A PLANT:

1. *Botanical information—a description of the plant, with its distribution and location and a full-color illustration—is given in the Plant Lexicon (pp. 33–112).* Standard English names *of the Lexicon's 247 plants are indexed on pages 36–37. If a name does not appear there, it can be looked up in the English-Latin Plant Index at the end of the book, where many* alternative English names *for the 247 healing plants are listed and cross-referenced.*

2. *Medical information on plants is found in Reference Section I (pp. 17–32): a listing of the ailments and complaints for which each plant can be used. For further detail, see Reference Section III (pp. 161–184), in which the constituents of each plant and their healing properties are given.*

3. *Practical information on the gathering and processing of plants is also furnished in Reference Section III (pp. 161–184). For basic techniques of plant remedies, see the How-To section (pp. 151–160) on teas, decoctions, gargles, poultices, salves.*

TO FIND INFORMATION ABOUT A COMPLAINT OR ILLNESS:

1. *Common ailments and physical problems are listed and discussed in Reference Section II (pp. 113–136). For each ailment the reader is told whether prompt professional care is needed, whether a prescription or patent medicine based on plants is available, and whether he can use the homemade plant remedies given in detail here. The physician's preliminary word of caution (p. 113) should be observed.*

2. *For additional guidance in the treatment of ailments, the reader can refer to the chapter on basic techniques for the preparation of herbal teas, gargles, poultices, salves (pp. 151–160).*

Background information on healing plants can be found in the chapters beginning on pages 7, 137, and 185.

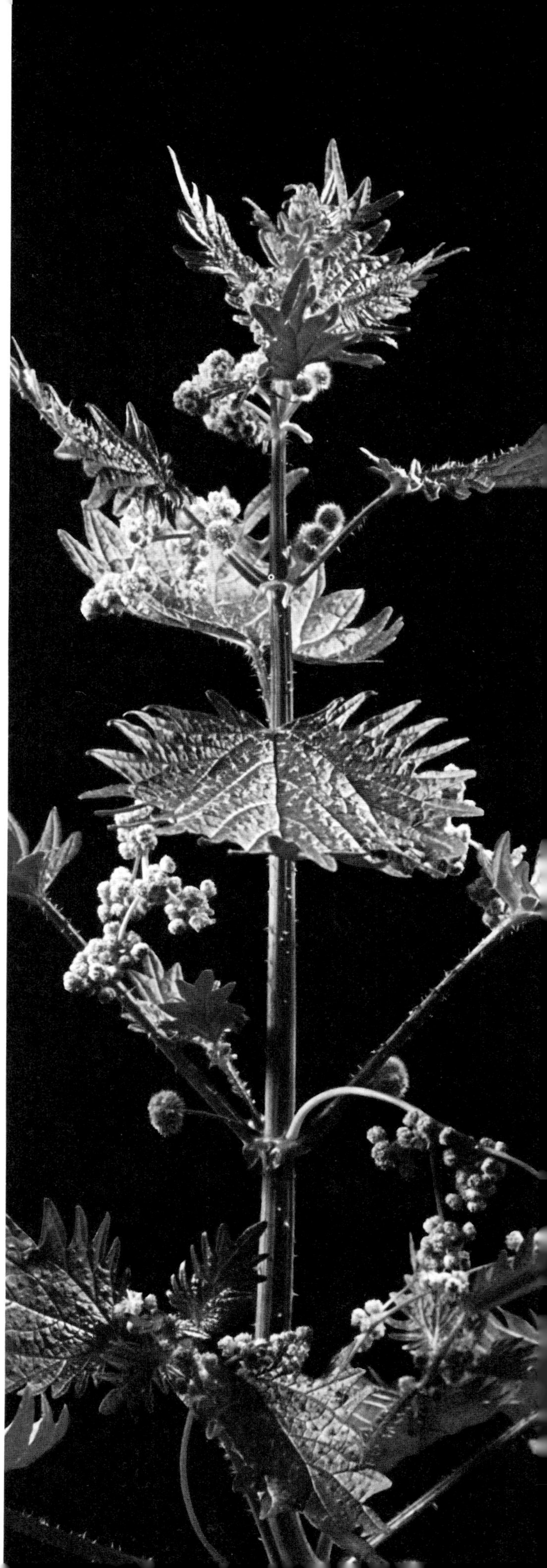

THE KINGDOM OF PLANTS

...god of his goodnesse that is creatour of all thynges
hath ordeyned for mankynde (whiche he hath created to his owne lykenesse)
for the grete and tender love,
which he hath unto hym to whom all erthely he hath ordeyned to be obeysant,
for the sustentacyon and helthe of his lovynge creature mankynde
whiche is onely made egally of the foure elementes
and qualities of the same,
and whan any of these foure haboundc or hath more domynacyon,
the one than the other it constrayneth ye body of man to grete infyrmytees or dyseases,
for the whiche ye eternall god hath gyven of his haboundante grace,
vertues in all maner of herbes to cure and heale
all maner of sekenesses or infyrmytes
to hym befallyng thrugh the influent course of the foure elementes beforesayd,
and of the corrupcyons and
ye venymous ayres contrarye ye helthe of man....
O ye worthy reders
or practicyens to whome this noble volume is present
I beseche yow take intellygence and beholde ye workes and operacyons of almyghty
god which hathe endowed his symple creature mankynde
with the graces of ye holy goost
to have parfyte knowledge and understangynge of the vertue of all maner
of herbes and trees in this booke comprehendyd.

The grete herball whiche geveth parfyt knowlege and understandyng of all maner of herbes and there gracyous vertues...
Colophon: Peter Treveris. London, 1526.

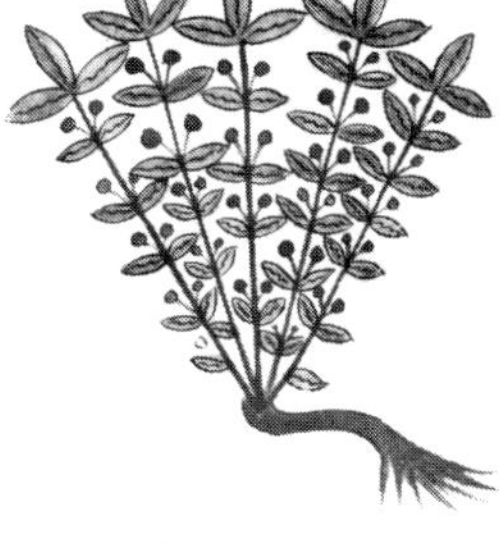

Throughout the development of human cultures, the relationship between man and his ambient vegetation has been intimate and vital. Man truly has lived with and depended on his green plants. It therefore is understandable that throughout all of prehistory and most of history, *botany* and *medicine,* for practical purposes, have been synonymous fields of knowledge. The shaman or medicineman—usually an accomplished botanist—represents probably the oldest professional man in social evolution. Most of the medicines, as well as foods, which we now use from the Plant Kingdom were not discovered by the sciences of modern, sophisticated societies, but by trial and error over millennia in unlettered cultures. Archaeology tells us that some of today's most highly prized drugs are heritages from the dim past of preshistory.

WHAT ARE HEALING PLANTS?

How did man ever learn of healing plants? With the intense experimentation that early man certainly practiced with plants, it had to be inevitable.

Man probably put most plants into his mouth. Many were innocuous, a few nourished him, and a number made him ill or killed him. Some, however, relieved symptoms of discomfort or sickness and a very few, through hallucinations, took him from this mundane existence to the realms of ethereal wonder. The plants in the last two categories became his medicines.

Every culture had individuals ready to take advantage of the gullibilities of their fellow men. At an early period, knowledge of the presumed medicinal properties and virtues of plants became associated with certain individuals: the medicine men. They rose to exalted positions, thanks to their actual knowledge of healing herbs, and exercised a form of primitive blackmail resulting from a fear of their supposed powers. The use of healing plants gradually became linked with superstition and magic and, finally, with the Doctrine of Demonology. This doctrine exploited the concept that health could not be restored until the demon causing the disease was expelled. Consequently, what was bad for the demon was good for the patient. Often, the more nauseous the drug, the more efficacious it was believed to be. It is no coincidence that the earliest medicinal plants were direct action drugs (e.g., emetics, purgatives).

Very early, however, man discovered plants with curious psychic effects: the hallucinogens. These "super-medicines"—usually tools of the shaman—became his medicines *par excellence* and enabled him to diagnose the cause and treat the disease through contact with the supernatural.

Primitive societies believed in healing by similarity. A red resin, for example, meant that the plant was good for the blood. This curious notion came down through classical Greece and Rome to Europe where, in medieval times, it was formulated as the Doctrine of Signatures by Paracelsus. All plants, it was believed, were placed on earth for man's benefit. The Creator had put

A HOLY STORY

Told by Chief Maza Blaska (Flat-Iron, meaning a piece of flat iron). Maza Blaska is one of the oldest living chiefs of the Ogallalla band.

From Wakan-Tanka, the Great Mystery, comes all power. It is from Wakan-Tanka that the Holy Man has wisdom and the power to heal and to make holy charms. Man knows that all healing plants are given by Wakan-Tanka; therefore are they holy.

To the Holy Man comes in youth the knowledge that he will be holy. The Great Mystery makes him to know this. Sometimes it is the Spirits who tell him. The Spirits come not in sleep always, but also when man is awake.

With the Spirits the Holy Man may commune always, and they teach him holy things.

The Holy Man goes apart to a lone tipi and fasts and prays. Or he goes into the hills in solitude. When he returns to men, he teaches them and tells them what the Great Mystery has bidden him to tell. He counsels, he heals, and he makes holy charms to protect the people from all evil. Great is his power and greatly is he revered; his place in the tipi is an honored one.

The people were encamped in a circle with the opening towards the east. In the middle of the circle they set up a great tipi made of several tipis put together. On one side of the tipi sat the women, on the other side the men. And they made ready a great feast. Beyond the central fire, opposite the doorway, the Holy Man made mystery. With a stick like an arrow he made a line of holes in the ground a finger's-length deep. Then he

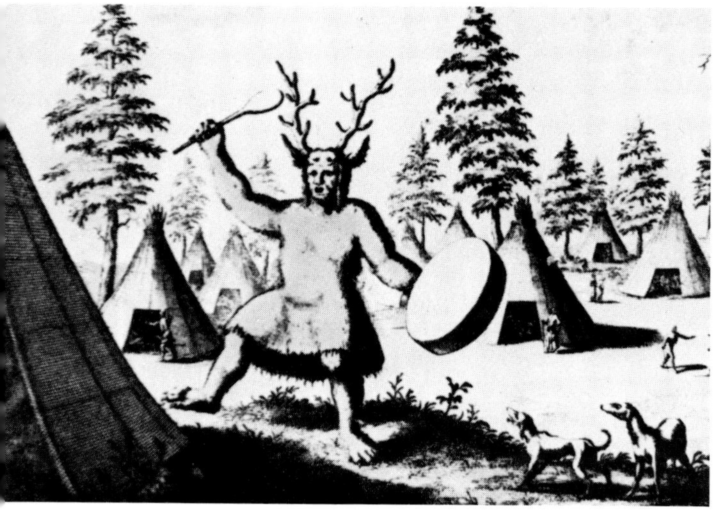

The shaman, or holy man, served as doctor in many so-called primitive societies, because of his thorough knowledge of the effects of plants. The illustration shows a Siberian shaman.

touched the ground in front of all the people and came back to the doorway and sat down. And he bade the people hasten to prepare the mystery. So they took clay and filled the holes with it and covered the holes with earth. When they had done this the Holy Man touched the ground. Then he came back to the doorway and was about to sing. And the people watched the ground where the clay was buried, and behold, young plants began to sprout. Then, before he sang, the Holy Man said:

Far to the west,
Far by the sky
Stands a blue Elk.
That Elk standing yonder
Watches o'er all the females
On the earth.

Thus he spoke; then he said, "Now I will sing," and beating on his drum he sang a holy song. When he had sung he bade the people pull up the sprouts, and they did so; one by one they pulled them up. And behold, the roots were holy mystery-power. And the people took the mystery-power and laid it on sprigs of sage, for sage is holy because it will heal. This mystery would protect the warriors in war. No arrow could pierce them, no arrow could strike them, unharmed would they pass through every danger.

So have I told of how a Holy Man made mystery to help the people. Now may Wakan-Tanka help me, because I have spoken truly of how Wakan-Tanka bade the Indians to do in the olden times.

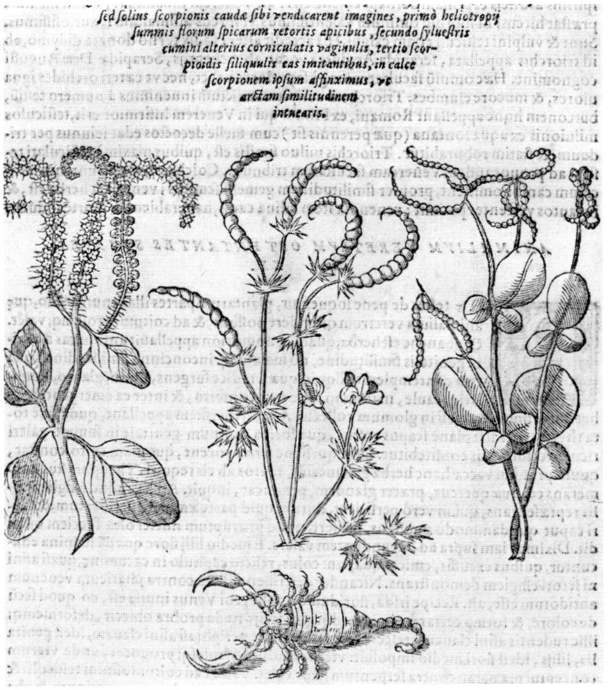
sed solius scorpionis caudæ sibi vendicarent imagines, primò heliotropij
summis florum spicarum retortis apicibus, secundo syluestris
cumini alterius corniculatis vaginulis, tertio scor-
pioidis siliquulis eas imitantibus, in calce
scorpionem ipsum affinximus, vt
arctam similitudinem
intuearis.

According to the Doctrine of Signatures elaborated in the sixteenth century, a plant's external appearance offered clues to its effectiveness. Thus the "scorpion-tail" heliotrope and similar plants were believed to cure scorpion bites: drawing from Giambattista della Porta's *Phytognomica* (1558).

a sign, or signature, indicating their use on plants not obviously valuable for food, fiber, etc. A heart-shaped leaf signaled its cardiac properties; a liver-shaped leaf was a sign of efficacy against jaundice. This doctrine was taken to even more absurd lengths by Porta, who discovered the most recondite of signatures and associated medical botany with astrology. Modern concepts of healing plants began in Europe with the appearance of herbals in the sixteenth century, resulting in great volumes of true and false information about the healing properties of plants. Progress was only slow and gradual, but a good percentage of our currently esteemed drug plants go back to this era and, in many cases, to even earlier times and more primitive societies.

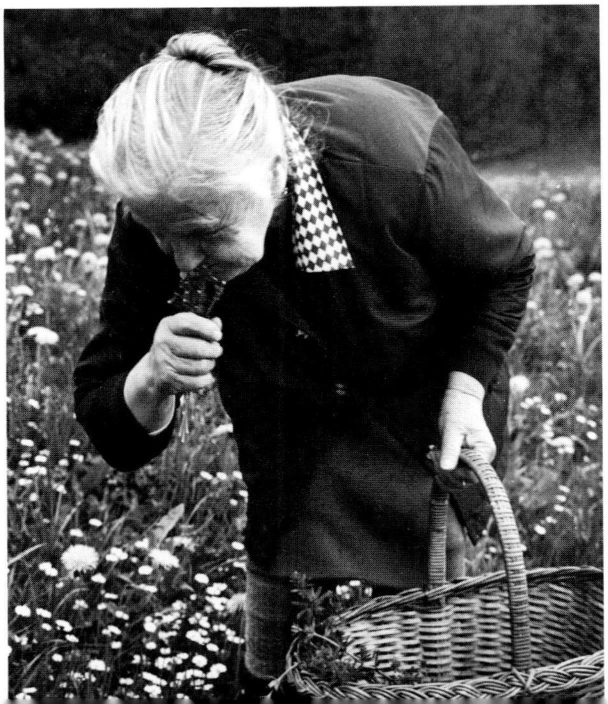

Women in some rural areas maintain the tradition of collecting medicinal herbs.

THE SIZE OF THE PLANT KINGDOM

No botanist, with certainty, can give an estimate of the size of the Plant Kingdom. Modern estimates vary between 250,000 and 500,000 species or more. Whichever figure is accepted, it represents a very large and heterogeneous assemblage of organisms—each different and each a distinct chemical factory; consequently, each of potential interest from the view point of utility. In 1753, Linnaeus, the Father of Systematic Botany, classified what he felt was the whole Plant Kingdom, stating that the "number of plants in the whole world is much less than is commonly believed," calculating that it "hardly reaches 10,000." A century later, in 1847, Lindley credited the Plant Kingdom with a total of 100,000 species in nearly 9,000 *genera.*

There has been a growing belief among botanists during the present century that previous estimates fall far short of the real extent of the Plant Kingdom and that a minimum of 500,000 species may give a truer picture of its size.

A few estimates by modern specialists in the different groups will indicate how far botanical knowledge has advanced since Lindley's estimate of 130 years ago. It is now believed that there are some 1,500 species of bacteria. The fungi are calculated at from 30,000 to 100,000; their study in the wet tropics, where they abound, has just begun and one contemporary mycologist has stated that even 200,000 might come nearer the grand total of species. An ancient group, the algae, are variously estimated at from 19,000 to 32,500 species, with one group—the diatoms—accounting for 6,000 to 10,000. The lichens are credited with 16,000 to 20,000 species. The bryophytes—mosses and liverworts—may have as many as 25,000 species, and the ferns and their allies 10,000. The gymnosperms are still a small group of some 700 species in 65 *genera.* The most extensive group of plants now dominant on land and man's principal source of healing plants, the angiosperms, comprise at least 250,000 species in 10,500 *genera* in 300 families. Of the angiosperms, one-quarter are monocotyledons; three-quarters dicotyledons.

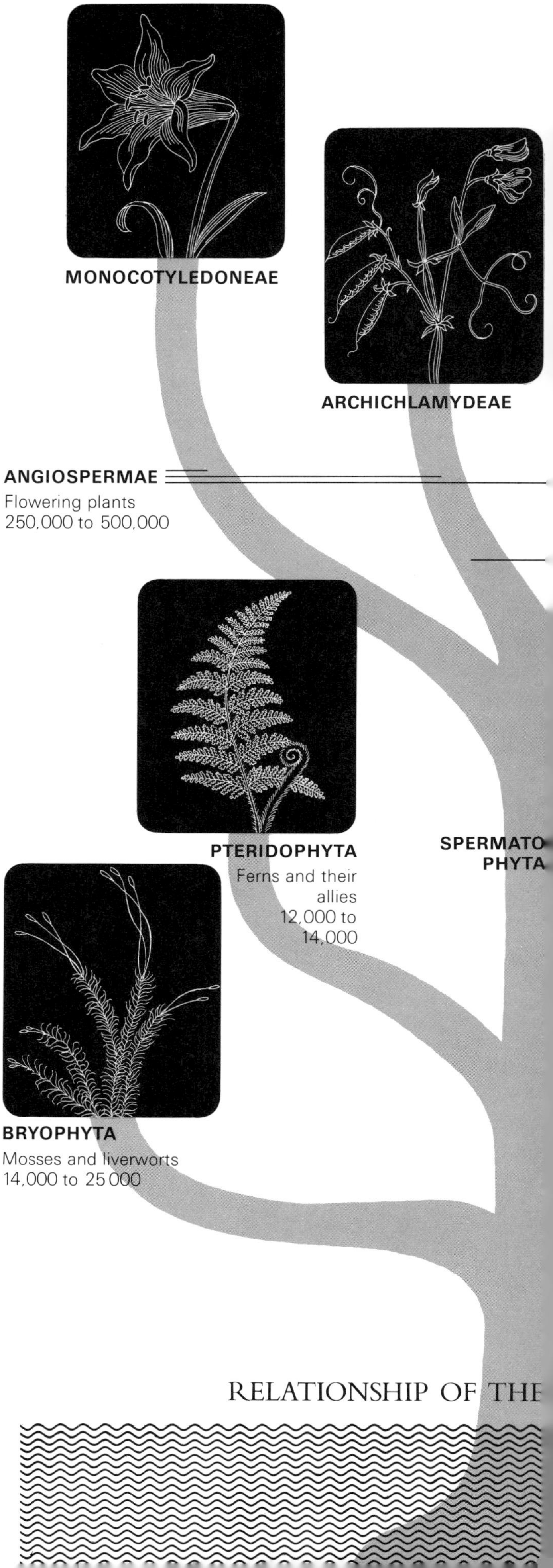
MONOCOTYLEDONEAE
ARCHICHLAMYDEAE
ANGIOSPERMAE
Flowering plants
250,000 to 500,000
PTERIDOPHYTA
Ferns and their allies
12,000 to 14,000
SPERMATO-PHYTA
BRYOPHYTA
Mosses and liverworts
14,000 to 25 000
RELATIONSHIP OF THE

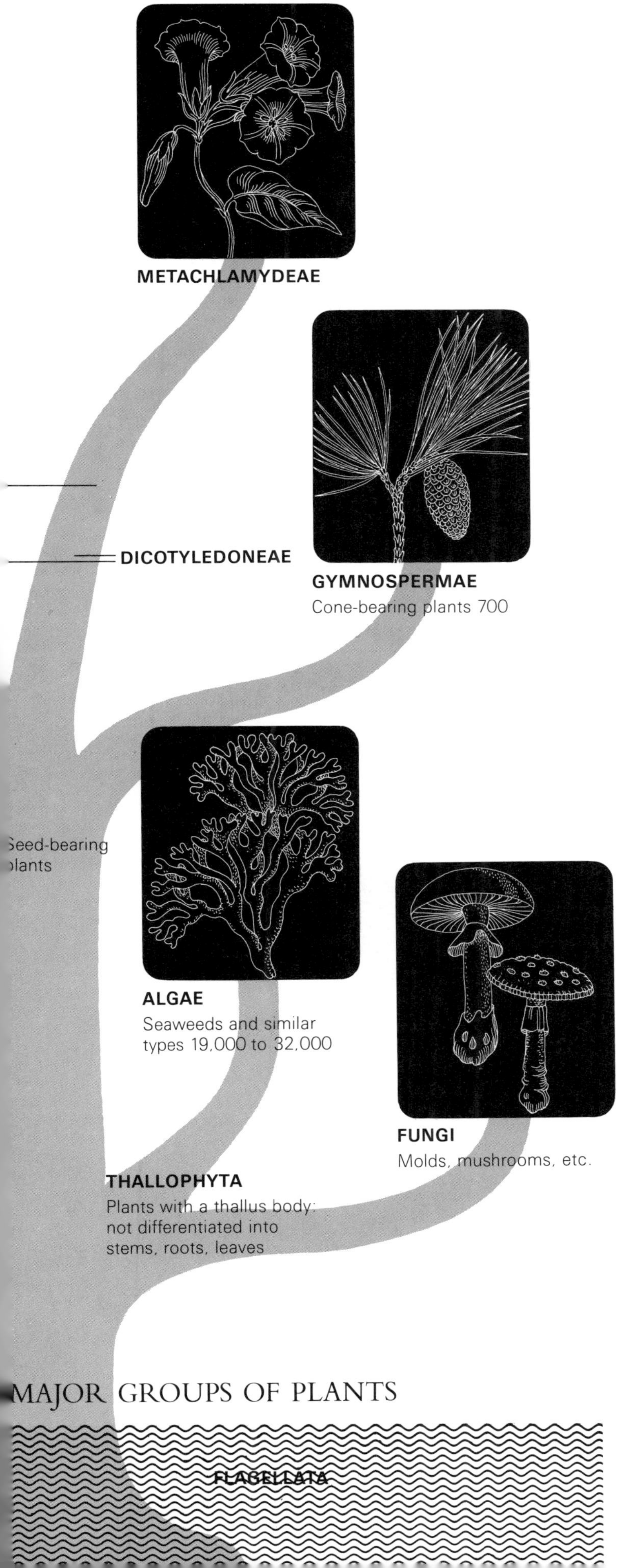

MAJOR GROUPS OF PLANTS

ACTIVE PRINCIPLES OF HEALING PLANTS

The medicinal value of drug plants is due to the presence in the plant tissue of a chemical substance—an active principle—producing a physiological effect. Many of the active principles are highly complex and their exact chemical nature occasionally is still unknown; others have been isolated, purified, and even synthesized or simulated. They most commonly fall into one of six categories: alkaloids, glycosides, essential oils, gums and resins, fatty oils, and antibiotic substances.

Alkaloids and glycosides are defined elsewhere (see p. 14). Essential oils usually have various chemical constituents; usually terpene derivatives or aromatic compounds. They rarely consist of a single constituent, but often contain alcohols, ketones, aldehydes, phenols, ethers, esters, and other compounds, as well as, sometimes, nitrogen and sulphur. Many are highly germicidal, this property being due to their volatility and ability to penetrate into proto-

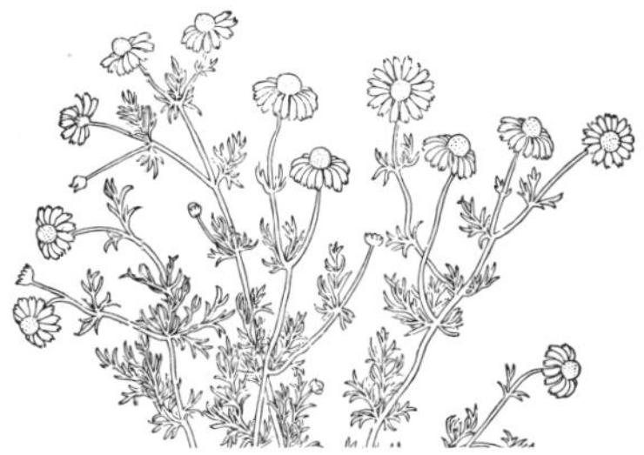

plasm, but they usually are too insoluble in water to be important in medicine as antiseptics. They are valuable as carminatives, in cough drops, mouth washes, gargles, sprays, and healing ointments. Gums are polymers of various rarer sugars and resins are oxidation products of essential oils; both are employed as purgatives and in ointments. Fatty oils or lipids—esters of fatty acids—are used in emulsions and as purgatives. Antibiotic substances are various complex organic compounds—usually from molds, actinomycetes, and bacteria—capable, in small amounts, of inhibiting life processes of microorganisms.

Healing plants may act in a great variety of ways. Many (e.g., carminatives) exert a soothing action. A large number act on the nervous system (e.g., belladonna). Others have neuromuscular (e.g., digitalis) or muscular (e.g., false hellebore) activity. The antibiotics heal by killing or inhibiting pathogenic microorganisms, especially bacteria.

THE IMPORTANCE OF HERBARIA, BOTANICAL GARDENS, AND EXPLORATION

Rare herbs and new fruit and vegetable varieties from all over the world have been studied and cultivated in the botanical gardens and *herbaria* that were constructed in Europe. The Physical Garden in Chelsea, England *(right),* founded in the mid-eighteenth century, is still in use. Shown at bottom right: the botanical garden in Leyden, Holland, around 1610.

The 150 years from Linnaeus's time throughout the nineteenth century was a period of intensive botanical exploration in many virgin territories. Even today, botanists are delving into ever more distant regions, especially the tropics, and are describing upwards of 5,000 new species and varieties of plants a year.

Many causes contributed to this post-Linnaean upsurge in plant exploration. Newer and faster methods of travel, population pressures in Europe, the growing need for exotic products from the warmer parts of the world, colonialism, and other socio-political factors had their effect. Yet intellectual and commercial interest in the plant world must also be counted as a major factor. For, after the Linnaean period, great botanical gardens and herbaria were established and their function and purposes underwent changes from similar institutions that existed in the past.

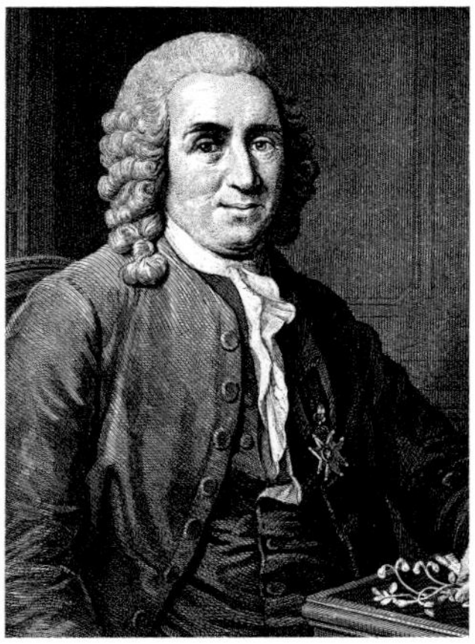

The Swedish naturalist Carl Linnaeus (1707–1778) established the binomial system of biological nomenclature and laid the groundwork for the study of ecology. In 1905 his pioneering botanical classification system was adopted internationally, and zoologists accepted his *Systema Naturae* (1758) as an authority in the scientific naming of plants and animals.

Botanical gardens usually are not recognized as a vital element in the study of medicinal plants. Quite generally they are considered solely in terms of horticulture: the introduction into cultivation and improvement of plants for their beauty. From earliest times, however, botanical gardens, which gradually grew out of olive groves and temple gardens, have played a major role in medical botany. The Egyptians had a utilitarian garden at Karnak in 1500 B.C. A botanical garden in Athens, of which Theophrastus was director in 350 B.C., received seeds of useful plants—many being medicinal—sent by Alexander the Great from his conquests as far east as India. Throughout the Dark Ages and early Middle Ages, monks in Europe maintained herb gardens. Beginning with the appearance of the herbals in Europe, many herbalists—the botanists of their time—maintained their own gardens. John Gerard of London had one of the most famous gardens in the seventeenth century. One such garden, the Chelsea Physic Garden in London, is still in operation.

In the New World, the ancient Aztecs had their garden outside of Mexico, devoted partially to medicinal herbs, but it disappeared after the Spanish conquest. Charles III established a botanical garden in Mexico in 1788 and, during this period, three famous botanical expeditions were sent from Spain to several parts of the Spanish possessions in America for a study of the flora, with special reference to useful plants: Sessé and Mociño to Mexico, the Royal Expedition to New Granada (Colombia and Ecuador) under the direction of Mutis, and the Royal Expedition to the Kingdom of Peru and Chile conducted by Ruíz and Pavón. The two royal expeditions to South America devoted very special attention to a study of Cinchona, the source of antimalarial quinine.

There are now more than 400 botanical gardens throughout the world, in many of which research is in progress on some aspect of medicinal plants.

The vital importance of botanical gardens in the establishment and study of medicinal and other economic plants is best illustrated by recalling several examples. Coffee, native to Abyssinia, was first introduced to Brazil, now the source of 75 percent of the world's supply, during the 1700s from the Jardin des Plantes in Paris. Botanical gardens maintained by the British and Dutch played major roles in the establishment of plantation quinine trees in Asia from wild material collected in the Andes of South America. Without a chain of efficient botanical gardens, such as those at Kew and in Ceylon, the introduction of the rubber tree from the Amazon to the Old World would never have been effected successfully.

Linnaeus made several contributions to botany, but two seem to be of fundamental importance: the establishment of a binomial system of nomenclature, and the establishment of an *herbarium* to authenticate the system of nomenclature.

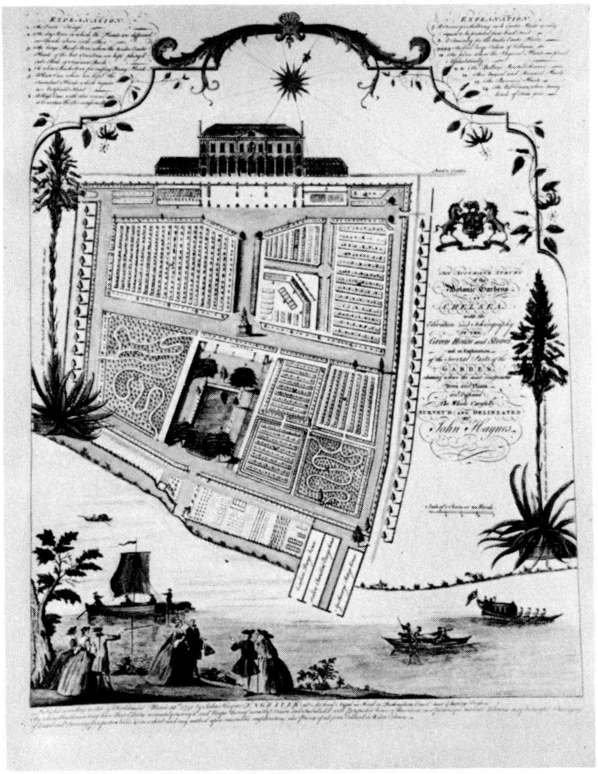

The *herbarium*—an archival collection of pressed, dried plant specimens—changed botanical classification from an inexact art to an exact science. For the first time in scientific history, the naming of plants could be standardized, leading to the use of one name for a species around the world. Vouchered specimens, upon which the name and first description of the species were based, filed away in permanent collections, could be available to research scholars of future generations.

In pre-Linnaean times, plants often were not known by a short word or two, but by long descriptive phrases of several or many words in different languages. Linnaeus, who employed Latin as the scientific language of the period, adopted the custom of describing a species and assigning each species to a higher category of related organisms—the *genus*. Each plant was given a species name and a generic name. Thus, the foxglove, belonging to the *genus Digitalis* and representing the species *purpurea*, was known as *Digitalis purpurea* and easily could be set apart nomenclaturally from the related woolly-leafed member of the *genus* known as *Digitalis lanata*. By international agreement, Latin—a dead language not subject, like living languages, to changes in meaning of words—is still the official language of botanical classification.

Linnaeus was not the first to create an *herbarium*, but he used his plant specimens as a basis for describing and naming species. His book *Species Plantarum*, published in 1753, is accepted universally as the starting point of modern botanical nomenclature. Although botanists are still actively classifying and naming plants new to science, they generally follow the parameters established by Linnaeus. Linnaeus's own *herbarium*, preserved in the Linnaean Society of London, can be consulted by contemporary botanists to clarify the use of a binomial or historical background in classifying large groups of plants.

The *herbarium* is now an essential adjunct of botanical institutions, not only for theoretical research into plant classification and evolution, but also as an almost untapped resource into collectors' notes on the uses of plants in primitive societies around the world. This information is not only firsthand, but the data concerning locality, people, and time are precise. Furthermore, unlike many citations of native uses in literature, there exists the voucher specimen for authentication of the identity of the plant. Several "*herbarium* searches" for aboriginal medicinal uses of plants recently have been carried out with very promising results. One search yielded more than 7,500 reports, many of which bear investigation by modern phytochemical and pharmacological methods.

The size of several of the larger *herbaria* illustrates how vast may be the potentiality for discovery from collectors' notes of ethnopharmacological hints. Among the largest are the Paris *herbarium* with 7.2 million specimens; Leningrad and Geneva, each with 5 million; the Royal Botanic Gardens in England with 4 to 5 million; and Harvard University with approximately 4 million.

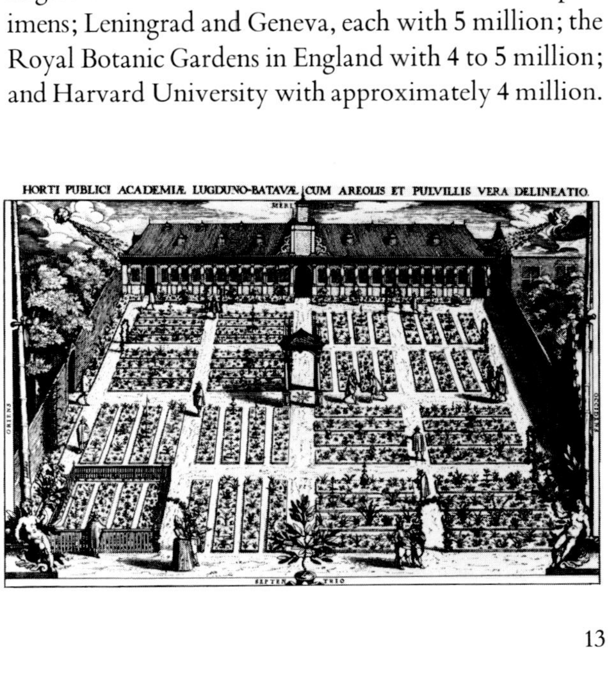
HORTI PUBLICI ACADEMIÆ LUGDUNO-BATAVÆ CUM AREOLIS ET PULVILLIS VERA DELINEATIO.

PLANTS AS CHEMICAL FACTORIES

A plant is the site of intense activity: photosynthesis turns carbon dioxide and water into sugars by means of solar energy, and metabolic action then creates many secondary organic compounds from the sugar.

More than 12,000 of these secondary organic plant principles have been isolated, and many of them have proved useful in medicine. The most important principles from the medical viewpoint are the alkaloids and glycosides.

Alkaloids are a diverse group of alkaline compounds with marked physiological activity; their ring structure is usually complex and always contains nitrogen. The alkaloids include morphine (first isolated in 1805), cocaine, nicotine, and quinine, and more than 5,500 others; more than 90 percent of the known alkaloids are found in flowering plants.

The plant families richest in alkaloids are the Nightshade, Pea, Madder, Logania, Lily, and Amaryllis Families and above all the Dogbane Family, which alone contains 18 percent of all known alkaloids. The richest genera are *Nicotiana, Vinca* (source of the antileukemic compounds vincristine and vinclastine), and *Strychnos;* rich single species include the poppy, *Papaver somniferum* (source of opium), with 25 alkaloids, and the Indian snakeroot, *Rauvolfia serpentina* (source of the tranquilizer reserpine), with approximately 30.

Glycosides are compounds which, when hydrolized, yield a component of one or several sugars (i.e., glycone) and a nonsugar component (aglycone).

There are 11 types of glycosides, classified according to their aglycone moiety. Among the most important in modern medicine are the cardiac glycosides (in the Dogbane, Milkweed, Lily, Mulberry, Buttercup, Figwort Families). *Digitalis,* one of our most widely prescribed drugs of plant origin, owes its activity to cardiac glycosides. Cyanogenic glycosides yielding hydrocanic acid have been reported from some 2,000 species in 112 angiosperm families. Recently, steroidal sapogenins (in the Pea, Figwort, Nightshade, Caltrop, Amaryllis, Lily, and Yam Families), have been reported from some 2,000 species in 112 angiosperm families.

To anyone working in the ethnopharmacology and phytochemistry of the Plant Kingdom, it must appear obvious that our discoveries of Nature's wonder drugs have only just begun.

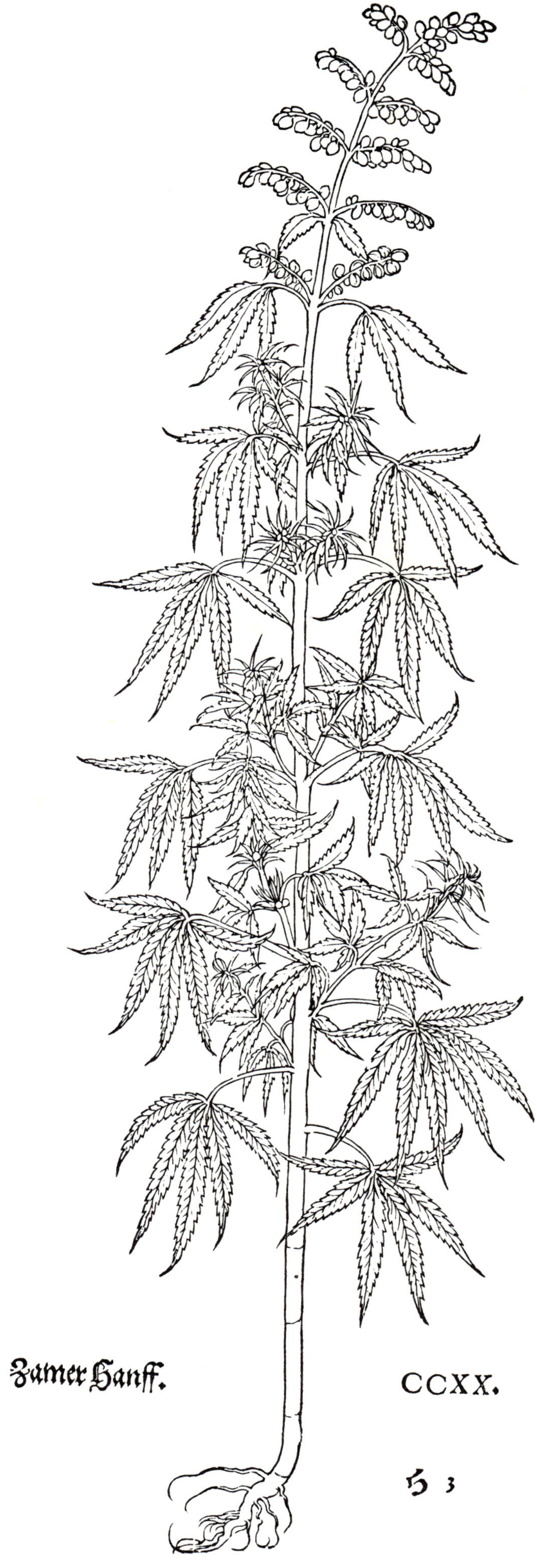

THE VERSATILE BENEFITS OF PLANTS

MEDICINE

Cannabis has been valued from earliest times for its powerful psychoactive and physical effects. In lands that possessed Cannabis, the plant was credited with healing properties. Throughout medieval Europe, it was very important as a medicinal herb, and was included in the United States Pharmacopoeia as a tranquilizer until 1937. Today, approximately 50 cannabinolic constituents have been discovered, of which some are promising as medicinally valuable compounds.

FOOD

In times of scarcity or famine, the akene (fruit) of Cannabis, though not very palatable, has been used as food for both animals and man. Today, it is a major constituent of bird feed in the United States. Cannabis fruits may have been domesticated originally for use as a food plant.

OIL

The fruit of Cannabis is very oil-rich. In central Asia, the oil has been extracted and used for centuries for domestic purposes (e.g., oil lamps). The greenish-yellow oil is excellent for paints, varnishes, and soap-making and in the leather industry. It resembles cottonseed oil, with 75 percent unsaturated and 25 percent fatty acids.

FIBER

Hempen fibers, one of the most useful products of the Plant Kingdom, have been found in some of the earliest archaeological sites from China to Asia Minor. Many strains of this plant were developed for long and strong fibers throughout history since they are well suited for cordage. The fibers are processed by retting.

NARCOTIC

In some areas of Asia, the narcotic influence of Cannabis placed it, very early, as a sacred plant for ceremonial use. It was known in India and China as early as 1500 B.C., but apparently was unknown in classical Mediterranean countries and medieval Europe. The ancient Scythians, who used it in a narcotic vapor bath, spread its use from central Asia.

CHEMICAL COMPOUNDS FROM PLANTS

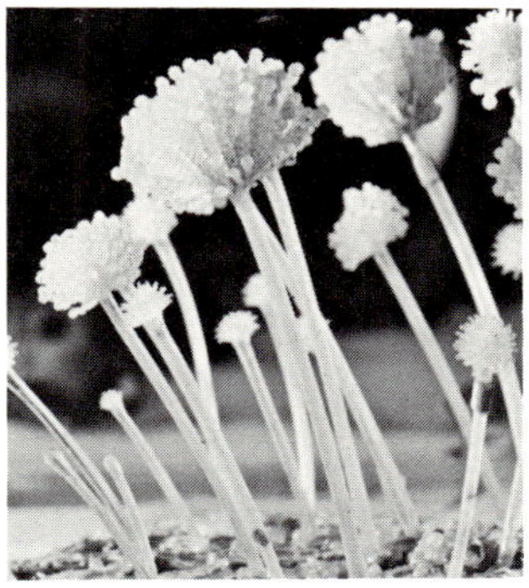

Mold *(Aspergillus herbariorum)*

ANTIBIOTICS

One-quarter of the prescriptions written in the United States call for antibiotics. The word means "against life" and describes the destructive or inhibiting activity to life processes of microorganisms by interfering with the metabolism of the organisms. They are complex chemical compounds. Penicillin, the first discovered and still one of the most important, produced by *Penicillium notatum* and *P. chrysogenum*, is not a pure compound but a mixture of several fractions.

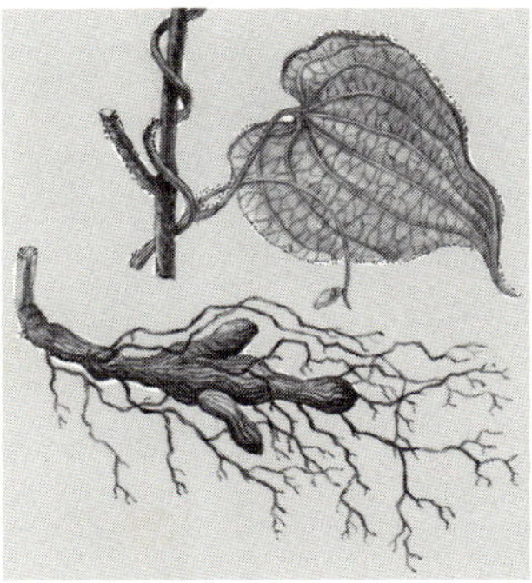

Yam *(Dioscorea villosa)*

STEROIDS

Steroids are found in plants and animals and may be synthetic. They have complex structures, but all have a 4-membered hydrocarbon ring system: *perhydrocyclopenta phenanthrene*. They are colorless, crystalline solids differing in the substitution of groups attached to the nucleus.

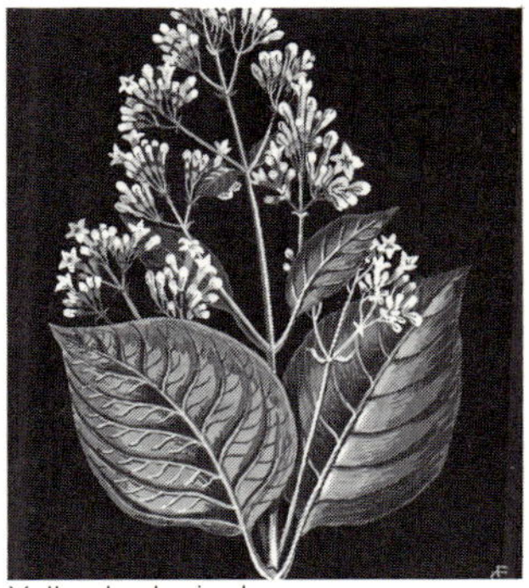

Yellowbark cinchona
(Cinchona succirubra)

ALKALOIDS

The bark of several species of *Cinchona*, Andean trees of the Madder Family, contains some 25 related alkaloids with a quinoline nucleus: principally quinine, quinidine, cinchonine, and cinchonidine. These alkaloids have febrifugal properties and have been employed for many years in treating malaria—especially quinine. Totaquine is a mixture of all cinchona alkaloids (cheaper to produce) sometimes used instead of the purified quinine or quinidine.

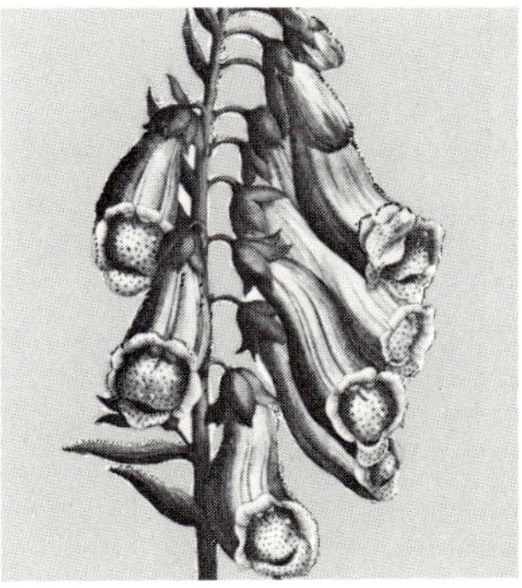

Foxglove *(Digitalis purpurea)*

GLYCOSIDES

Foxglove—*Digitalis purpurea*—owes its cardiotonic activity to a number of glycosides: principally digitoxin, a microcrystalline white powder that increases the tone of the cardiac muscle, causing the heart to be more effectively emptied, and is extremely toxic. The same and other glycosides—gitalin, digoxin, lanatoside C, deslanoside, etc.—occur in other species, especially the commercially valuable *D. lanata*. Digitonin, a glycoside from foxglove, combines with cholesterol.

THE FUTURE OF PLANTS IN MEDICINE

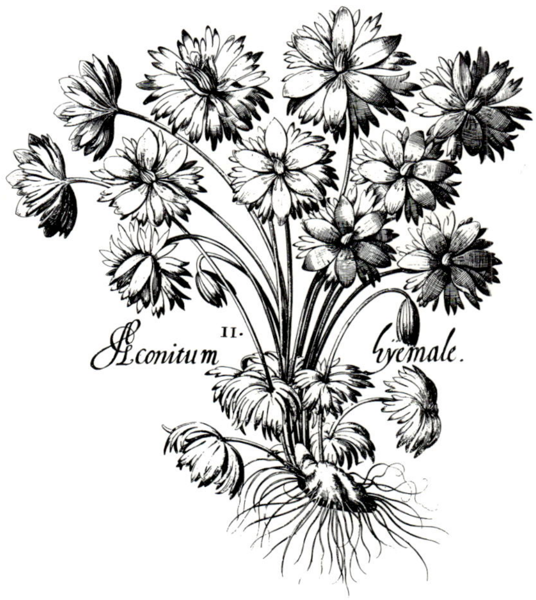

It has been estimated that only 10 percent of the organic constituents in the Plant Kingdom have been discovered. Modern phytochemistry, with extraordinarily new sophisticated techniques, must assure astonishing new finds in the next few years, when larger segments of the Plant Kingdom are thoroughly examined. For, to date, chemical studies have been desultory, erratic, and incomplete.

For the future of medicine, more intensive studies are imperative. Even though former times saw a great percentage of medicaments come from plants, a few statistics about the present will indicate the bright future that looms ahead for medical botany. In 1973, 38 percent of the 1.5 billion prescriptions filled in the United States contained active constituents from higher plants or employed microbial products, and drugs from the higher plants amounted to a $3 billion business.

The period of 1930 through 1960 was remarkable in medical botany, characterized by the successive discovery of many startlingly effective "Wonder Drugs," almost all of which were of vegetal origin. Beginning with the muscle relaxing alkaloids derived from South American arrow poisons and the discovery of penicillin and many other antibiotics from molds, actinomycetes, bacteria, lichens, and other plants, the series continued unabated. There came cortisone precursors from sapogenins; hypotensive agents from *Veratrum;* cytotoxic principles from *Podophyllum, Vinca,* and other sources; khellin from *Ammi Visnaga;* reserpine from the Indian snake root; and others, not to mention the numerous psychoactive compounds of potential value in experimental psychiatry. Not only have new drugs been discovered, but studies have led to novel uses of older drugs.

If so many revolutionary discoveries have come about within the past few years, why assume that, with ever more sophisticated chemical and pharmacological techniques, the future will see an end to such progress? The chemical examination of the Plant Kingdom—as Linnaeus prophesied two centuries ago—truly has only just begun.

RICHARD EVANS SCHULTES

Man, ever desirous of Knowledge, has already
explored many things; but more and greater
still remain concealed; perhaps reserved for far
distant generations, who shall prosecute
the examination of their Creator's work in remote
countries, and make many discoveries for
the pleasure and convenience of life.
Posterity shall see its increasing Museums, and
the knowledge of the Divine Wisdom,
flourish together; and at the same time all
the practical sciences ... shall be enriched;
for we cannot avoid thinking, that what we know
of the Divine works are much fewer than those
of which we are ignorant.

Linnaeus

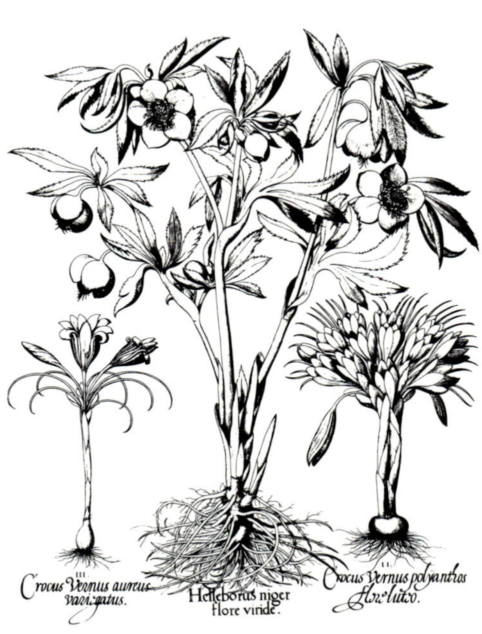

The 247 Most Beneficial Plants

Reference Section I

On the following pages the reader will find an alphabetical list of the 247 major medicinal plants. Beside each plant is a list of complaints or minor illnesses (such as sore throat, cough, headache) for which the plant has been found helpful. This section also gives information on the value of plants as preventive medicine: the raising of resistance to colds, the taking of a tonic, and so forth. NOTE: Such self-medication must be practiced with caution. If symptoms persist or become worse in spite of self-treatment, or if the condition becomes at all acute, such as high fever or severe pain, then medical advice must be sought forthwith.

Some of the many uses of plants are illustrated in the woodcut *(right)* of an herbal entitled *Das Kreuterbuch oder Herbarius,* from Augsburg, Germany, 1543. Fruit is being grown and picked outside, while indoors we see persons drying herbs in a chest, eating, and shampooing.

Opposite page: Two examples from the *Hortus Eystettensis,* a plant atlas by the apothecary Basilius Besler (Nuremberg, 1613). The work contains nearly 1,100 engravings (each 55 by 47 centimeters) and descriptions of medicinal plants. Above, *Aconitum hyemale,* an Aconite. Below, *Helleborus niger,* Black hellebore, between crocuses.

This selection of only a few of the many healing herbs provides a fascinating overall picture of the wealth of nature's healing power. The information provided here is based on the cumulative experience of the ages. Much of this wisdom was acquired the hard way, by trial and error, and handed down from generation to generation. As today's medical profession began to evolve from protagonists of the healing art, information about herbal remedies was incorporated in pharmacopoeias—official publications dealing with recognized drugs—which gave their doses, preparations, sources, and tests for purity and activity.

We tend to forget in our modern science-oriented age that, to almost the turn of the century, herbal or "natural" remedies occupied a leading place in the official pharmacopoeias of the world. Aspirin, for example was only synthesized and introduced in 1899.

Unfortunately, on more than one occasion in recent years, clever scientists have produced a drug that is less effective and more toxic than the original herbal remedy. For this reason, an increasing number of doctors feel that herbs and plants have a useful place in modern medicine.

We must not automatically reject, therefore, the old wives' tales and traditional herbal remedies of the past. Many have a sound medical basis and have stood up to the test of time.

Herbs still have a useful place in coping with many of the ills to which mankind is heir. This is particularly true in the case of the so-called minor ailments of life such as indigestion, coughs, and pains. Inevitably, therefore, it is these minor ills which predominate in the accompanying reference table. Minor, however, is something of a misnomer. What may be "minor" to the doctor may be anything but minor to the patient, for whom it may make life unbearable. Nature has many remedies for our ailments and only a few of these are listed in this section. Tested in many cases through the ages, these natural remedies still claim attention as herbs that heal.

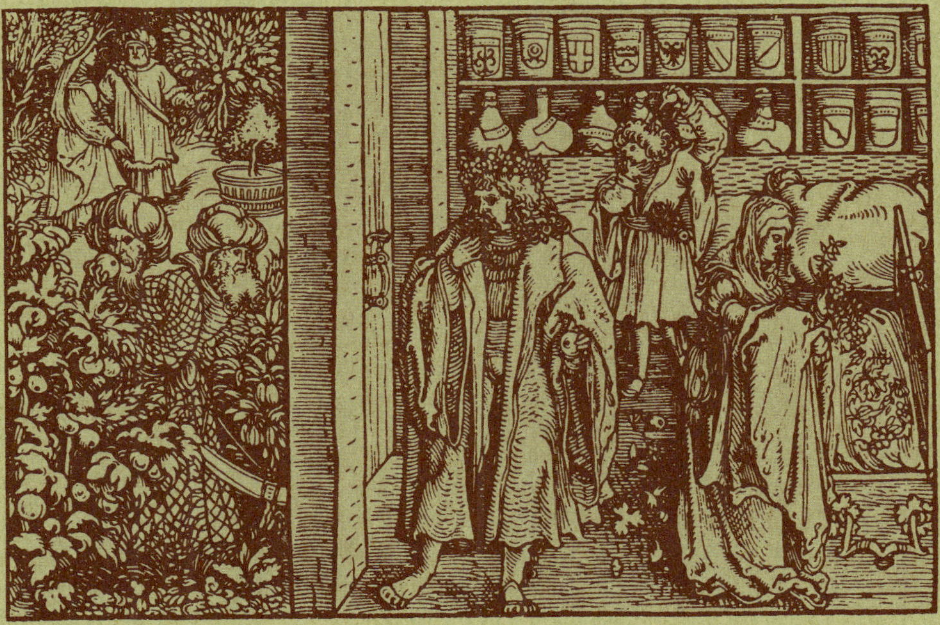

William A.R. Thomson, M.D.

Plant number (see Lexicon, page 38)	Plant name	Principal medicinal uses
103	AGAR AGAR	Chronic constipation Gelatin substitute Pharmaceutical adjuvant for the production of pills, suppositories, and lotions
6	AGRIMONY	Diarrhea Diseases of the liver and gall bladder Indigestion Sore throat Laryngitis
190	ALDER BUCKTHORN	Chronic and spastic constipation
213	ALPINE RAGWORT	Menstrual disorders Bleeding of nose and gums
158	AMERICAN GINSENG	Low blood pressure Depression Exhaustion and weakness
116	AMERICAN PENNYROYAL	Flatulence Digestive disorders
16	ANGELICA	Loss of appetite Flatulence Rheumatism Exhaustion
169	ANISE	Bronchitis Dry coughs Flatulence
27	ARNICA	Bruises Rheumatism Sprains Inflammation of the gums Neuralgia Sore throat Phlebitis Slowly healing wounds

Plant number (see Lexicon, page 38)	Plant name	Principal medicinal uses
74	ARTICHOKE	Gallstones Disorders of the liver Nausea
95	ASH	Bladder and kidney disorders Fever Rheumatism Constipation Dropsy
67	AUTUMN CROCUS	Gout
107	AVENS	Diarrhea Nausea and vomiting Gingivitis Toothache
148	BALM	Flatulence Gastric disorders Migraine Neuralgia Insomnia Restlessness
179	BALSAM POPLAR	Rheumatism Fever Hemorrhoids Diseases of the bladder
35	BARBERRY	Fever Liver and gall bladder disorders Kidney stones Gallstones Constipation
135	BAY	Anorexia Digestive disorders Skin diseases Rheumatic complaints Spice

Plant number (see Lexicon, page 38)	Plant name	Principal medicinal uses
165	BEAN	Arthritis Dropsy
23	BEARBERRY	Cystitis Pyelitis
236	BEARDED USNEA	Chills Influenza Pharyngitis Tonsillitis Intestinal diseases
10	BEAR'S GARLIC	Flatulence Digestive disorders High blood pressure
101	BEDSTRAW	Diseases of the bladder Diseases of the skin Dropsy
32	BELLADONNA	Eye diseases Biliary colic Peptic ulcers Excessive sweating Parkinsonism Kidney stones Asthma
24	BETELNUT PALM	Betel chewing (a widespread custom throughout southeast Asia; indulged in for the pleasure it induces and as a stimulant for salivary secretion) Intestinal worms
227	BIGLEAF LINDEN	Chills and colds Influenzal infections
237	BILBERRY	Inflammation of the mouth Sore throat Digestive disorders in children Diarrhea

Plant number (see Lexicon, page 38)	Plant name	Principal medicinal uses
36	BIRCH	Cystitis Rheumatism Dandruff Loss of hair
183	BITTER ALMOND	Cough Gastritis and enteritis Earache Production of emulsions
61	BITTER ORANGE	Nausea Nervous gastric complaints Sleeplessness Nervous restlessness
170	BLACK CARAWAY	Bronchitis Laryngitis Sore throat
184	BLACK CHERRY	Bronchitis Catarrh of upper respiratory tract Whooping cough
58	BLACK COHOSH	Coughs and colds Bronchitis Indigestion Loss of appetite
193	BLACK CURRANT	Vitamin C deficiency Colds Sore throat
241	BLACK HAW	Painful menstruation Asthma
119	BLACK HELLEBORE	Heart failure Dropsy

Plant number (see Lexicon, page 38)	Plant name	Principal medicinal uses
37	BLACK MUSTARD	Bronchitis
		Pleurisy
		Arthritis
		Sciatica
		Rheumatism
185	BLACKTHORN	Constipation
		Bladder disorders
		Skin ailments
63	BLESSED THISTLE	Anorexia
		Indigestion
		Flatulence
		Diseases of the liver and gall bladder
205	BLOODROOT	Bronchitis
		Skin ailments
186	BLUE LUNGWORT	Bronchitis
		Hoarseness
		Catarrh of the upper respiratory tract
164	BOLDO	Gall bladder disorders
		Gallstone colic
76	BROOM	Disorders of cardiac rhythm
		Dropsy
34	BUCHU	Cystitis
		Pyelitis
150	BUCKBEAN	Migraine
		Indigestion
		Diseases of the liver and gall bladder
		Fever
		Anorexia
141	BUGLEWEED	Nervous heart complaints
161	BUTTERBUR	Bronchitis
		Inflammation of urinary passages

Plant number (see Lexicon, page 38)	Plant name	Principal medicinal uses
161	*(Continued)*	Gall bladder and liver disorders
		Skin ailments
		Menstrual disorders
31	BUTTERFLY WEED	Bronchial catarrh
		Fever
166	CALABAR BEAN	Glaucoma
87	CALIFORNIA POPPY	Insomnia
		Restlessness and overexcitability
		Nervousness
		Bed-wetting
11	CAPE ALOE	Constipation
46	CARAWAY	Flatulence
		Intestinal disorders
		Inadequate lactation
45	CARLINE THISTLE	Urinary complaints
		Cleansing and healing of wounds
191	CASCARA SAGRADA	Constipation
194	CASTOR BEAN	Constipation
		Purgative
53	CELANDINE	Inflammation of gall bladder
		Gallstones
		Gastric pains
		Warts
50	CENTAURY	Heartburn
		Digestive disorders
245	CHASTE TREE	Bleeding disorders
		Painful menstruation
		Insufficient lactation

Plant number (see Lexicon, page 38)	Plant name	Principal medicinal uses
124	CHAULMOOGRA	Leprosy
57	CHICORY	Indigestion Gallstones Coffee substitute (chicory coffee)
219	CHINESE PAGODA TREE	Diseases of the veins Hemorrhage (capillary)
222	CHIRATA	Digestive disorders
60	CINNAMON	Flatulence Digestive disorders
86	COCA	Local anesthetic Stimulant
65	COFFEE	Fatigue Headache Dropsy Circulatory disorders
66	COLA	States of fatigue and weakness Circulatory insufficiency Migraine Stimulant (countries of origin)
232	COLTSFOOT	Bronchitis Chronic cough Catarrh of upper respiratory tract Skin inflammation
223	COMFREY	Bronchitis Coughs Rheumatism Neuralgia Phlebitis Chronic ulcers Slowly healing wounds
230	COMMON NASTURTIUM	Bronchitis Influenzal infections Colds
69	CORYDALIS	Parkinsonism (paralysis agitans) Preparation for anesthesia
110	COTTON	Production of bandage material
182	COWSLIP	Bronchitis Colds and chills Coughs Headache, nervous Insomnia
199	CURLED DOCK	Constipation Skin ailments
231	DAMIANA	Weakness and exhaustion Nervousness
224	DANDELION	Rheumatism Chronic skin disorders Liver and gall bladder disorders Digestive disorders Kidney stones Dropsy
15	DILL	Seasoning Flatulence Hemorrhoids
195	DOG ROSE	Vitamin C deficiency Bladder disorders
203	DWARF ELDER	Kidney and bladder disorders Constipation

Plant number (see Lexicon, page 38)	Plant name	Principal medicinal uses
145	EAGLE VINE	Gastric disorders
130	ELECAMPANE	Loss of appetite
		Asthma
		Chronic bronchitis
		Manufacture of diabetic foods (sugar substitute)
117	ENGLISH IVY	Bronchitis
		Whooping cough
		Rheumatism
174	ENGLISH PLANTAIN	Bronchitis
		Insect stings
		Catarrh of upper respiratory tract
		Indigestion
		Contusions
		Bleeding superficial wounds
242	ENGLISH VIOLET	Bronchitis
		Cough
		Catarrh of upper respiratory tract
131	ENGLISH WALNUT	Eczema
		Blepharitis
		Indigestion
83	EPHEDRA	Bronchial asthma
		Bronchitis
		Hay fever
		Nettle rash
		Whooping cough
		Circulatory insufficiency
		Eye diseases
		Low blood pressure
62	ERGOT	Migraine
		Obstetrics
		Uterine bleeding
		Menstrual disorders

Plant number (see Lexicon, page 38)	Plant name	Principal medicinal uses
88	EUCALYPTUS	Colds
		Sore threat
		Nasal catarrh
		Bronchitis
		Chills
		Rheumatism
217	EUROPEAN BITTERSWEET	Chronic eczema
		Psoriasis
		Rheumatism
		Chronic itching
198	EUROPEAN BLACKBERRY	Domestic tea
		Vitamin C deficiency
		Diarrhea
		Indigestion
204	EUROPEAN ELDER	Chills and influenza
		Fever
		Neuralgia
		Rheumatism
		Constipation
128	EUROPEAN HOLLY	Chills and influenzal infections
		Fever
244	EUROPEAN MISTLETOE	High blood pressure
		Chronic rheumatism
178	EUROPEAN POLYPODY	Bronchitis
		Hoarseness
		Coughs
		Constipation
25	EUROPEAN SNAKEROOT	Suppuration
		Fistulae
		Boils and ulcers
		Burns

Plant number (see Lexicon, page 38)	Plant name	Principal medicinal uses
118	EVERLASTING FLOWER	Gall bladder disorders
90	EYEBRIGHT	Blepharitis Conjunctivitis Eyestrain Styes Black eyes
239	FALSE HELLEBORE	High blood pressure Heart disease
93	FENNEL	Flatulence Digestive complaints Bronchitis Coughs Conjunctivitis Inflammation of the eyelids
228	FENUGREEK	Chapped hands and lips Indigestion Stimulates lactation
91	FIG	Constipation Coughs Coffee substitute (fig coffee)
210	FIGWORT	Chronic skin diseases, particulary facial eczema
139	FLAX	Shingles Hoarseness Boils and ulcers Inflammation of the mouth Sore throat Gallstones Gastric hyperacidity Constipation Rheumatic pains Psoriasis

Plant number (see Lexicon, page 38)	Plant name	Principal medicinal uses
85	FLEABANE	Bronchitis Diarrhea
78	FOXGLOVE	Control of the failing heart Dropsy
54	FRINGE TREE	Gall bladder and liver disorders Slow healing wounds
97	FUMITORY	Gallstone colic Constipation Migraine Skin ailments
17	GARDEN CHAMOMILE	Digestive disorders Inflammation of the mouth Nasal catarrh Sore throat Menstrual disorders Healing of wounds
202	GARDEN SAGE	Sore throat Inflammation of mouth Hoarseness Smoker's cough
9	GARLIC	Arteriosclerosis High blood pressure Dyspepsia Increases resistance to infection Worms

Plant number (see Lexicon, page 38)	Plant name	Principal medicinal uses
146	GERMAN CHAMOMILE	Insomnia Indigestion Inflammation of the eyes Eczema Inflammation of the mouth Nasal catarrh Sore throat Hemorrhoids Menstrual disorders Healing of wounds
225	GERMANDER	Indigestion Slowly healing wounds
247	GINGER	Appetite loss Diarrhea Indigestion Flatulence Used in veterinary medicine
108	GINKGO	Cerebral circulatory disorders Peripheral arterial circulatory disorders
98	GOAT'S RUE	Insufficient lactation
218	GOLDENROD	Inflammation of the bladder Kidney gravel and stones Healing of wounds
125	GOLDENSEAL	Intestinal hemorrhage Uterine hemorrhage Menstrual disorders
246	GRAPE	Liver disorders Constipation Obesity
115	GRAPPLE PLANT	Painful joints Liver and gall bladder disorders
22	GREAT BURDOCK	Rheumatism Skin ailments Seborrhea Dandruff Healing of wounds Ulcers
42	GREEN PEPPER	Arthritis Rheumatic complaints Indigestion Spice
114	HARONGA TREE	Inflammatory diseases of the pancreas Biliary domplaints Dyspepsia
70	HAWTHORN	Angina pectoris Heart failure High blood pressure Nervous disorders of heart and circulation in old age
111	HEDGE HYSSOP	Gout Skin ailments Menstrual disorders Constipation Dropsy
89	HEMP AGRIMONY	Chills Skin ailments Liver complaints Dropsy
99	HEMPNETTLE	Bronchitis Bronchial asthma

Plant number (see Lexicon, page 38)	Plant name	Principal medicinal uses
126	HENBANE	Asthma Bronchitis Neuralgia Rheumatism
106	HERB ROBERT	Inflammations of mouth and throat Diarrhea Skin ailments Nosebleeds
143	HIGH MALLOW	Bronchitis Inflammation of the mouth and throat Laryngitis Eczema Indigestion
123	HOPS	Nervous anxiety Nervous gastric disorders Sleeplessness
144	HOREHOUND	Slowly healing wounds Chronic bronchitis Gall bladder disease
5	HORSE CHESTNUT	Diarrhea Rheumatism Diseases of the veins
26	HORSERADISH	Spice Indigestion Bladder and kidney disorders Bronchial catarrh Neuralgic and rheumatic complaints
84	HORSETAIL	Chilblains Rheumatic complaints Skin diseases Local circulatory disorders Bladder and kidney disorders

Plant number (see Lexicon, page 38)	Plant name	Principal medicinal uses
84	*(Continued)*	Dropsy Healing of wounds
75	HOUND'S TONGUE	Rheumatic and neuralgic complaints Irritating cough Phlebitis Diarrhea Healing of wounds Ulcers
52	ICELAND MOSS	Bronchitis Irritative cough Catarrh of the upper respiratory tract States of exhaustion and weakness Gastritis Anorexia
20	INDIAN HEMP	Heart failure High blood pressure Dropsy
189	INDIAN SNAKEROOT	Anxiety Depression High blood pressure
140	INDIAN TOBACCO	Bronchial asthma (Production of asthma cigarettes and asthma smoking powder) Bronchitis Whooping cough
51	IPECACUANHA	Bronchitis Amoebic dysentery
55	IRISH MOSS	Bronchitis Whooping cough Catarrh of the upper respiratory tract Indigestion Constipation

Plant number (see Lexicon, page 38)	Plant name	Principal medicinal uses
168	JABORANDI	Glaucoma
		Dropsy
157	JAVA TEA	Pyelitis
		Dropsy
132	JUNIPER	Arthritis
		Muscular rheumatism and neuralgia
		Bladder and kidney disorders
		Dropsy
172	KAVA	Skin diseases
		Sleeplessness
		Nervous restlessness
		Bladder complaints
14	KHELLA	Angina pectoris
		Bronchial asthma
		Biliary colic
		Renal colic
		Whooping cough
		Menstrual disorders
19	KIDNEY VETCH	Gastric complaints
		Injuries
		Slow healing wounds
8	LADY'S MANTLE	Diarrhea
		Climacteric complaints
		Menstrual complaints
		Inflammation of the mouth and pharynx
		Suppuration
136	LAVENDER	Cardiac complaints
		Circulatory insufficiency
		Migraine
		Nervousness
		Neurasthenia
		Neuralgia
		States of exhaustion
		Sleeplessness

Plant number (see Lexicon, page 38)	Plant name	Principal medicinal uses
12	LEMON VERBENA	Indigestion
		Flatulence
		Nervous insomnia
109	LICORICE	Gastric ulcers
		Cough
112	LIGNUM VITAE	Bladder and kidney disorders
		Gout
		Rheumatism
		Skin diseases
68	LILY-OF-THE-VALLEY	Cardiac insufficiency
		Dropsy
138	LOVAGE	Spice
		Diseases of the bladder and kidney
		Dropsy
		Rheumatism and gout
		Indigestion
197	MADDER	Bladder and kidney stones
		Bedwetting
81	MALE FERN	Tapeworms
40	MARIGOLD	Bruises
		Contusions and strains
		Slow healing wounds
		Ulcers
		Skin diseases
		Indigestion
		Gall bladder complaints
156	MARJORAM	Coughs
		Inflammation of the mouth
		Sore throat
		Indigestion
		Menstrual pain

Plant number (see Lexicon, page 38)	Plant name	Principal medicinal uses
13	MARSH MALLOW	Bronchitis Coughs Sore throat Inflammation of the mouth Indigestion Diarrhea
163	MASTERWORT	Anorexia Bronchial asthma Bronchial catarrh Indigestion
175	MAYAPPLE	Gall bladder disease Constipation Cancer of the skin
215	MILK THISTLE	Biliary complaints
2	MONKSHOOD	Arthritis and fibrositis Sciatica Neuralgia
211	MOSSY STONECROP	Hemorrhoids Slow healing wounds
137	MOTHERWORT	Nervous heart disorders Climacteric complaints
29	MUGWORT	Loss of appetite Kitchen spice (better tolerance of fatty foods; "roast goose spice")
240	MULLEIN	Bronchitis Inflammation of upper respiratory tract Irritative cough
49	NEW JERSEY TEA	Sore throat Inflammation of the mouth

Plant number (see Lexicon, page 38)	Plant name	Principal medicinal uses
212	NIGHT-BLOOMING CEREUS	Heart disorders
221	NUX-VOMICA	General tonic Loss of appetite
188	OAK	Eczema Sweating of the feet Chilblains Diarrhea Hemorrhoids Indigestion Bleeding of the gums
33	OATS	Eczema Indigestion Diarrhea Kidney and bladder disorders Neuralgia Rheumatic complaints Disorders of sleep
153	OLEANDER	Heart failure Circulatory disorders
154	OLIVE	Gallstones Diseases of the gall bladder Indigestion Constipation High blood pressure
159	OPIUM POPPY	Severe diarrhea Painful conditions
151	OSWEGO TEA	Flatulence Digestive complaints Diuretic Menstrual disorders Tea substitute

Plant number (see Lexicon, page 38)	Plant name	Principal medicinal uses
243	PANSY	Eczema
44	PAPAYA	Diseases of the gall bladder and liver Disorders of fat digestion Dyspepsia
129	PARAGUAY TEA	Tea drink (national drink in South America) States of fatigue Rheumatism
162	PARSLEY	Inflammation of bladder and kidneys Digestive disorders
187	PASQUE FLOWER	Diseases of the eye Menstrual disorders
149	PEPPERMINT	Flatulence Nausea and sickness Gall bladder complaints
133	PERUVIAN KRAMERIA	Sore throat Inflammation of the mouth Laryngitis Diarrhea Chilblains
167	POKE	Skin diseases Rheumatism Constipation
155	PRICKLY RESTHARROW	Kidney and bladder disorders Bladder and kidney stones Dropsy
173	PSYLLIUM	Bronchitis Coughs Soothing skin application Indigestion Constipation

Plant number (see Lexicon, page 38)	Plant name	Principal medicinal uses
71	PUMPKIN	Worms
82	PURPLE CONEFLOWER	Abscesses Colds, chills, and influenza Mild burns Slow healing wounds
142	PURPLE LOOSESTRIFE	Diarrhea Indigestion Healing of wounds
229	PURPLE TRILLIUM	Skin disorders Slow healing wounds Menstrual disorders
7	QUACK GRASS	Bladder disorders Skin ailments Indigestion Rheumatism
92	QUEEN-OF-THE-MEADOW	Diseases of the bladder and kidney Fever Headache Rheumatism Dropsy
73	QUINCE	Inflammation of mouth and throat Irritating cough Constipation
39	RED BRYONY	Bronchitis Whooping cough Diuretic
192	RHUBARB	Diarrhea (small doses) Constipation (larger doses)
96	ROCKWEED	Source of iodine (for prevention and treatment of endemic goiter) Obesity

Plant number (see Lexicon, page 38)	Plant name	Principal medicinal uses
121	ROSELLE	Domestic tea Constipation
196	ROSEMARY	Low blood pressure Weakness and exhaustion Circulatory disorders Nervous heart complaints Indigestion Rheumatic and neuralgic complaints
200	RUE	Varicose veins Phlebitis Nervous anxiety Nervous dyspepsia
120	RUPTUREWORT	Kidney and bladder disorders Kidney and bladder stones Psoriasis
127	ST. JOHN'S WORT	Neuralgic and rheumatic pain Varicose veins Gastritis Climacteric complaints Menstrual disorders
216	SARSAPARILLA	Skin disorders Rheumatism
208	SASSAFRAS	Skin dirorders Rheumatism
214	SAW PALMETTO	Bladder complaints Bronchitis
209	SCOPOLIA	Biliary upsets Constipation Sleeplessness
171	SCOTCH PINE	Bronchitis Catarrh of the upper respiratory passages Sinusitis Neuralgia Rheumatism Sleeplessness
64	SCURVY GRASS	"Spring cures" Bleeding of the gums
122	SEA BUCKTHORN	Tonic
234	SEA ONION	Heart failure Dropsy
43	SEDGES	Arthritis Skin diseases
176	SENECA SNAKEROOT	Bronchitis Catarrh of upper respiratory tracts
47	SENNA	Constipation
41	SHEPHERD'S PURSE	Menstrual disorders Uterine hemorrhage
180	SILVERWEED	Inflammations of the mouth Diarrhea Hemorrhoids Indigestion Healing of wounds
177	SMARTWEED	Hemorrhoids
233	SMOOTH-LEAF ELM	Diarrhea Hemorrhoids Eczema Inflammations of the mouth Sore throat Slow healing wounds

Plant number (see Lexicon, page 38)	Plant name	Principal medicinal uses
206	SNAKEROOT	Slow healing wounds Contusions Bronchitis Sore throat
207	SOAPWORT	Bronchitis Coughs Skin disorders
48	SPANISH CHESTNUT	Bronchitis Whooping cough Rheumatism Diarrhea
21	SPIKENARD	Coughs Flatulence Rheumatism
4	SPRING ADONIS	Low blood pressure Cardiac insufficiency Functional heart complaints
235	STINGING NETTLE	Rheumatism Lumbago Loss of hair Bladder disorders Dropsy Skin diseases
94	STRAWBERRY	Diarrhea Bladder and kidney stones
220	STROPHANTHUS	Heart failure
80	SUNDEW	Bronchial asthma Bronchitis Hoarseness Irritative cough Whooping cough
3	SWEET FLAG	Loss of appetite Indigestion Biliary upsets Exhaustion and weakness
18	SWEET VERNAL GRASS	Sciatica Rheumatism Colic
100	SWEET WOODRUFF	Insomnia Nervous anxiety Digestive complaints
56	TANSY	Digestive disorders Intestinal worms
77	THORNAPPLE	Bronchial asthma Parkinsonism
226	THYME	Bronchitis Whooping cough Hoarseness Chills and colds Digestive disorders
181	TORMENTIL	Minor burns Diarrhea Inflammation of the gums Sore throat
72	TURMERIC	Spice Gall bladder and liver diseases Indigestion
238	VALERIAN	Nervous exhaustion Nervous dyspepsia Headaches of nervous origin Nervous heart disorders Insomnia
152	WATERCRESS	Chronic rheumatism Kidney and bladder stones Metabolic disorders Skin blemishes

Plant number (see Lexicon, page 38)	Plant name	Principal medicinal uses
134	WHITE DEADNETTLE	Skin sores Bladder disorders
201	WHITE WILLOW	Chills and influenza Fever Rheumatic and neuralgic pain Headache and migraine
30	WILD GINGER	Sore throat Laryngitis Dropsy
160	WILD PASSIONFLOWER	Sleeplessness Nerve sedative Nervous heart complaints
38	WINTER CABBAGE	Peptic ulcers Rheumatic and neuralgic ailments Slowly healing wounds
102	WINTERGREEN	Sciatica Lumbago Rheumatism Neuralgia
113	WITCH HAZEL	Hemorrhoids Contusions and sprains Slow healing wounds Nose bleeds
28	WORMWOOD	Flatulence Indigestion Biliousness General weakness

Plant number (see Lexicon, page 38)	Plant name	Principal medicinal uses
79	YAM	Bronchial asthma Whooping cough Neuralgia Rheumatism Biliary colic Manufacture of hormones
1	YARROW	Anorexia Flatulence Indigestion Diarrhea Billiary colic Hemorrhoids Menstrual disorders Healing of wounds Ulcers
59	YELLOWBARK CINCHONA	Disturbances of cardiac rhythm Fever, chills Muscle cramps Indigestion
105	YELLOW GENTIAN	Loss of appetite Indigestion
104	YELLOW JESSAMINE	Facial neuralgia Cramp Migraine Bronchial asthma
147	YELLOW SWEETCLOVER	Contusions Joint pains Gall bladder complaints Indigestion Varicose veins Phlebitis

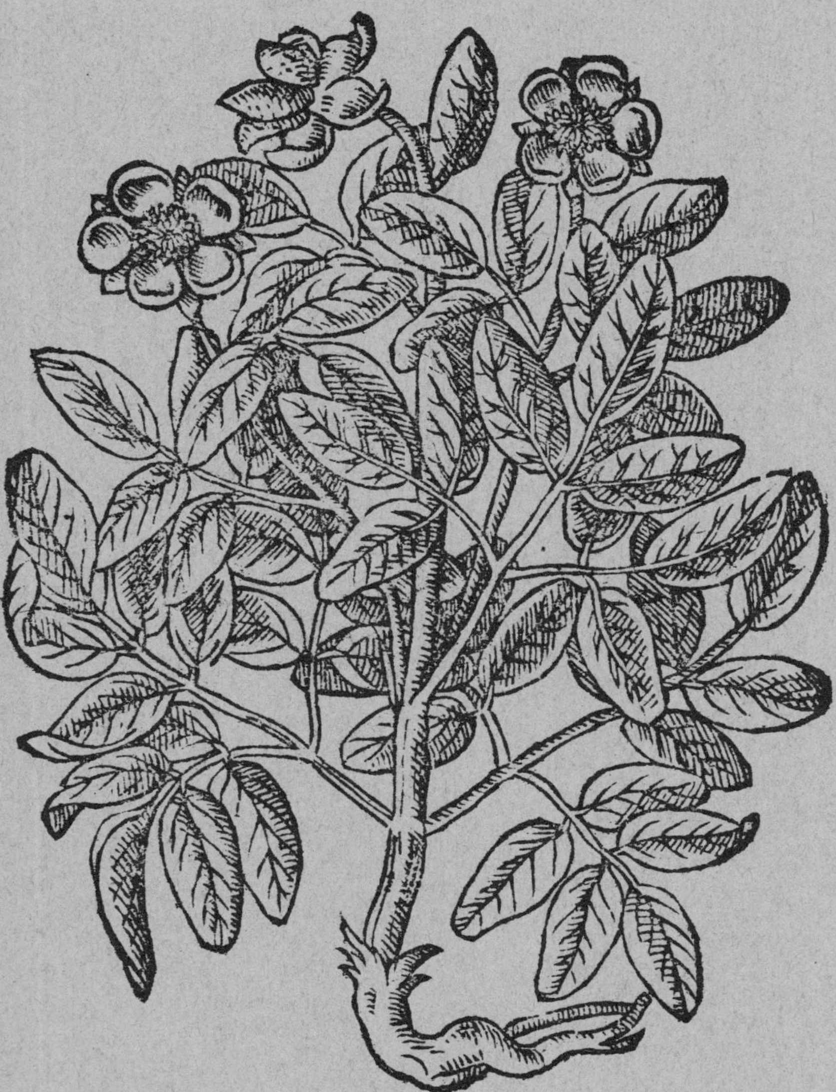

Many a time and oft
have I bethought within
myself of the
wondrous works of the
Shaper of the
Universe. . . . While considering
these matters
I likewise recalled
that the Shaper of Nature,
who has set us
amidst such perils, has
granted us a remedy
with all manner of herbs,
animals, and
sundry other created
things. . . . I thank Thee,
O Shaper of heaven
and earth . . . that
Thou hast granted to me
grace of revealing
this treasure,
which has until now
lain hidden
and buried from the sight
of common men.

Peter Schoeffer,
Der Gart der Gesundheit, 1485

Drawing of a peony, *Paeonia mascula,* from the *Herbarium* by Bartholomaeus Zornn, published in Cologne in 1673, a work of nearly 500 pages containing descriptions of some 2,000 plant genera. The peony is recommended by Zornn in the treatment of brain disorders and epilepsy, for biliary weakness, and as a diuretic, among many other uses—although modern herbal medicine does not agree.

Lexicon of the Healing Plants

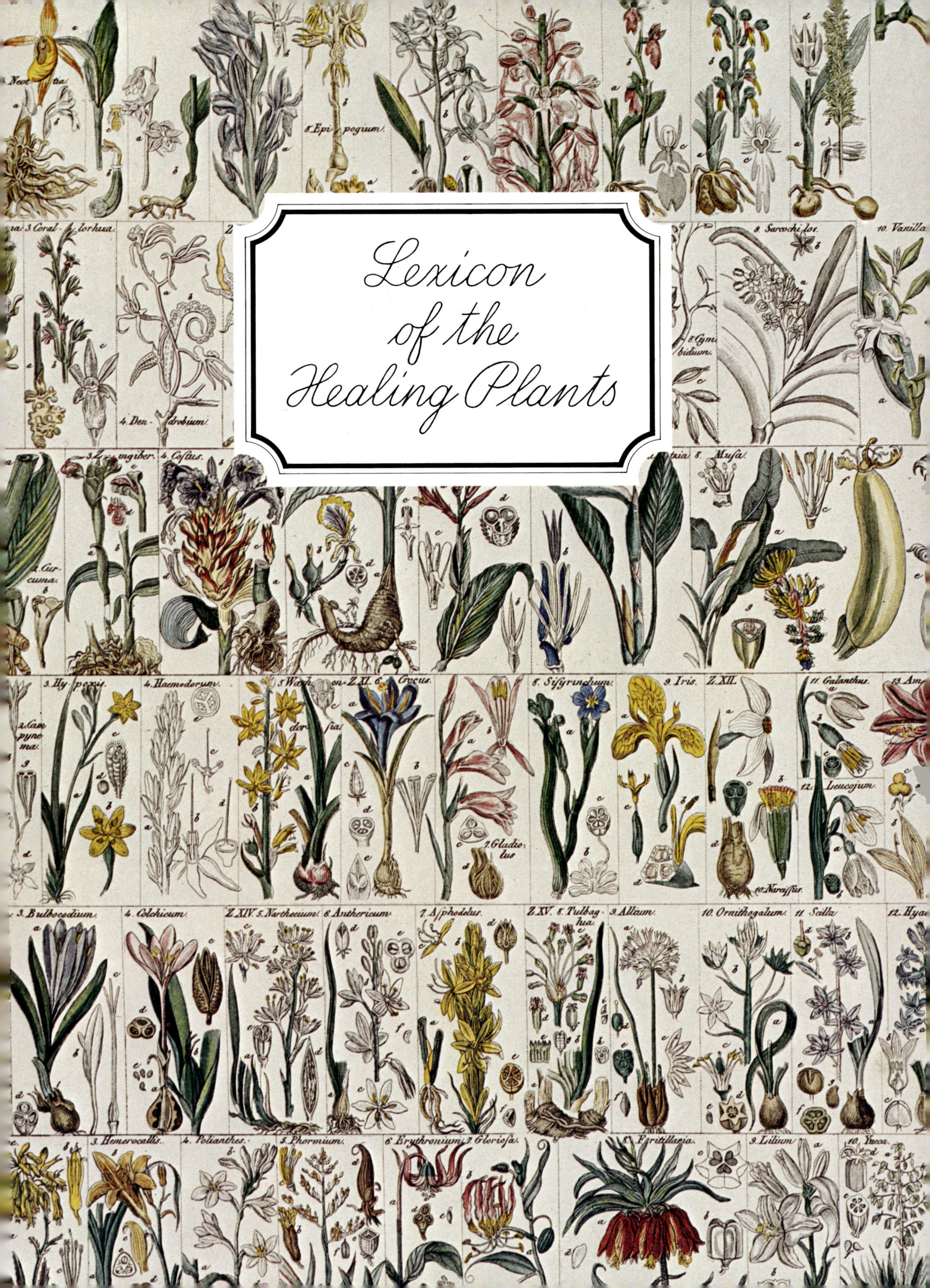

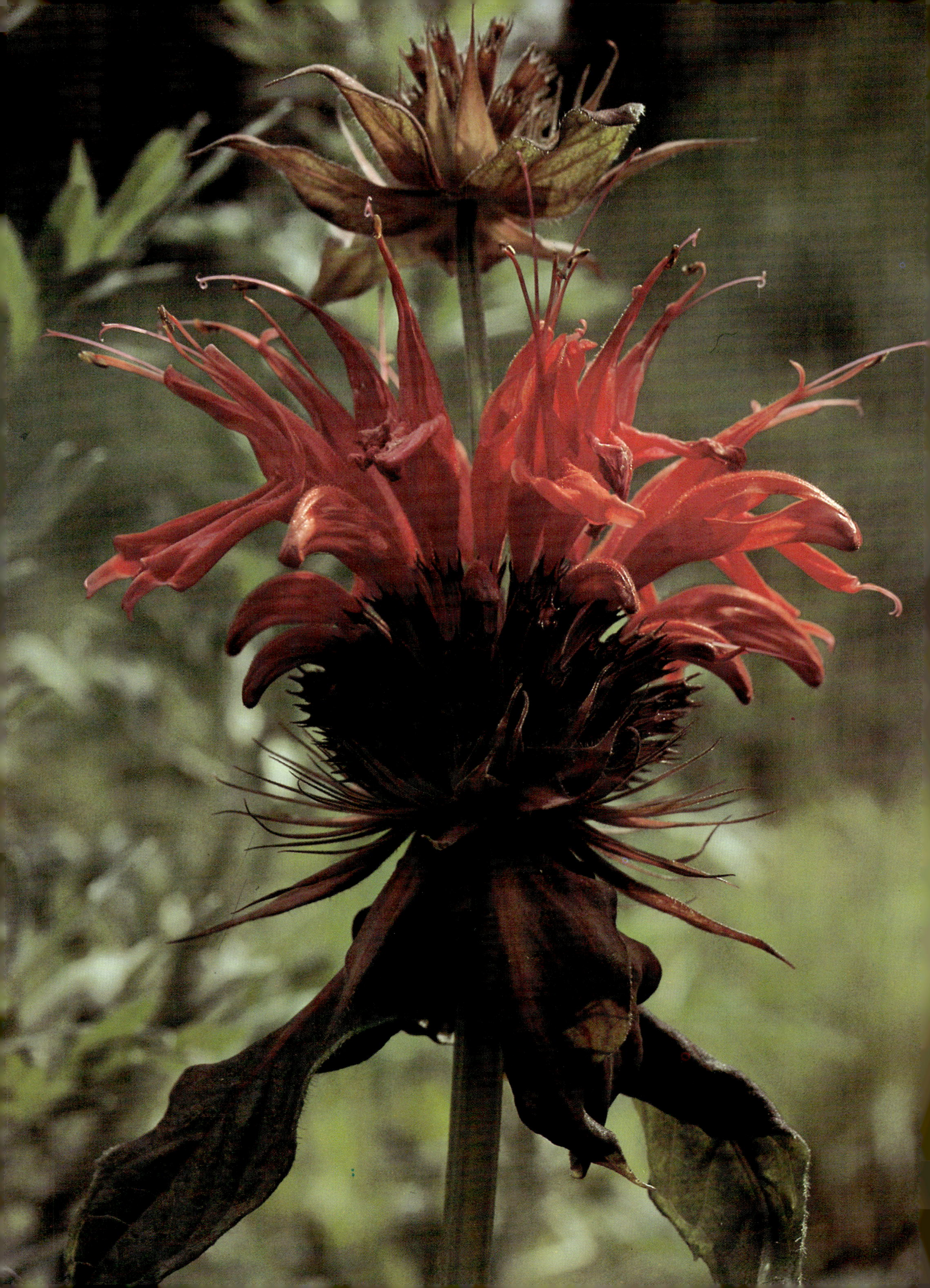

Plant Lexicon

The old herbals continue to exert a charm and fascination, while their meticulously drawn and hand-painted illustrations (by anonymous artists) are often clearer and more informative than many modern diagrams. The picture on p. 33 is a composite of plates from *Oken's allgemeine Naturgeschichte für alle Stände,* a natural history text published in Stuttgart in 1843.

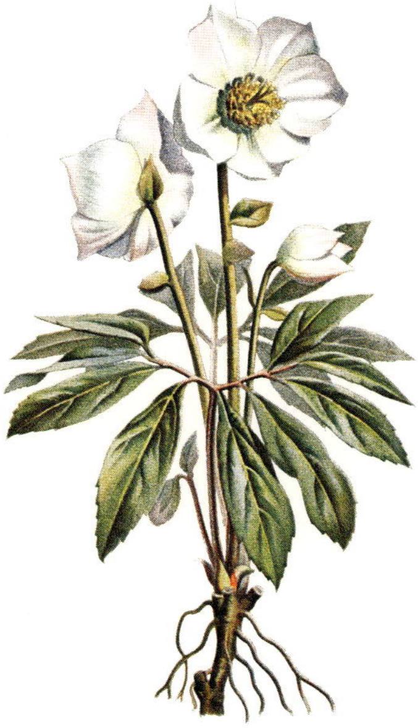

Other paintings from old herbals. Black hellebore *(Helleborus niger),* above, and rose *(Rosa centifolia),* right, in paintings from *Les Plantes Medicinales,* by Dr. F. Losch, published in Bienne, Switzerland, in 1888.

Left: Oswego tea *(Monarda didyma),* an important American medicinal herb.

This section includes basic descriptions, primarily botanical in nature, of the 247 medicinal herbs that constitute basic material of the book.

SELECTION CRITERIA FOR THE 247 PLANTS

- Priority was given to plants of proven effectiveness.
- Added to this group of plants were those with an empirically proven effectiveness even though the how and the why of their functioning still elude us.
- Poisonous plants were excluded except when no substitute for their beneficial effects could be found.
- As a rule, plants were excluded whose extracts are available only in commercial or pharmaceutical preparations; but exceptions were made in cases where no substitute was available.
- Plants primarily used as food or spice, with only minor or secondary medicinal value, were also omitted.
- Some plants, even though they continue to be used in folk medicine, were ruled out because of the tenuousness of their claims, and because they could be replaced by other, more effective plants.

CONTENTS OF THE PLANT LEXICON

For each plant we provide the Latin name, common English names, the plant family to which it belongs, and indications of its geographical distribution. Classification of plants is by no means as simple as it was in the day of Linnaeus. An attempt has been made to adhere as closely as possible to his classification, but other systems of nomenclature are also used at times (their authors are cited in the Latin-English Plant Index at the back of the book).

The text on each plant explains its name and gives a detailed account of its appearance and characteristics (growth, blooming, seed-bearing, and so on). Indications of the plant's *active principles* (i.e., active constituents) and medicinal uses are also given. The reader will find further information in Reference Sections I and III.

Indispensable to any plant description is, of course, an illustration that can guide us in recognizing and identifying the healing plant in its natural site. Particular care has been given to the selection of photographs, and of hand-painted illustrations from herbal guidebooks of the last century, which are both accurate and beautiful.

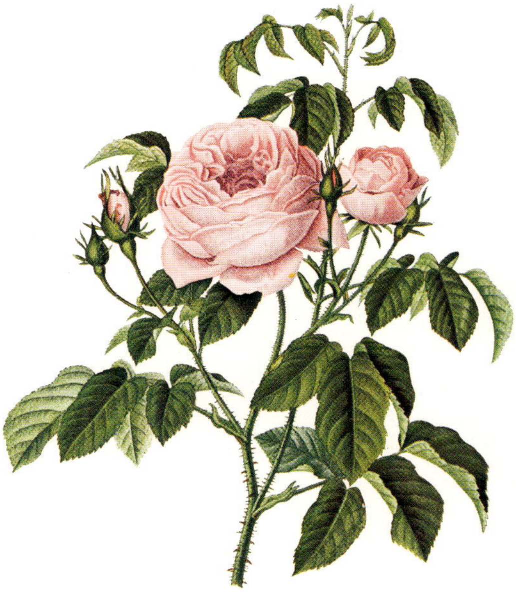

HOW TO LOCATE A PLANT IN THE LEXICON

Because English common names of the plants are so unstandardized and variable, the 247 plants of the Lexicon have been arranged in alphabetical order according to their standard *Latin names* and each plant has been assigned a number from 1 to 247. This number can be located in the list of English names on the next two pages. The reader can look up the more common English names in this list; if a particular name is not listed, it can be sought in the English Plant Index at the end of the book, where a further range of alternative English names are given, with cross-references to their number in the Lexicon.

Index and Key

Common English names of the 247 plants are listed here with the number designating each plant's location in the Lexicon.

Each text in the Plant Lexicon includes the following information in its heading:

Latin name, English name, plant family, plant number (in a blue box), and references to the plant's geographical distribution. The distribution is indicated in two lines. The first line gives the plant's original habitat or place of provenance; the second, in italics, indicates areas in which the plant has been introduced by man and grows either wild or cultivated. The following geographical abbreviations are used:

Af	Africa
Aus	Australia
Eur	Europe
N Am	North America
S Am	South America
C-S Am	central parts of South America
C+SW-N Am	central and southwestern parts of North America
E-N Am	eastern parts of North America
N-N Am	northern parts of North America
NE-N Am	northeastern parts of North America
S-N Am	southern parts of North America
SE-N Am	southeastern parts of North America
W-S Am	western parts of South America

ACHILLEA MILLEFOLIUM

YARROW, MILFOIL

Asteraceae/Compositae

1 Eur, N Am, N Asia
S Aus

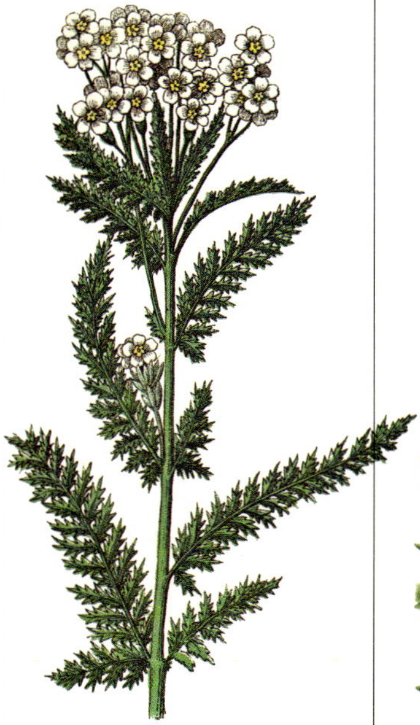

The Ancient Greeks greatly valued this medicinal herb and named it after the heroic warrior Achilles. The byname, *millefolium*, means "a thousand leaves" and refers to the feathery appearance of the finely divided leaves. These are not very noticeable, however, compared to the great numbers of small florets gathered in flattened umbel-like clusters. From a creeping underground root grow tough, angular stems bearing the snow-white flowers. The plant needs light and warmth to produce in its leaves and particularly in the flowers the bitter essential oil that can bring healing in many ways.
Yarrow is commonly found on roadsides, in meadows, and on dry, sunny slopes. It grows also in the mountains, sometimes with a pink or pale lilac color. At higher altitudes up to 3000 meters, one finds the musk milfoil *(Achillea moschata)*.

ACONITUM NAPELLUS

MONKSHOOD, ACONITE

Ranunculaceae

2 Eur, N Asia, N Am

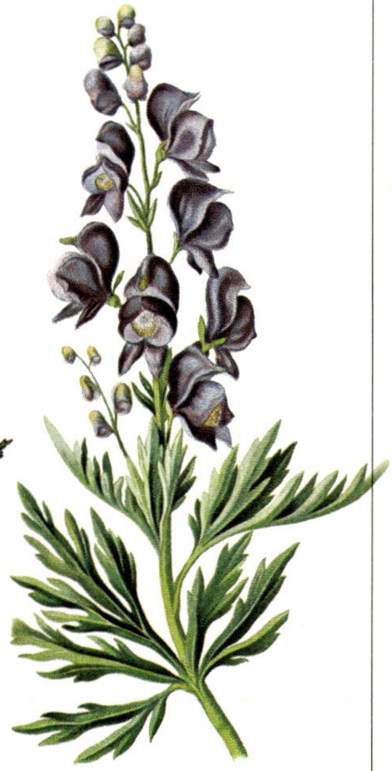

In mountain regions, large colonies of monkshood are often found in damp, rich meadows, an adornment to the landscape. Other varieties are the yellow aconite and the blue English monkshood *(Aconitum anglicum)*. Monkshood is one of the most poisonous medicinal plants. The shape of the deep blue flower resembles the helmet of a medieval knight, and one of the old names for this plant was helmet-flower. The strong stem does not branch much at the top. It grows up to 150 cm high, bearing the characteristic dark green deeply divided leaves and terminating in a handsome spike of flowers, the most striking feature of the plant. Root growth is unusual, with a new tuber formed each year, next to the old one which dies. The root also has the highest concentration of active principles (alkaloids). To obtain these, the plant is cultivated in the Balkans, Spain, and Italy.

ACORUS CALAMUS

SWEET FLAG, CALAMUS

Araceae

3 SE Asia
Eur, E Af, E-N Am

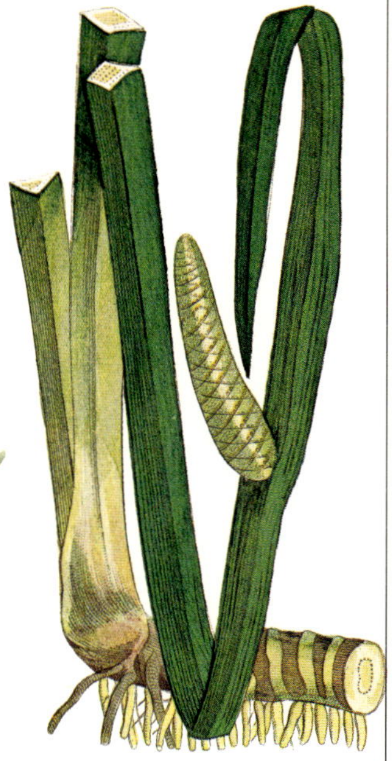

This is an aquatic plant found mostly in ditches filled with stagnant water. The underground shoot may reach a length of 1.5 m, with long roots growing downward from it. It is constantly producing new runners, thus ensuring continuance of the species. From the shoot, erect fleshy sword-like leaves grow in solid sheaves up to a meter high. The tip of the underground shoot produces a flowering stem bearing a solid cylindrical spike, 10 cm in length, which is closely covered with small greenish-yellow flowers. Seeds are not formed in central European regions. The underground root contains the fragrant, bitter volatile oil to which the drug owes its aromatic taste and healing properties.

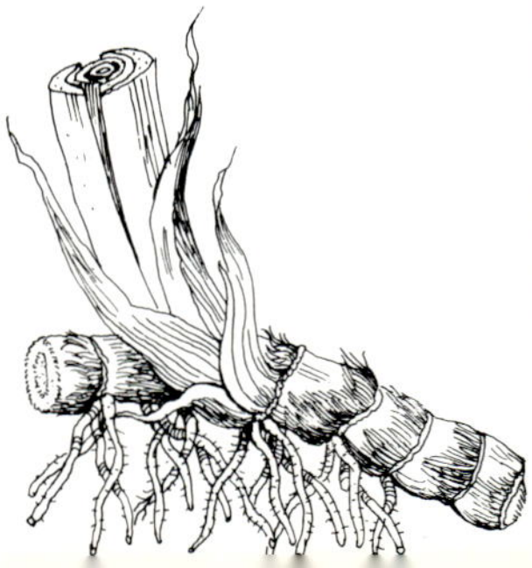

ADONIS VERNALIS

SPRING ADONIS, PHEASANT'S EYE

Ranunculaceae

4 SE Eur, W Asia
N-N Am

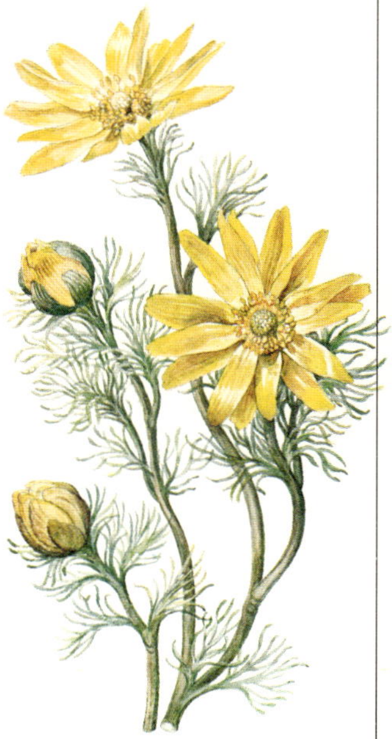

An Adonis among plants, this harbinger of spring is unfortunately becoming increasingly rare; it is protected. The downy flower buds on their short, upright stems first appear in April, on sunny rock valley slopes. They open as soon as the sun appears, always facing the light. The bright yellow star-shaped flowers have a silky sheen and are 4–7 cm in diameter. The pale green, finely divided feathery leaves with their thread-like tips do not appear until the stems have reached a height of 20–30 cm. Ants distribute the tiny nut-like seeds in autumn. The active principles contained in the whole plant have an action on the heart similar to that of *Strophanthus*. *Adonis vernalis* cannot be cultivated. It is frequently used for medicinal purposes in eastern Europe. It is an important remedy in homeopathic medicine but is very poisonous.

AESCULUS HIPPOCASTANUM

HORSE CHESTNUT

Hippocastaneae

5 SE Eur, W Asia
C Eur, N-N Am

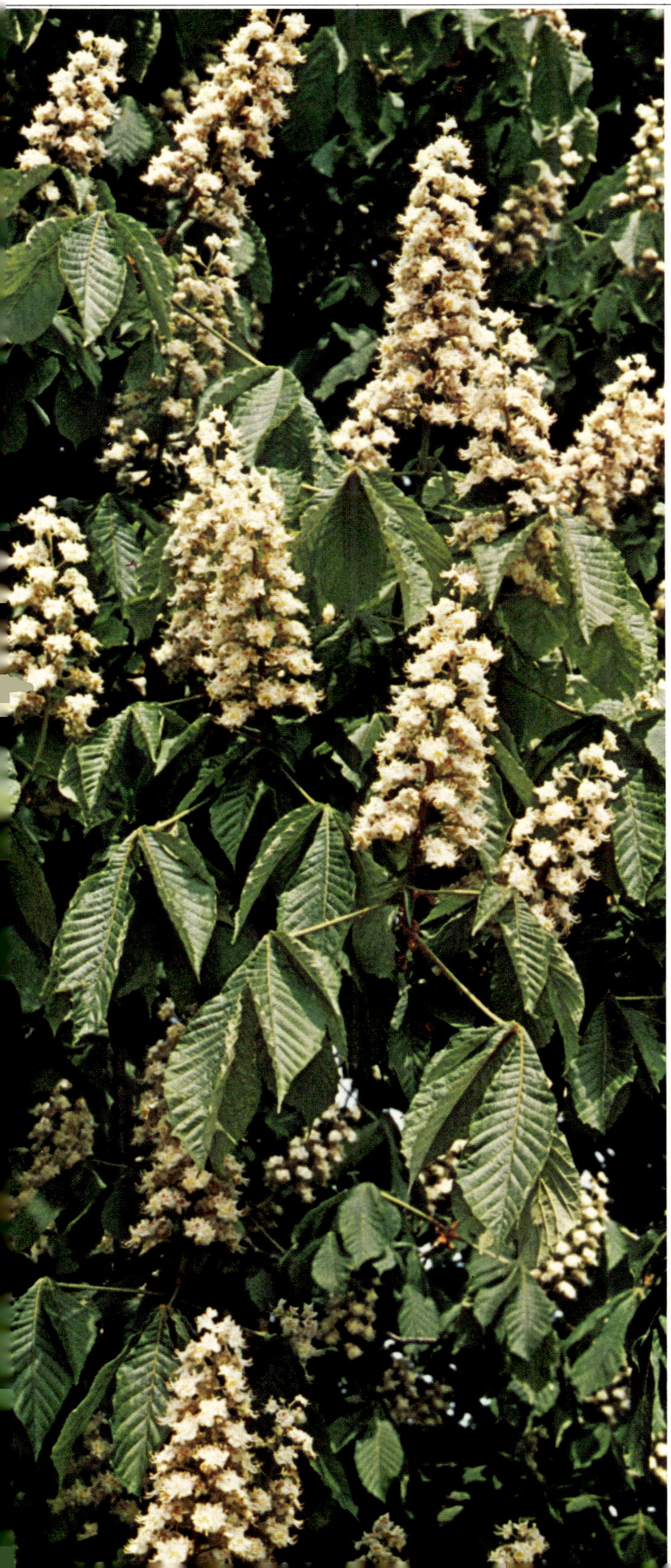

It will always remain a mystery at what point in history this tree found its way from western Asia, its original home, across the Caucasus to Europe, and on to North America. One may assume that crusaders, or perhaps Venetian merchants, brought the strange shiny brown chestnuts with them as a curiosity, for that is what happened also with other plants. Grown first as an ornamental tree in palace gardens, the horse chestnut was known in Vienna in the sixteenth century. Today the shade-giving tree is popular everywhere. In early spring the brown sticky buds open to release small, downy, tender green leaflets that develop into dark green long-stemmed parasols of leaves spreading like fingers from the palm of a hand. The upright spikes of white and pink flowers stand out like candles against the rich green in May or June. Their scent is heady. The fruits ripen in fleshy, spiny capsules, tumbling out, dark brown and shiny, when ripe In hard times they have been used to feed horses.

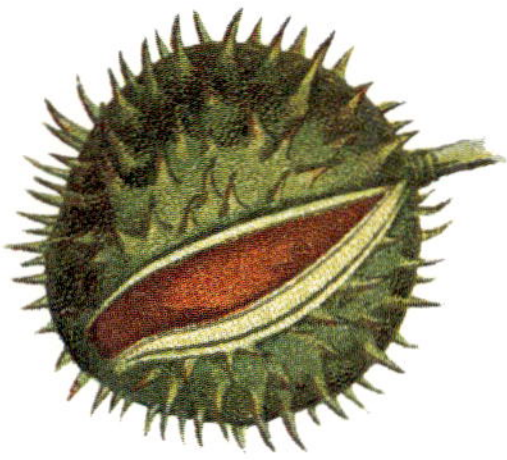

A number of active principles (saponins), concentrated in the fruit, are important healing factors for damaged blood vessels. Nowadays the bark from young trees, which is rich in tannins, is used in the manufacture of bath products.

AGRIMONIA EUPATORIA

AGRIMONY, COCKLEBUR

Rosaceae

6 Eur, N Af, W Asia
N Am

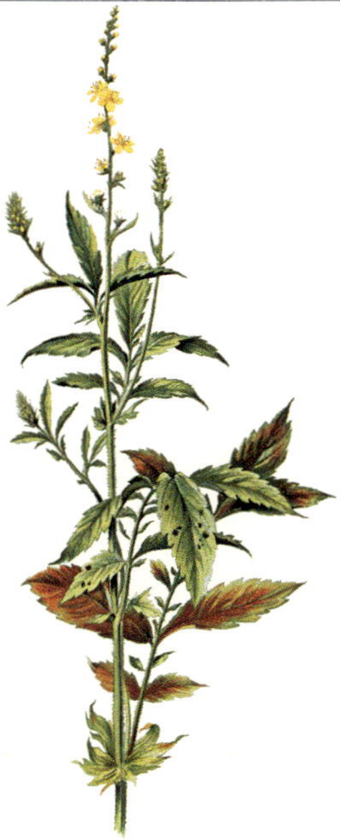

Agrimony may be found in sunny, lean meadows and waste places. The downy stem of this perennial does not branch much as it grows to a height of 40–90 cm, bearing long, divided leaves that are very hairy and often sticky. It terminates in a spike bearing numerous flower buds which, starting from below, continue to open, one starry yellow flower after another, from June right into autumn. The bitter, aromatic principles of this herb stimulate liver activity. Agrimony presents a rather unusual appearance for a member of the rose family. This comprises more than 2000 species in a wide range of forms. Certain active principles are characteristic of the rose family: sugars in fruit, tannins in flowering plants, and the highly poisonous prussic acid in some stone fruits (sweet and bitter almond). Rich scents are also typical.

AGROPYRON REPENS

QUACK GRASS, COUCH GRASS

Poaceae/Gramineae

7 Eur, N Af, Asia
Temperate Zones

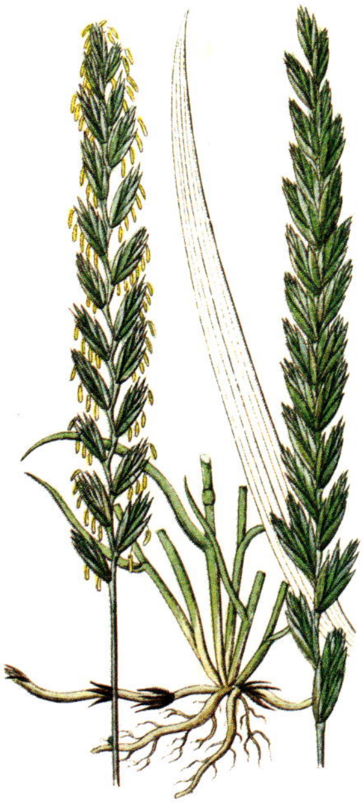

The creeping *(repens)* quack grass and its relatives belong to the large family of grasses that also provides the majority of our cereal plants. As a weed, quack grass is a persistent nuisance. It grows in fields where the soil is clayey, in uncultivated ground, and along walls anywhere, including in mountain regions. The slender white creeping underground stems hold fast to the soil with bunches of thin brown rootlets. Stems 50–80 cm high rise from them vertically, with very narrow bright green lancet leaves. The flowers and fruit are arranged in flattened, loose spikes. Wheat, a close relative, concentrates its reserves in the seed, but in the quack grass one finds them in the creeping root. This contains various carbohydrates and silicic acid, as well as antibiotics, and is frequently used in phytotherapy.

ALCHEMILLA VULGARIS/ ALCHEMILLA ALPINA

LADY'S MANTLE, LION'S FOOT

Rosaceae

8 Eur, N Af, Asian, N Am

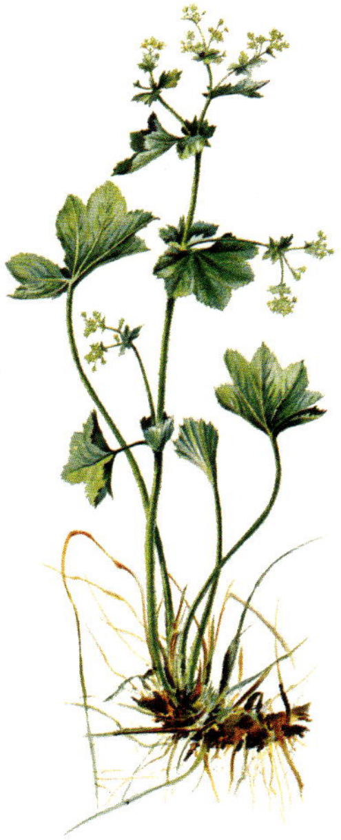

The beautifully shaped leaf cups of the lady's mantle collect droplets of water that are exuded at the rib ends and mix with the dew.
In damp pastures, open woodland, and in mountain regions also on bands of rock, the lady's mantle or its alpine variety (above 1000 m) often forms whole carpets. A woody rootstock produces branching flower shoots, 10–30 cm in height, with small, inconspicuous, greenish-yellow flowers. A notable feature is the soft, rounded green leaves, which have 7–11 semicircular, gently pleated lobes with toothed margins. The leaves are hairy, and those of the alpine variety (5–7 lobes) have a silky, silvery sheen.

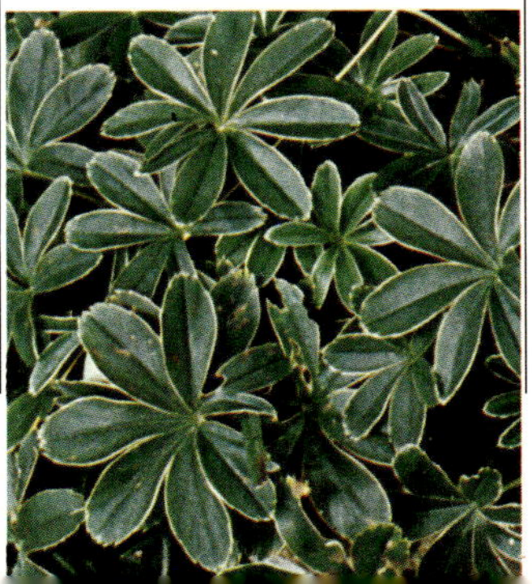

ALLIUM SATIVUM

GARLIC

Liliaceae

9 C Asia
Warm Temperate Zones

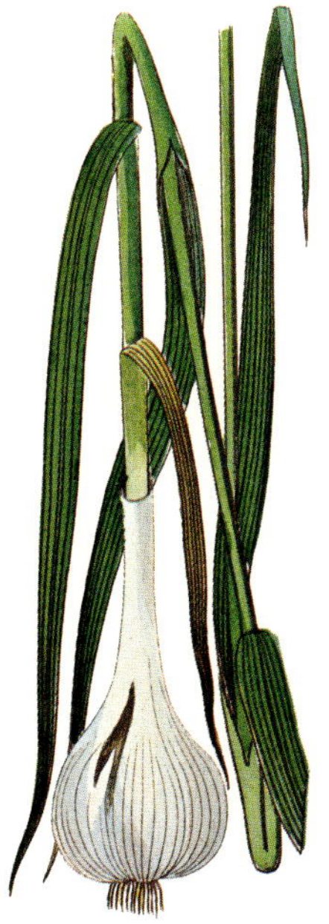

The bulb of garlic is widely used for flavoring and forms part of the staple diet in eastern countries; it is also greatly valued for its medicinal properties. The elongated oval parent bulb sits on a flat root base surrounded by independent bulblets (cloves). In spring, a round, hairless flower stalk rises up to a meter high. It is supported at the lower end by the tubular leaf sheaths of the long, narrow, pointed flat green leaves. The terminal flowers grow in a purplish-white tassel enclosed in a papery bract. The seeds do not mature in cultivated plants. The pressed juice of the bulb contains a number of valuable active principles. The onion *(Allium cepa)* grows to a larger size than garlic. The bulb and flower stalk are fleshier, and the medicinal properties are less marked. Onions are used in popular medicine for local applications and in diets based on juices.

ALLIUM URSINUM

BEAR'S GARLIC, RAMSONS

Liliaceae

10 Eur

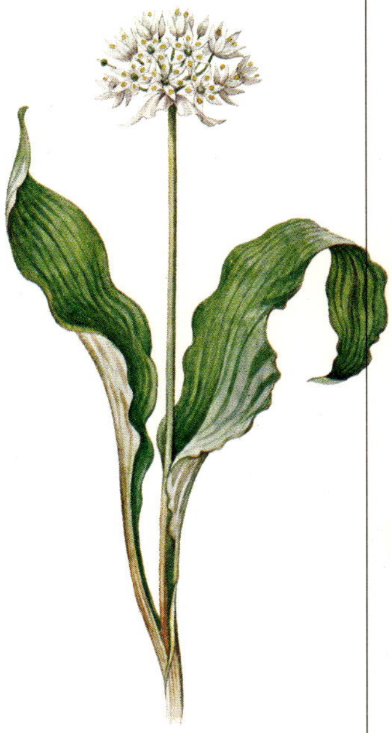

In the moist humus-enriched soil of deciduous forests and river valleys, bear's garlic may grow in large colonies. From the composite bulb, two or three elliptical, lance-shaped basal leaves rise in early spring. Their fresh green color and pungent smell attract attention, and they are gathered to be used in spring salads and for their gentle garlic falvor. The flowering stalk with its terminal umbel of numerous snowy white six-petaled flower stars does not appear until later. Ants carry off the small black seeds, ensuring the continuing distribution of this valuable medicinal plant. It is most effective when used fresh, either in spring, or throughout the year in the form of freshly pressed juice. The dried leaves quickly lose their medicinal powers.

ALOE FEROX

CAPE ALOE

Liliaceae

11 S Af
S Eur, E Af, N-S Am

This huge succulent is designed to survive in hot, dry climates. The stem is short, though in some species it may reach 2 or 3 m in height. The stem is marked with numerous leaf scars and bears a huge rosette of fleshy pointed leaves, each about 50 cm long, their margins and underside beset with dark red or pale spines. In January–April the flowering stem grows from the center of the rosette. It is about 1 m long and closely covered with cylindrical clusters of flowers. Depending on the species, the glowing colors of the flowers range from a fiery purple to pale red or orange. The resinous, milky juice is collected by letting it drain from the cut-off leaves.

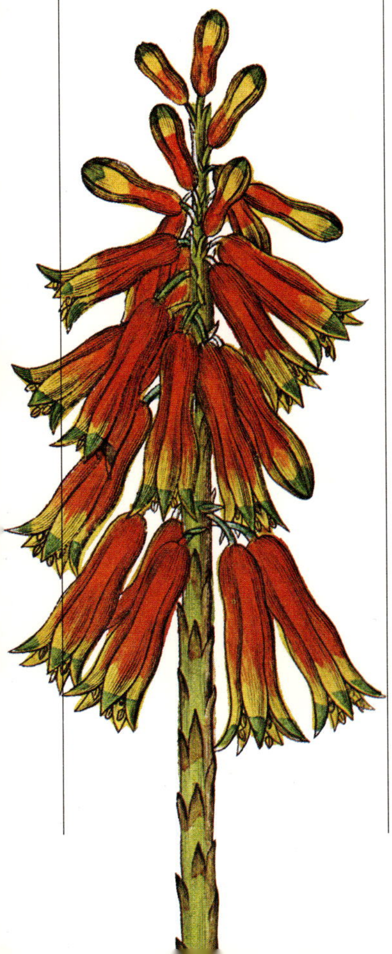

ALOYSIA TRIPHYLLA, LIPPIA CITRIODORA

LEMON VERBENA

Verbenaceae

12 S Am
S Eur, N Am

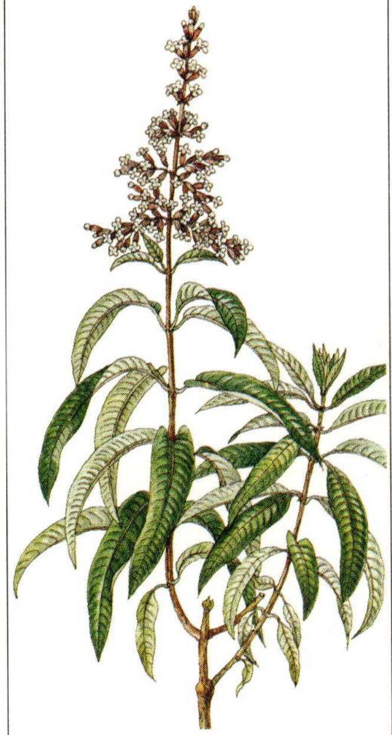

This shrub, which may be up to 2 m high, comes from South America and was introduced to northern countries as an exotic garden plant. The lemon verbena is sometimes confused with vervain *(Verbena officinalis)*, another member of the family, though the two have little in common. The vervain is a small, not very striking perennial, the only English native of the family, and is not much used for medicinal purposes nowadays. The lemon verbena shrub bears handsome whorls of narrow leaves 6–8 cm in length, with marked veins. These are a yellowish green and tend to be bent back. A delicious, refreshing lemon-like scent arises when they are rubbed between the fingers. Small pale pink flowers grow on the shoots in slender terminal spikes. The aromatic volatile oil with its refreshing scent is concentrated in the leaves, as is often the case with labiate flowerers of this kind.

ALTHAEA OFFICINALIS

MARSH MALLOW

13 SE Eur
S+W Eur, W Asia, NE-N Am

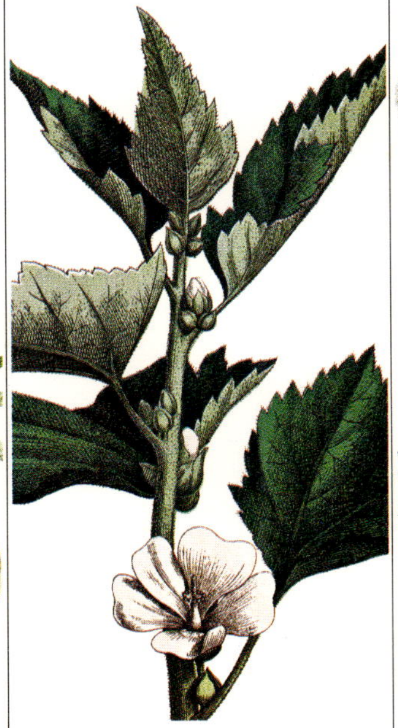

Originally a native of salty soils, the marsh mallow thrives in moist uncultivated ground. It is also frequently cultivated. From the strong, pale yellow root grows a fleshy stem, often woody at the base, which does not branch much. The leaves are short-stemmed, broadly egg-shaped, with 3–5 lobes and toothed margins. Stem and leaves are covered with a velvety down. The flowers with their five delicate reddish-white petals sit in the leaf axils (The flowers of the related hollyhock are white to mauve, those of the tree mallow purple to deep mauve.) The numerous stamens have yellow or mauve anthers. The leaves and particularly the root contain much mucilage and are widely used as a demulcent and emollient. The pigments found in the dark purple flowers of the hollyhock *(Althaea rosea)* up also have healing properties.

AMMI VISNAGA

KHELLA, VISNAGA

Apiaceae/Umbelliferae

14 S Eur, N Af, W Asia
Warm Temperate Zones

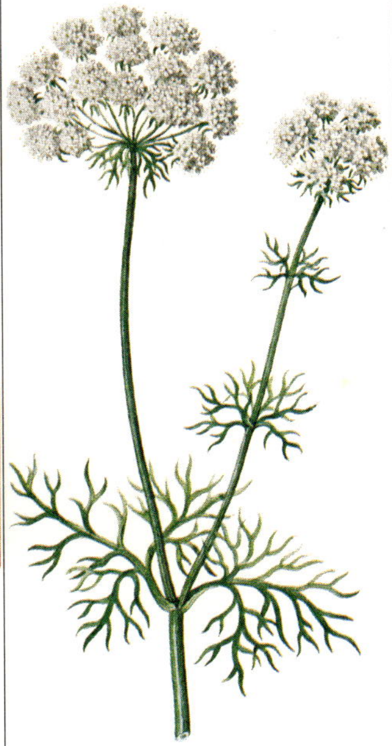

Known to the Arabs for centuries, this medicinal herb was mentioned by Fuchs in the sixteenth century. It was then forgotten, taken up again at the end of the last century, and its active principles isolated at a later date. The plant is an annual, with a longish white root producing an erect, fluted round stem. This branches at the top, reaching a height of 80–120 cm. The delicate leaves are repeatedly divided into thin wisps, similar to those of the hog's fennel or the carrot. The large, many-rayed umbel arises from a thickly branching base, quite often consisting of more than 100 rays or stalks 4–5 cm in length, each bearing a small umbel of numerous white flowers. When the flowering is over, the rays dry up and become woody, like toothpicks. The small, egg-shaped elliptical fruits are smooth and grayish brown; they break up into two as they dry. The fruits and leaves have a bitter aromatic scent.

ANETHUM GRAVEOLENS

DILL

Apiaceae / Umbelliferae

15 SE Eur, SW Asia
Temperate Zones

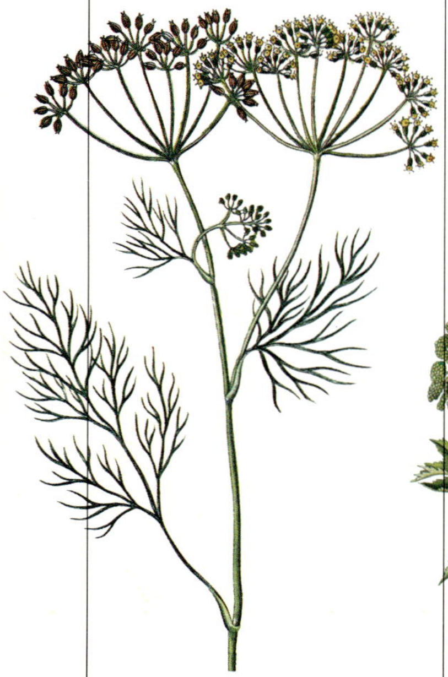

Dill is cultivated as a culinary herb in many countries; it grows wild as an escape in southern countries and was introduced to the northern regions at an early date. It is one of the many herbs mentioned in Egyptian papyri. Its name is derived from the Norse *dilla*, "to soothe," on account of its reputation as a healing herb.

Dill is an annual, growing from a thin, spindle-shaped root. The hollow, finely grooved stem with green and white longitudinal stripes reaches a height of 60–100 cm. The very finely divided leaves are like threads and emerge from a sheath clasping the stem, similar to fennel, but more luxuriant. The stems terminate in large many-rayed domed umbels with small yellow flowers. The elliptical brown fruits have prominent ribs. They divide into two. Dill is one of the warmth-giving herbs, particularly the seeds, which taste different from the leaves.

ANGELICA ARCHANGELICA

ANGELICA

Apiaceae / Umbelliferae

16 N + E Eur, N Asia
N-N Am

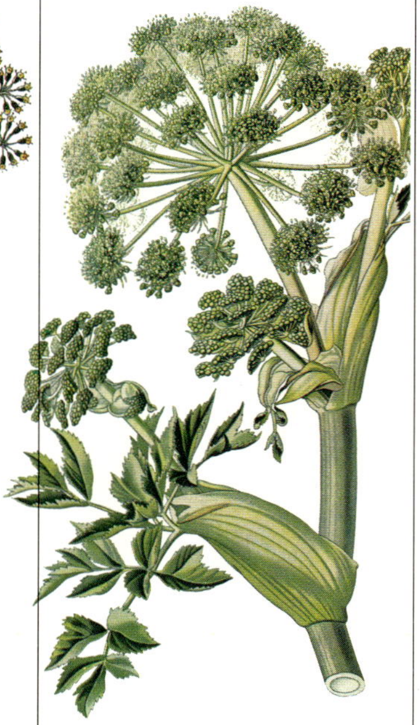

Angelica likes to grow in moist places, in ravines, woods, and coastal regions. It is also widely cultivated. The rootstock develops as the roots are growing, and cultivated angelica in particular produces a good root system. A flourishing rosette of leaves is produced in the first year. In the second or third year, a hollow fluted stem rises up to a height of 2 m. The leaves, triangular in shape, are up to 50 cm long lower down, growing smaller as they go higher up the stem. They are divided and subdivided 2–3 times, with sharply toothed margins. The upper leaf axils are enclosed within inflated leaf sheaths. The umbel is a hemisphere of small, greenish-white flowers, constantly visited by insects. The roots contain the bitter, aromatic medicinal principles. In the Middle Ages angelica was thought to have supernatural powers against contagious diseases.

ANTHEMIS NOBILIS

GARDEN OR ENGLISH CHAMOMILE

Asteraceae / Compositae

17 SW Eur, NW Af
Eur, N Am

Garden chamomile prefers a dry, sandy soil rich in silica. The wild-growing variety has single flowers; the cultivated variety, double flowers. The plant has a small rootstock that produces runners and upright, freely branching flowering stems. The leaves are very finely divided and light green in color. The flowers are most striking; they grow in great numbers on strong stems, with white or faintly yellow ray florets and a solid cone at the center. The plant grows to a height of 30–40 cm and has a strong, pleasantly aromatic scent. The volatile oil concentrated in the flower is medicinal and similar to that found in German or wild chamomile *(Matricaria chamomilla)*.

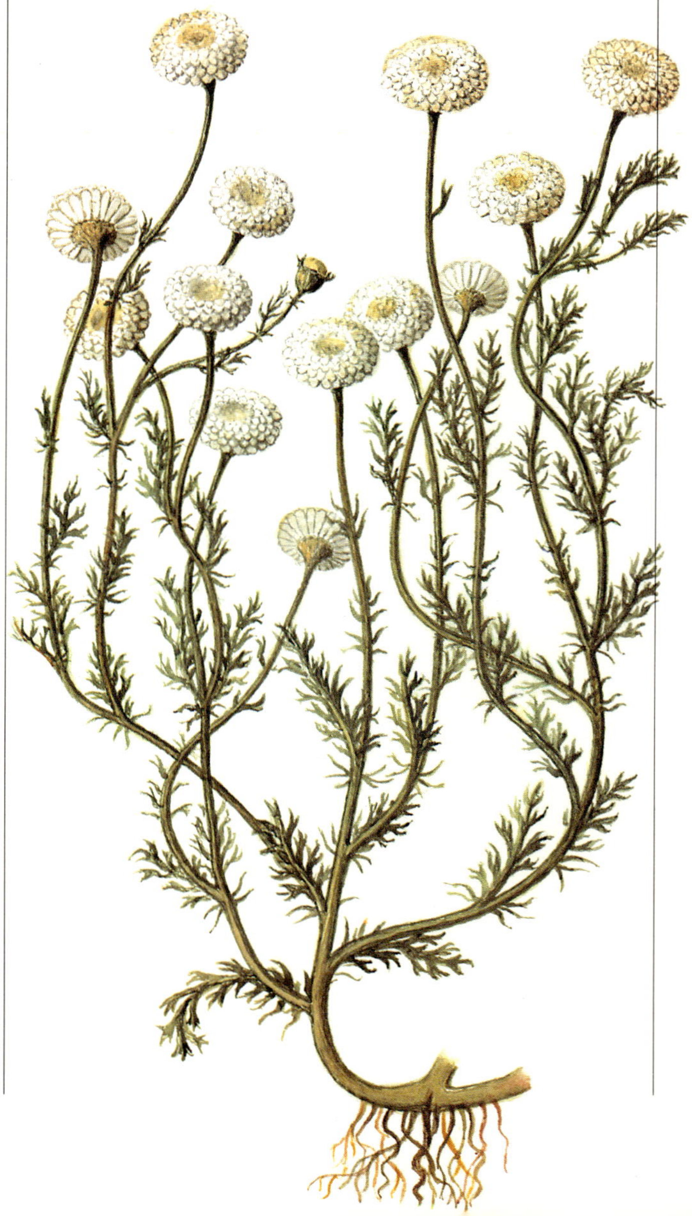

ANTHOXANTHUM ODORATUM

SWEET VERNAL GRASS

Poaceae / Gramineae

18 C+N Eur, N Asia
Temperate Zones

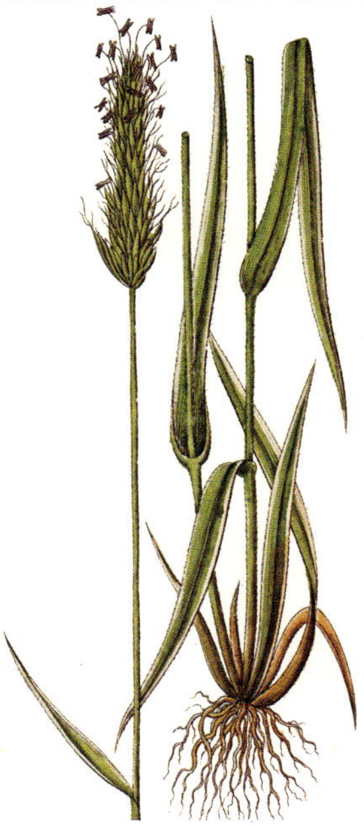

The vernal grass occurs in a variety of species. Like many other grasses, it contains coumarin, a substance liberated only on drying (as in the case of the woodruff), which is responsible for the scent of hay. Included in the fodder given to animals, vernal grass stimulates digestion. The slender stalks, 25–40 cm in height, grow from a persistent, branching root. The stalks bear short narrow leaves running down into the stem. The terminal spike of flowers is pointed like an ear of corn and brownish-green in color. The flowers are sterile and arranged laterally, each an awn covered with hairs on the outside and bearded on the back. This grass may serve as the representative of the many grasses which make up *Flores graminis* (hayseed). Baths and compresses prepared with *Flores graminis* are widely used in continental Europe to treat rheumatic complaints and stimulate the circulation.

ANTHYLLIS VULNERARIA

KIDNEY VETCH, WOUNDWORT

Fabaceae / Papilionaceae

19 Eur, N Af, W As
N Am

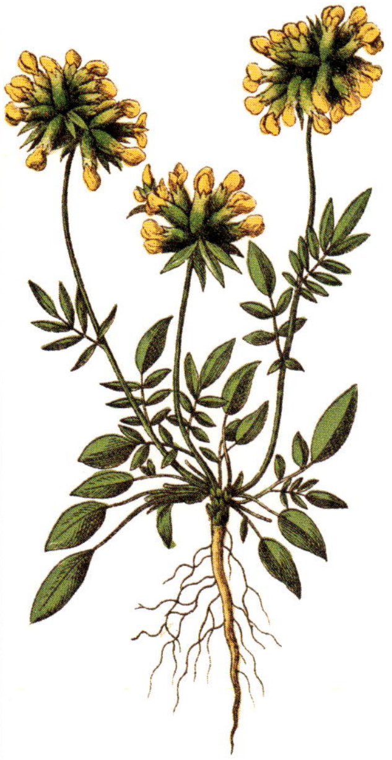

The kidney vetch is very common on lean, dry soils rich in chalk, in meadows and uncultivated ground up to an altitude of 2500 m. The root, which tends to be perennial, produces stems with a reddish tinge, 10–30 cm long. The base leaves are a rich green and undivided; those borne on the stem are divided into pairs of leaflets on an axis with one terminal leaflet. The stem ends in a head of 5–8 vivid yellow peaflowers, visited by honey-gathering bees and bumblebees. The byname *vulneraria* refers to the traditional use of the plant in popular medicine for healing wounds. Recent investigations have shown that the floral pigment contains flavonoids, very interesting active principles with a wide range of medicinal actions that are found in many species and in different plant organs.

APOCYNUM CANNABINUM

INDIAN HEMP, HEMP DOGBANE

Apocynaceae

20 N Am

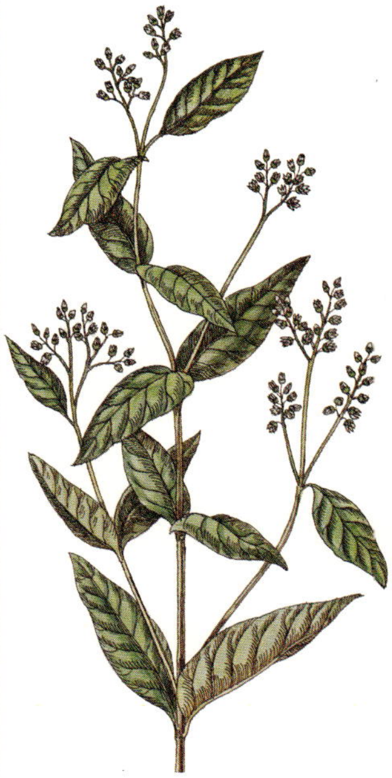

The Apocynaceae include climbing plants, with long branches the thickness of an arm, growing in tropical forests. In northern forests they are represented by the humble periwinkle *(Vinca minor)*. Strong fibers, and in some species milky juice, are characteristics of the family. *Apocynum cannabinum* owes its name "Indian hemp" to the fibrous nature of its stems, although it does not belong to the hemp family. Indian hemp is frequently found in the prairies and open woodlands and along river banks in the northeastern parts of the American continent. The powerful rootstock, furrowing the soil in any and every direction, annually produces slender stems, about 1 m in height, with opposite branches. The leaves are linear, pointed, and up to 10 cm in length; prominent veins indicate their fibrous nature. The stems terminate in white lilac-like flowering structures. The plant is poisonous.

ARALIA RACEMOSA

SPIKENARD

Araliaceae

21 E-N Am

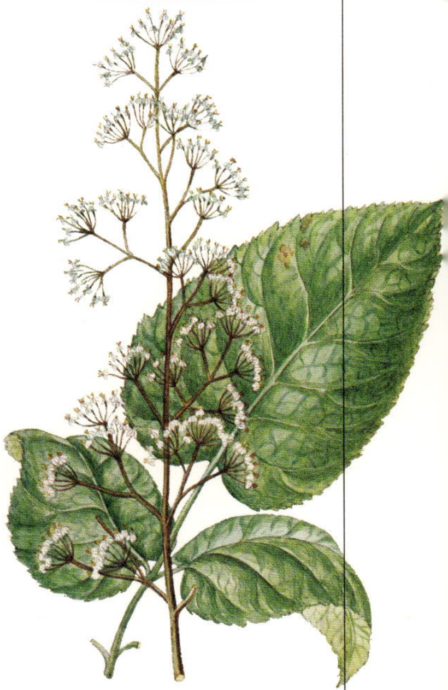

In northern regions, the ivy *(Hedera)* is the only representative of the Araliaceae (ivy family). In America and Asia, they grow as shrubs or trees with strong branches, some of them spiny. Some species are popular as house plants. A perennial, herbaceous plant, it grows from a thick, nodular rootstock. Its partly woody stems, 120–150 cm long, form a bush. The large, dark green, leathery leaves are divided 3 to 5 times into thin, oval leaflets 10–20 cm in length and usually heart-shaped at the base. The greenish-white flowers grow in clusters of 10 to 20. The fruits are dark red or purple berries. The active principles of the spikenard (chiefly saponins) are contained mainly in the root. This is a fleshy rootstock, 3–5 cm thick, its spongy white tissues filled with a yellow milky juice. The juice gives the root its aromatic, balsamic odor and taste. It has been used as a substitute for sarsaparilla.

ARCTIUM LAPPA

GREAT BURDOCK

Asteraceae / Compositae

22 Eur, NW Asia
Temperate Zones

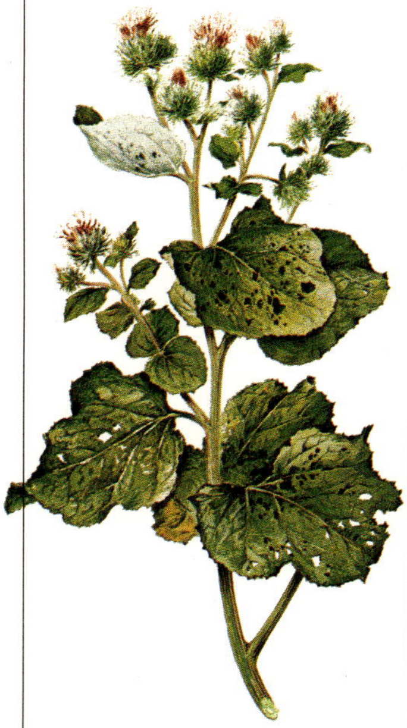

The thistle-like fruit heads with their hooked prickles cling to anything, hence the byname *lappa,* which derives from the Greek word meaning "to seize." In the first year the root, which may be a meter long, produces only a large rosette of leaves. The following year, the solid herbaceous stems, grooved and downy, grow to a height of 150 cm. The leaves are alternate, stalked, and broadly ovate with prickly tips. Their upper surface is green, and the underside is covered with matted downy hairs. The tubular florets in the flower heads are reddish-purple, divided into five at the top, and surrounded by narrow green hooked bracts that are usually longer than the florets. The great burdock prefers a heavy soil rich in nitrogen and is found in alpine meadows, glades, and along roadsides. The medicinal properties are concentrated in the root. It has antiseptic properties.

ARCTOSTAPHYLOS UVA-URSI

BEARBERRY

Ericaceae

23 Eur, N Asia, N Am

Bears certainly relish the berries, and it seems likely that the Greeks based their name for this plant on observations in nature. The bearberry is an evergreen dwarf shrub. Like all the heath family, it prefers a soil rich in humus. It is often found covering large areas in alpine coniferous forests, up to a height of 3000 m. The short trailing branches bear small dark green leathery leaves, which are egg-shaped and broadest at the tip. The small reddish-white bell-shaped flowers appear in spring. The red berries, which ripen in autumn, are sour and astringent and not really edible, but reserved for the birds and the bears. In phytotherapy, the persistent leaves are greatly valued for their disinfectant properties on the urinary tract. Cranberries are very similar to the bearberry, but have upright branches and small dots on the underside of the leaves. More than 100 species of bearberry may be found on the Pacific side of North America, some of them large shrubs. The leaves of the alpine bearberry, an arctic species growing at altitudes above 2000 m, are not leathery. They have toothed margins and a few hairs, and turn a bright scarlet before they drop off in the autumn. On northern heathlands, and also in lowlands, bearberry species form large carpets. They contribute much to humus production and thus help to create the conditions in which other plants can grow.

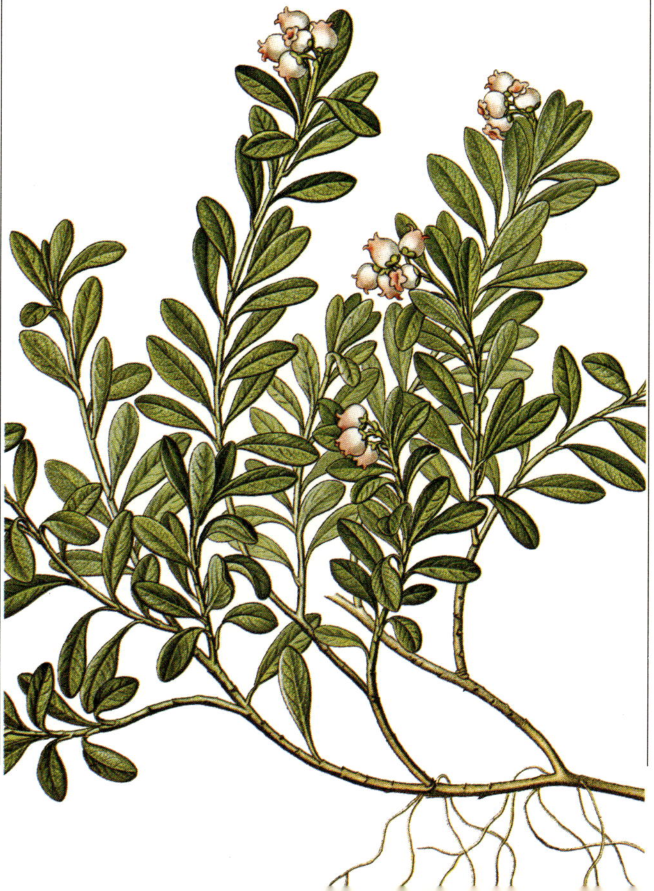

ARECA CATECHU

BETELNUT PALM, ARECA NUT

Arecaceae

24 S Asia

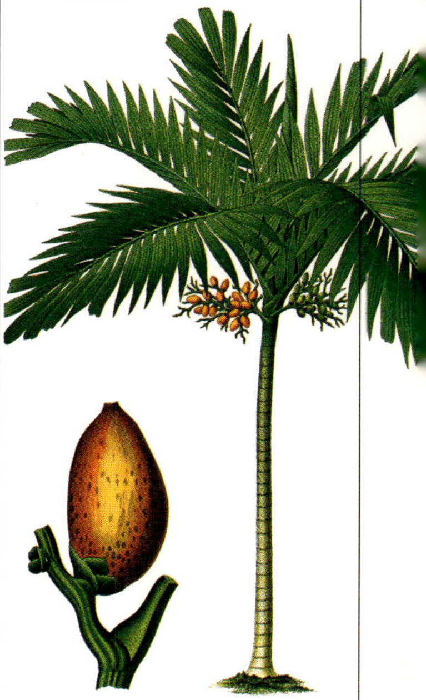

This is one of the handsomest palms. Its slender, utterly straight stem reaches a height of 15–25 m and a circumference of 50 cm. The stem terminates in palm fronds up to 150 cm long, with numerous blades 30–60 cm in length. The fronds have an inflated sheath. Slightly below are the branched flowering structures, with the scented whitish male flowers on the upper part of the branch and the larger female flowers forming the base of the cylinder. From the trigonal ovary develops an orange-yellow egg-shaped fruit, about 5 cm in length. The seeds are about 3 cm long, hemispherical or broadly conical. The Malay people have a long tradition of chewing the seeds. The active principles (alkaloids) promote the secretion of saliva, intestinal juice, and sweat. They have a toxic effect on intestinal parasites and are therefore used in veterinary medicine.

ARISTOLOCHIA CLEMATITIS

EUROPEAN SNAKEROOT, BIRTHWORT

Aristolochiaceae

25 C+S Eur, SW Asia
N Am

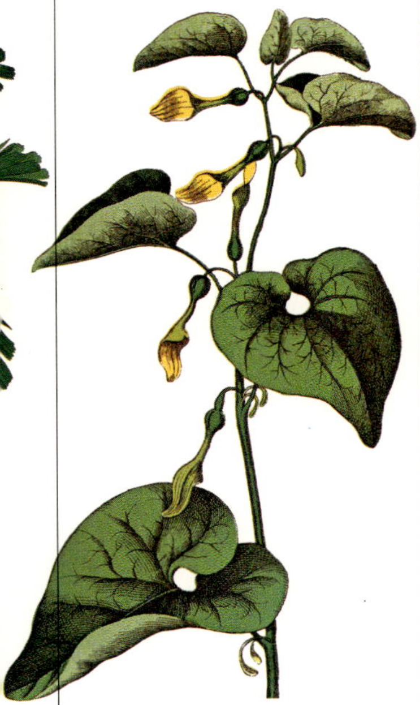

European snakeroot (Greek *Aristolochia* = promoting birth) was used as a female remedy in antiquity; forgotten for a long time, it has gained new favor in phytotherapy. Originally a native of southern Europe, it probably came north accidentally with the cultivation of vines. It is quite common in vineyards, along hedges, and on the edges of fields. The creeping underground stem spreads wide and produces upright shoots, 30–70 cm high, with pale green, deeply incised heart-shaped leaves. Clusters of yellow, elongated tubular flowers arise in the leaf axils. Pollination is by insects (flies), which crawl down the floral tube and are kept trapped by hairs pointing downward until pollination has occurred. The active principles of this medicinal plant can be utilized only in the form of pharmaceutical preparations. They have been found effective in assisting bodily defenses against organisms causing infection.

ARMORACIA RUSTICANA (=LAPATHIFOLIA)

HORSERADISH

Brassicaceae / Cruciferae

26 E Eur
Temperate Zones

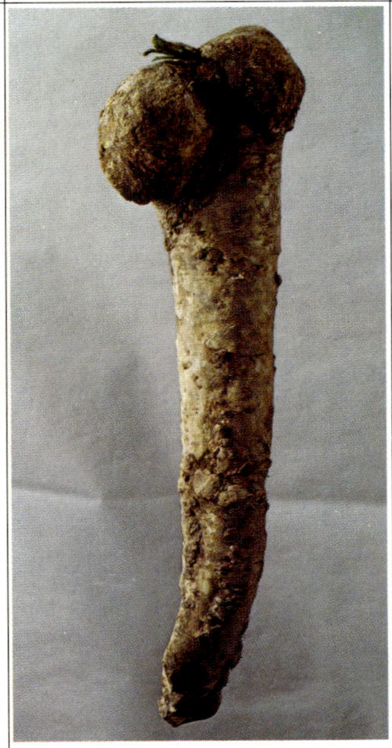

As a pungent condiment with a hot, mustardy flavor, horseradish is most widely used in the more northern countries. Its medicinal qualities are less well known The root may reach a length of 50 cm. It has several crowns and produces runners. The strong, dark green root leaves are large and may be as much as a meter long. They have long stems, are elongated, with a pointed tip, and have toothed margins. The stem leaves are much smaller and narrower and grow on very short stems. The flowering stem terminates in loose spikes of numerous clustered white flowers. Small pods develop immediately beside these, a characteristic feature of plants related to mustard. Propagation is usually through the root, however, and it is the fresh root that is used medicinally. The plant is cultivated for culinary purposes in northern Europe, and the leaves are also used in pharmaceutical preparations.

ARNICA MONTANA

ARNICA

Asteraceae / Compositae

27 Eur

Arnica is one of the most beautiful mountain plants and generally popular all over the world. It may be found in acid peaty soil and in mountain pastures left unmanured. It does not like chalk. The creeping underground stem first produces a ground rosette of yellowish-green egg-shaped downy leaves. The following year the flowering stems grow up to 60 cm high. They are slightly hairy and bear 1–3 pairs of opposite oval leaves. The stems terminate in single composite flowers with bright yellow ray florets on a conspicuous green calyx. Individual ray florets are bent back to a different degree. The whole plant has a pleasant aromatic scent. The volatile oil it contains and the floral pigments have many medicinal properties. It is said that Goethe used arnica drops to strengthen his faltering heart, and on the Continent many preparations designed to stimulate the heart and circulation contain extracts of arnica. Arnica shares its habitat with quite a number of similar daisy-type flowers such as the hawkweeds, red-veined dandelion, cat's-ear, doronicum, and several ragworts. Many of these have yellow composite ray flowers. Arnica may be safely distinguished from these by the few pairs of opposite leaves on the stem, and by the fact that the ray florets are irregularly turned back. The other members of the daisy family have alternate leaves.

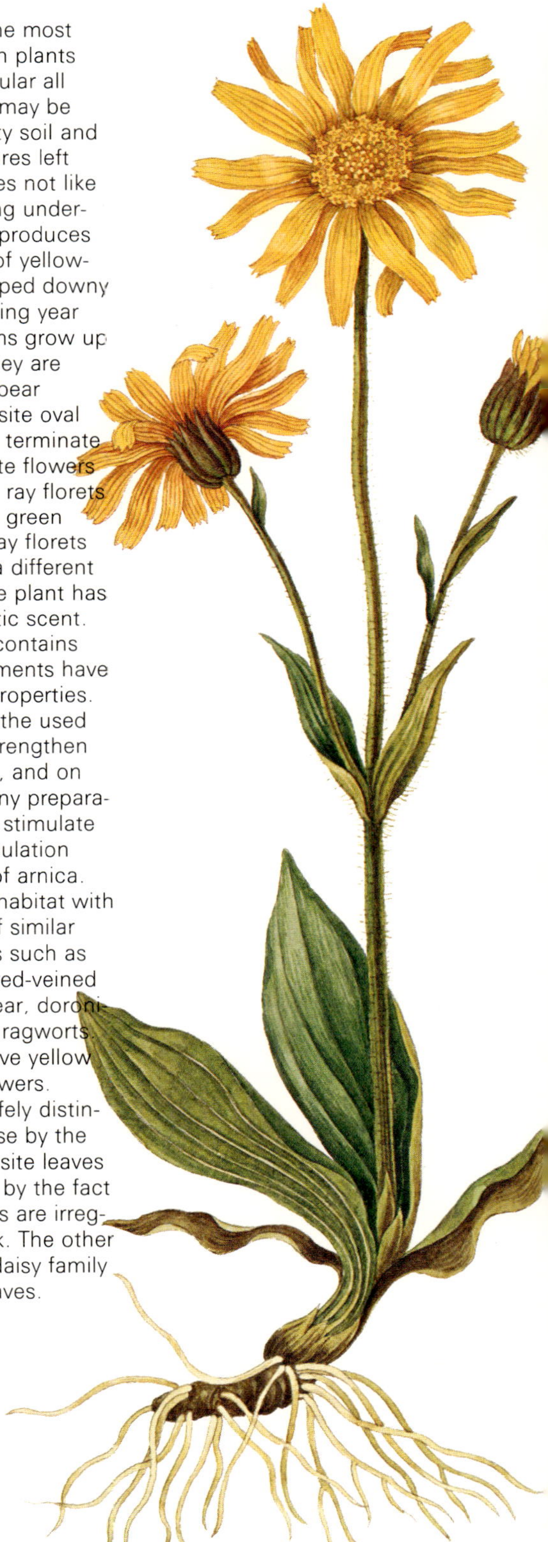

ARTEMISIA ABSINTHIUM

WORMWOOD

Asteraceae / Compositae

28 C+S Eur, N Af, C Asia
Temperate Zones

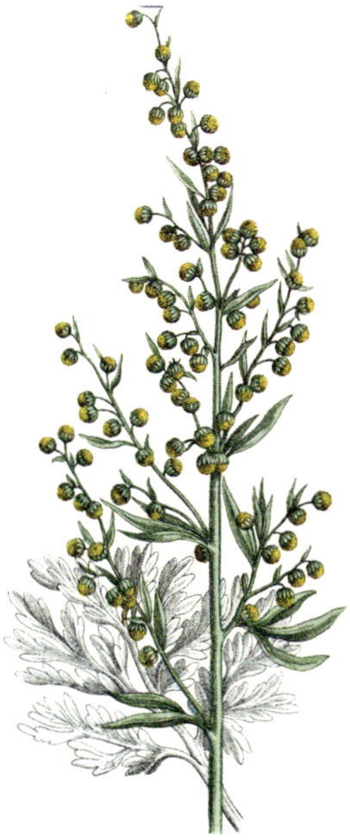

The ancient Greeks dedicated this medicinal plant to Artemis, goddess of fertility. It is a bitter herb. From a woody perennial root, which in the wild will flourish only on slopes getting the full sun and in dry rock steppes, this half-shrub grows up to 1 m high. The leaves, particularly the lower ones, are divided and feathery with pointed tips. The whole plant has a grayish-green appearance, being covered with fine hairs. The tiny yellow flowers growing in hemispherical heads on the upper side branches also have gray-green calyces. Wormwood grows in mountain valleys up to a height of 2000 m. Other *Artemisia* species may be found at higher altitudes. They all contain powerful bitters, but unfortunately also thujone, a substance that may affect brain function. Wormwood tea should therefore be taken only in small quantities and not too frequently.

ARTEMISIA VULGARIS

MUGWORT

Asteraceae Compositae

29 Eur, N Af, Asia
Temperate Zones

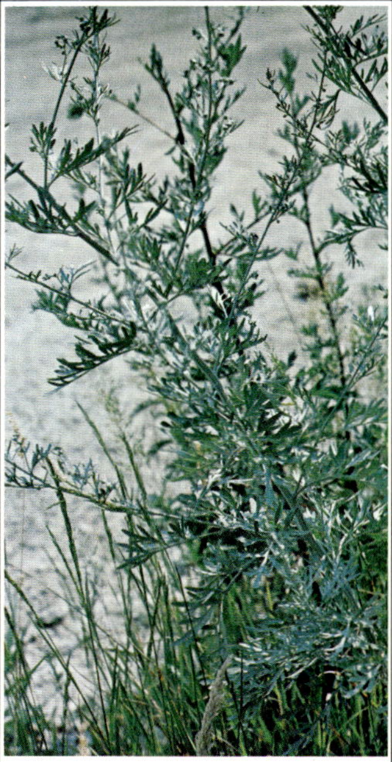

The mugwort, a relative of the wormwood, is a perennial shrubby herb to be found almost anywhere in waste places, along roadsides, on slopes of rubble, and on river banks. The tough, grooved stems often have a reddish hue; they bear dark green, deeply divided leaves and differ from wormwood in that they have only a few hairs. They terminate in long spikes of numerous small reddish or yellow flowerheads. The southernwood *(Artemisia abrotanum)* is a small species cultivated in Mediterranean countries and Asia Minor for its aromatic bitters. A small shrub similar to wormwood is *Artemisia mutellina,* which grows at high altitudes, while the sea wormwood *(Artemisia maritima)* populates the seashore. The flowerheads of the Levant wormseed *(Artemisia cina),* which contain santonin, used to be a popular remedy for worms. Other species *(Artemesia maritima)* also contain santonin.

ASARUM EUROPAEUM

WILD GINGER, ASARABACCA, HAZELWORT

Aristolochiaceae

30 Eur, W Asia

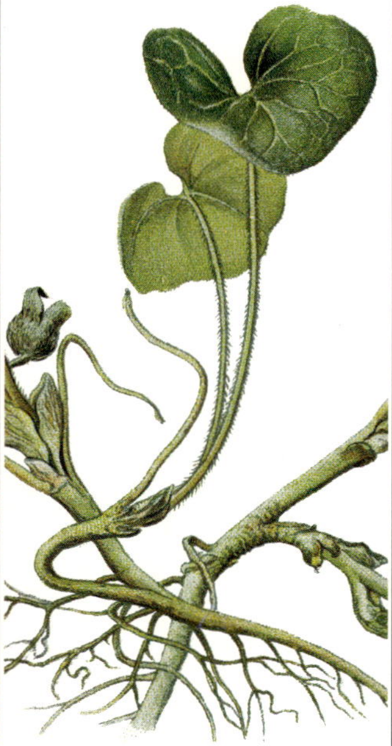

This small perennial, barely 15 cm high, forms large carpets in deciduous forests rich in humus, in hedges and bushes. In the soft ground the underground stem branches freely, producing many rootlets. The short creeping flowering stem bears 2 long-stemmed leathery kidney-shaped dark green leaves. These and the stem are covered with down. The young shoots produce inconspicuous 3-lobed bell-shaped flowers on short stems that offer welcome refuge to insects. Ants like to eat the seed capsules, and in this way distribute the tiny seeds. Wild ginger smells and tastes strongly of pepper. The underground stem and the leaves contain a volatile oil and other substances of medicinal interest, though caution is indicated in their use. The herb and root are still widely used in purgative powders given to animals.

ASCLEPIAS TUBEROSA

BUTTERFLY WEED, PLEURISY ROOT

Asclepiadeceae

31 N Am

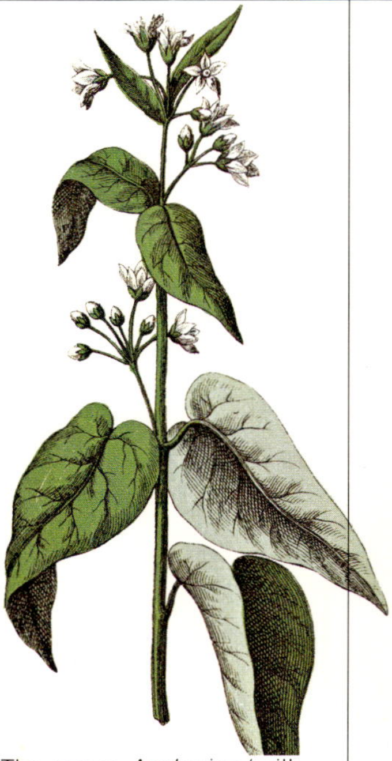

The genus *Asclepias* (milkweed) of the *Asclepiadaceae* family is represented by numerous species. They belong to the group of plants containing milky juice. Another feature of the genus is the tufts of silky seed hairs, to which one species, *A. syriaca,* owes its popular name, Indian paintbrush. In Europe, some species of *Asclepias* are grown as ornamental plants. The rootstock produces an erect stem about 1 m high. The narrow, lance-shaped leaves, 10–20 cm in length, are arranged in a spiral. The stem branches at the top and terminates in erect spikes of numerous 5-lobed flowers, generally orange-colored, but occasionally also red or yellow. The sepals turn downward. The fruit is an elongated hairy, pod-like follicle containing seeds with tufts of silky hair. The active principles found in the roots of various *Asclepias* species are similar to those of *Digitalis.*

ATROPA BELLADONNA

BELLADONNA, DEADLY NIGHTSHADE

Solanaceae

32 Eur, N Af, Asia
N Am

There is an air of mystery around this plant, which may be found in deciduous forests and in glades. In Greek mythology, Atropos, one of the three Fates, cut the thread of life. Belladonna, on the other hand, refers to beautiful ladies who used the juice of the berries to give their eyes greater brilliance. The plant is perennial and grows from a thick, branching root to a height of 50–150 cm. The stem is bluntly angular and branches freely; its upper part is downy. The large pointed oval leaves grow in pairs; they are dark green on the upper surface and a paler green on the underside. Single bell-shaped flowers, their crowns about 2 cm in length, grow in the leaf axils, their color a dingy brownish-purple. In late summer, cherry-sized berries develop. Green at first, they become black and glossy as they ripen, and contain numerous seeds and inky purple juice. The whole plant is extremely poisonous to man, but of great medicinal value. The active principles found in the leaves and root form a constituent of many pharmaceutical products. Poisoning from the berries is still quite common, and children should be expressly warned. First aid measures are to induce vomiting and give charcoal tablets.

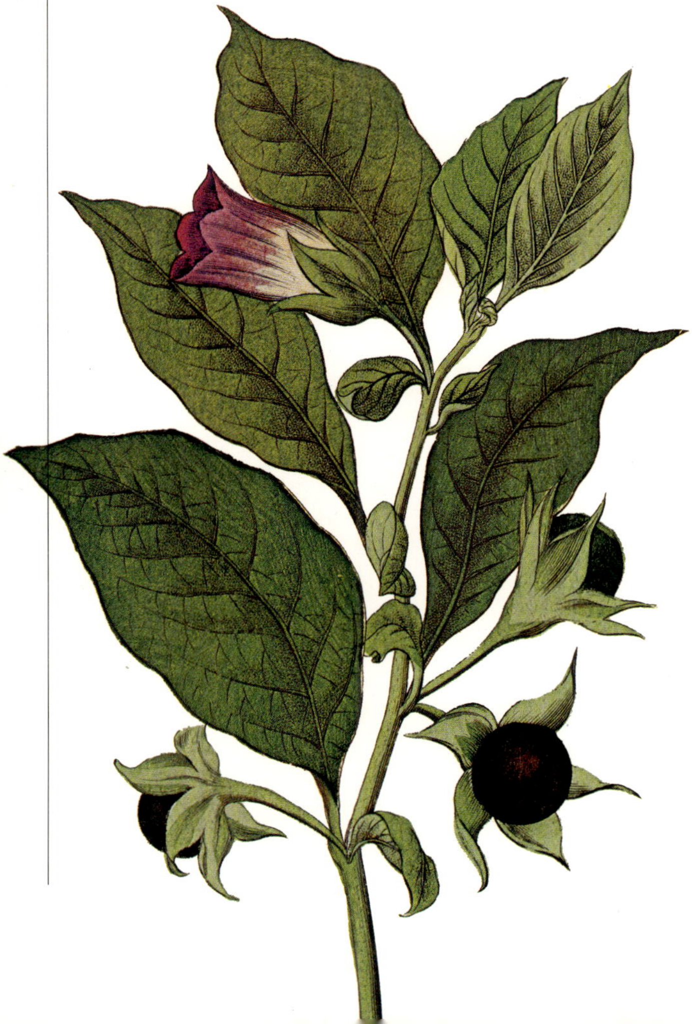

AVENA SATIVA

OATS, GROATS

Poaceae/Gramineae

33 *Temperate Zones*

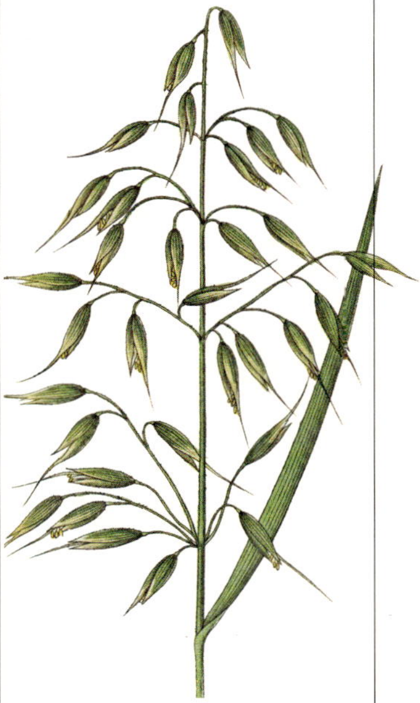

Oats are of major importance as a food plant. The plants cultivated for human consumption were often found to have medicinal properties, and this also proved true for the flowers and straw of the oat. Oats differ from rye and wheat in the arrangement of the fruits, and moreover the oat grain has a higher fat content. Oat straw is used medicinally, and homeopaths also make use of an essence prepared from fresh oat flowers. Gruel and porridge made from oats are popular as a food that is easily digestible. For a long time oatmeal porridge was the traditional meal of Scotland, and it still finds its place on the breakfast menu of many Scottish hotels. Oatmeal gruel is a useful nourishing dish during convalescence. Externally oatmeal is still used as a cleansing rub and, perfumed, as a cosmetic.

BAROSMA BETULINA

BUCHU

Rutaceae

34 S Af
S Am

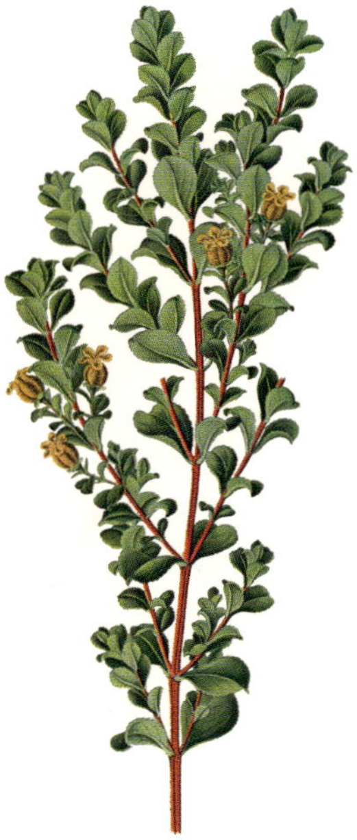

This shrub grows to about 2 m in height and bears inversely egg-shaped, almost stemless leaves about 2 cm in length that are similar to birch leaves. The leaf is stiff, slightly leathery, bluish to yellowish-green, somewhat shiny, and dotted with oil glands. The tips and part of the margins often curve backward. In the leaf axils grow white, 5-petaled flowers that give off a heavy, sweetish scent. The fruit is a capsule made up of 5 parts. The whole plant smells strongly of a mixture of peppermint and rosemary. It is widely cultivated in South Africa. Buchu taken in light doses can serve as a diuretic. Long used in orthodox medicine as a tincture and in herbal medicine as a tea, its medicinal properties have recently aroused fresh interest.

BERBERIS VULGARIS

BARBERRY

Berberidaceae

35 C+S Eur
N-N Am

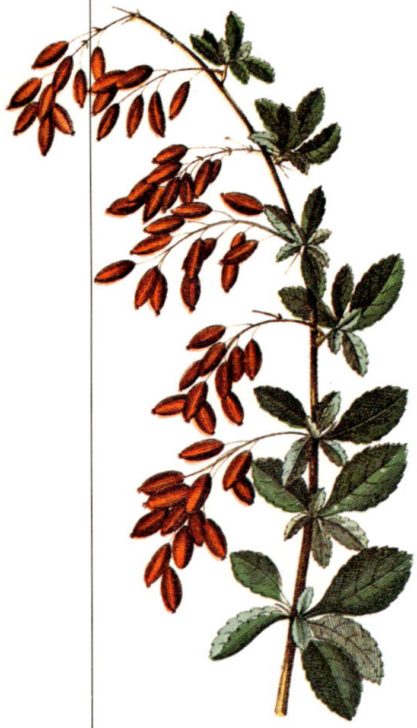

This thorny shrub, up to 2 m high, is often eradicated because it may be the intermediary host of a very dangerous rust fungus that attacks wheat. The densely growing bushes may still be found on the edges of woods and fields, in waste places, and in forest glades up to middle mountain heights. The bark of the branching root is a striking yellow. The long thin branches bear very sharp 3-pointed spines that may be regarded as stunted, contracted forms of leaves. Just above the spines grow short shoots bearing bunches of small, pale green leaves. Golden-yellow flowers hang down in grape-like clusters. They have a strong and rather unpleasant smell. The berries are small, bright red, and elongated and very sour to the taste. The leaves turn red in autumn. It contains a number of medicinal principles, not only in the berries, which are rich in vitamins, but also in the bark of the root.

BETULA PENDULA, BETULA PUBESCENS

BIRCH, WHITE BIRCH, DOWNY BIRCH

Betulaceae

36 Eur, W Asia
N-N Am

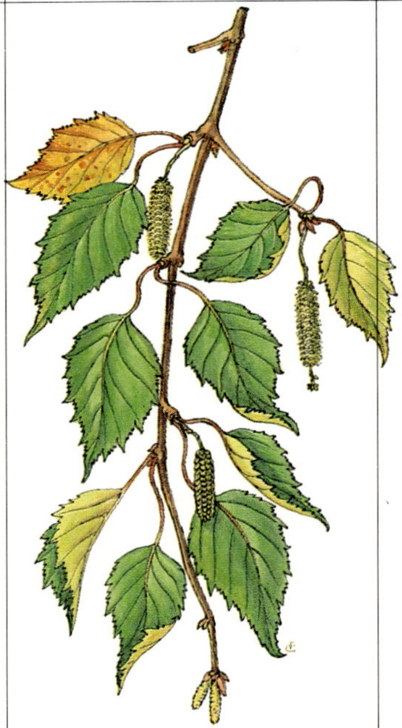

This beautiful tree, light green and up to 30 m in height, with its white and black bark and the hanging branches bearing bright leaves, enlivens otherwise somber heathlands, moors, and swamps, but it also grows on dry heaths at altitudes up to 2000 m. The pendent branches bear stalked triangular or rhomboid leaves with toothed margins. The wind carries the fine, dust-like pollen from the hanging male catkins to the upright female catkins. The absorption and transport of water is very active in birches. In spring, sap is collected by boring holes in the trunk or branches and inserting a tube through which the liquid runs into a collecting vessel. It has valuable medicinal properties, as do the leaves, the bark, and the wood. The birch was widely planted as an ornamental tree. Birch elixir is made from the sap and is popular in folk medicine as a spring cordial.

BRASSICA NIGRA

BLACK MUSTARD

Brassicaceae / Crucifera

37 S Eur, N Af, W Asia
Temperate Zones

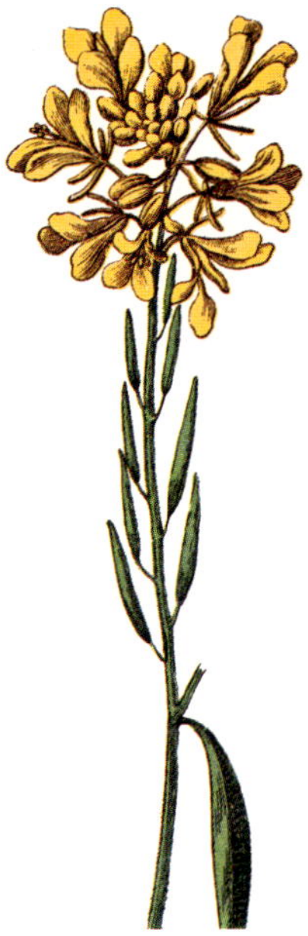

The first plant to appear on freshly broken fallow land is the charlock *(Brassica arvensis)*, which is very similar to black mustard. This, an annual herb, produces a branching, leafy stem up to 1 m high. The lower leaves are lyre-shaped and lobed; those higher up are smaller and narrower. Yellow flowers with their petals standing away form loose terminal spikes. The fruits are green pods standing upright close to the stem. They contain 4–8 black globular seeds. Mustard oil, a strongly irritant substance, is obtained from these. Like white mustard, black mustard is widely used as a condiment. It is also appreciated for its medicinal powers. Because of its strong irritant action on the skin and mucous membranes, it should be used with discretion, as it may cause serious inflammation. Concentrated mustard oil is poisonous.

BRASSICA OLERACEA

WINTER CABBAGE

Brassicaceae / Cruciferae

38 C+W Eur
Temperate Zones

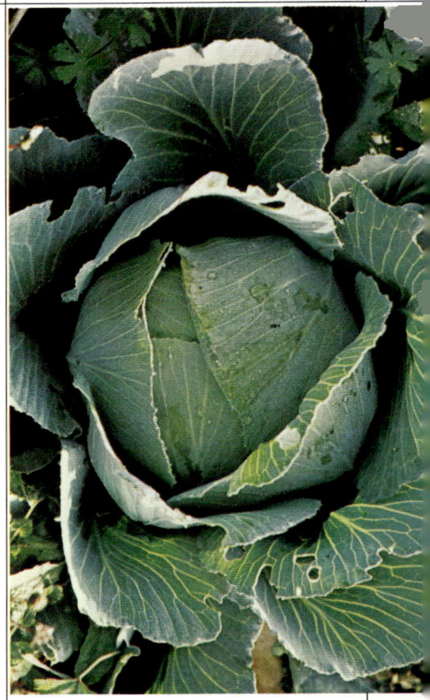

In antiquity, the Greeks and Romans regarded cabbage varieties as medicinal as well as food plants. Cabbage leaves have always been used to treat a variety of conditions in popular medicine, especially indigestion. The cabbages widely cultivated as garden vegetables produce round heads 20–25 cm in diameter growing close to the ground, on a round, fibrous rootstock. The fleshy leaves with their strong ribs and veins are closely interlaced, with large green leaves forming the outer cover. The many cultivated varieties, such as cauliflower, brussels sprouts, kohlrabi, often reveal their relationship only when allowed to flower. They then produce tall spikes of yellow flowers with 4 petals arranged crosswise, like those of the rape and charlock. The juices of most of the Cruciferae contain sulfur compounds, and the plants are able to concentrate organic iodine.

BRYONIA DIOICA

RED BRYONY, WILD HOP

Cucurbitaceae

39 S+W Eur, NE Af

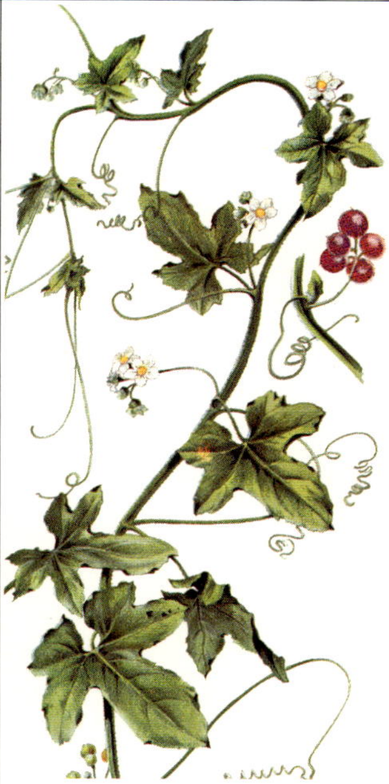

The red bryony is a climbing plant 3–4 m long found growing up the undergrowth in hedges, bushes, and at the edges of woods in the warmer regions of Central Europe. The root may grow as large as a sugar beet. In spring, pale green shoots emerge from the root; these hold on to stems and branches with their tendrils and produce 5-lobed leaves shaped like a hand on short stems, rather like those of the vine. The flowers are small and inconspicuous and grow on long stalks, male and female on different plants; the female flowers are yellowish, the male ones pale green. In autumn, bright red berries appear among the leaves. These are poisonous. The root contains some powerful principles used in medicinal preparations for the treatment of gout, rheumatism, and fevers. As the plant is extremely poisonons it should be given in homeopathic dilution only.

CALENDULA OFFICINALIS

MARIGOLD, POT MARIGOLD

Asteraceae / Compositae

40 S Eur, N Af, W Asia
Temperate Zones

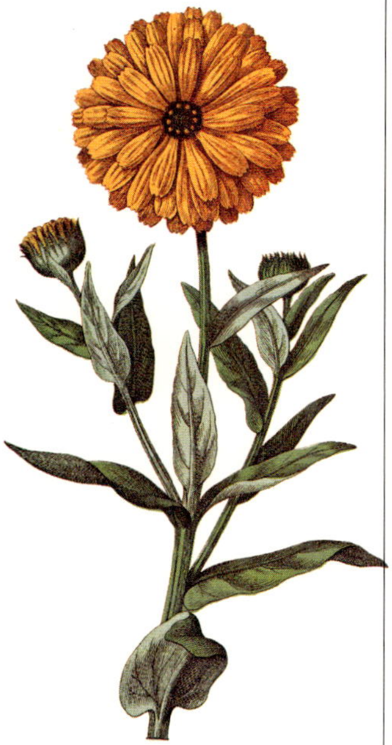

The marigold is a popular garden flower because it will grow in any soil. It seeds freely year after year, and flowers from July to September. Double varieties are grown for cut flowers. It has spread from gardens and become a wild plant, growing wherever it finds sufficiently friable soil. The plant is generally annual, with herbaceous branching stems that break easily and grow 30–60 cm high. The lower leaves are spatulate, hairy, and a juicy green; those higher up are smaller and narrower. The stems end in flower heads on well-developed green floral receptacles. For a long time the ligulate or strap florets of the marigold were used only to improve herbal tea mixtures. More recent investigations suggest that the floral pigments have medicinal properties. They promote the healing of skin tissue injuries, and stimulate secretion in certain organs.

CAPSELLA BURSA-PASTORIS

SHEPHERD'S PURSE

Brassicaceae / Cruciferae

41 Eur, N Af, W Asia
Temperate Zones

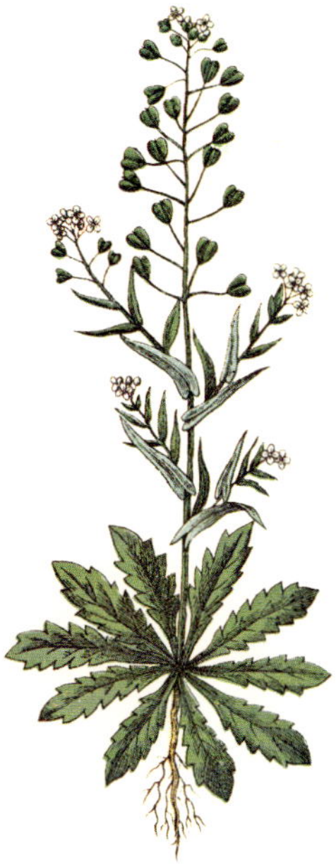

The unusual name derives from the small flat seed pouches which resemble the pouches worn by shepherds of old. The herb grows to a height of 20–40 cm and is found practically anywhere on wasteland and among the stones on railway embankments and river banks. The spindle-shaped root first produces a rosette of leaves similar to, though smaller than that of the dandelion. The stem is clasped by small narrow leaves. It ends in a cluster, wider at the top, of small white flowers. New flowers continue to open at the top, well into autumn, while those below are already forming fruits. One plant may produce up to 40,000 seeds. An indestructible weed, the whole plant contains useful medicinal principles. These have actions similar to those of ergot but far less powerful. They are best utilized in the form of medicinal preparations and not as a tea.

CAPSICUM ANNUUM

GREEN PEPPER, CHILI PEPPER

Solanaceae

42 C Am
Torrid + Warm Temperate Zones

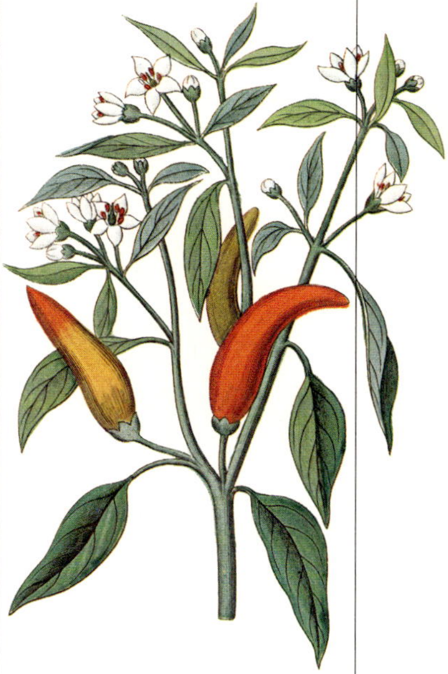

The nightshade family includes poisonous plants like the deadly nightshade and henbane, as well as many food plants such as the potato (the green parts of the potato are also poisonous), tomato, and paprika, many varieties of which are cultivated. From the taproot, which is usually straight, grows a perennial spiky shrub up to 1 m high. The luscious stalked dark green leaves are elliptical in form and toothed. The fruits are bright red air-filled pods, 6–10 cm in length, with numerous seeds on their fleshy inner partitions. The *Capsicum annuum* are used in pharmaceutical preparations, but the smaller fruits of cayenne *(Capsicum frutescens)* are preferred because they are more "fiery," with a higher concentration of active principles.

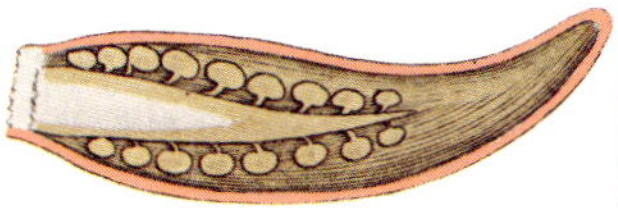

CAREX ARENARIA

SEDGES

Cyperaceae

43 N+W Eur, E-N Am

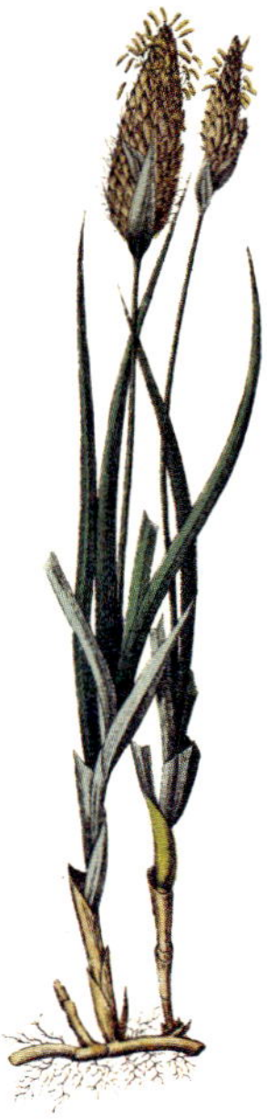

The sedges are a very large family of grasses. Sand sedges have the useful function of covering sand dunes and establishing vegetation on them. Other varieties of sedges serve the same function in mountain regions, holding together the topsoil and producing humus among the rocks. The nodular, branching, dark brown rootstock, its basal leaves dissolved into fibers, produces upright 3-cornered stems 20–50 cm in height. At the base, these are enclosed in brown leaf sheaths. The long, narrow, ribbed leaves, 2–4 mm wide, continue down into the stem; their margins and the central vein on the underside are rough. The flowering spike is 3–6 cm long; the top bends down slightly. It bears 4–16 male and female flower spikes. The haulm and flowers have a slight aromatic scent. The active principles are found in the rootstock, which in Germany has been used as a substitute for sarsaparilla.

CARICA PAPAYA

PAPAYA, MELON TREE

Caricaceae

44 C+N-S Am, C Am *Torrid Zones*

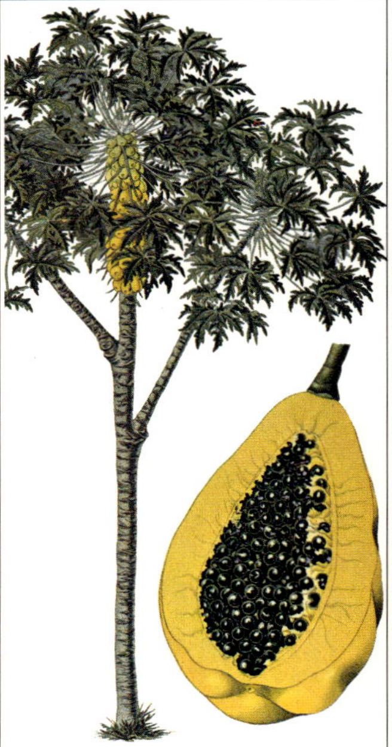

The papaya tree is similar to a palm tree. It is much cultivated in the tropics. The trunk reaches a height of 4–6 m. Only part of it grows woody, with the bark showing large leaf scars. The tree grows very rapidly and dies after 3 or 4 years. The trunk terminates in a head of large, long-stemmed leaves, each shaped like an outspread hand. Male and female flowers grow on different plants (dioecious), the male in spikes arising from the leaf axils, the female singly or in twos or threes in the leaf axils, yellowy white and 5-petaled. The ovary contains numerous ovules. The fruits, fleshy berries with projecting angles, rather similar to melons, are 5–30 cm in length and weigh up to 5 kg. The juicy, yellowish-red fruit flesh is sweet and aromatic and contains numerous shiny black seeds. The plant contains a milky juice, and a number of interesting enzymes have been found in the fruits, seeds, and leaves.

CARLINA ACAULIS

CARLINE THISTLE

Asteraceae/Compositae

45 C Eur

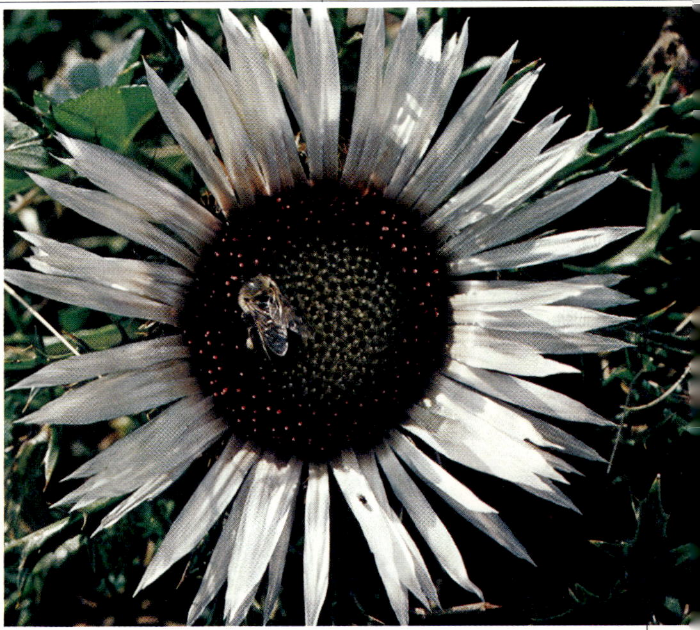

The stemless Carline grows on sunny stony slopes and in open woodland, from low-lying countries up to altitudes of 2000 m. It prefers chalky soil, sending down its taproot to a depth of about 20 cm. Close to the ground it spreads a rosette of deeply incised leaves with angular lobes ending in prickly points. This is indeed very much a thistle. Parchment-like bracts form a silver-white disk up to 12 cm in diameter around the actual flower head of closely packed yellow or reddish tubular florets. The whole of the flower disk opens only when the sun shines and serves as a barometer. Carline thistles do not wither and are used for floral decorations, like everlasting flowers. The active principles are found in the root. *Carlina acaulis* is protected in many countries and therefore no longer widely used.

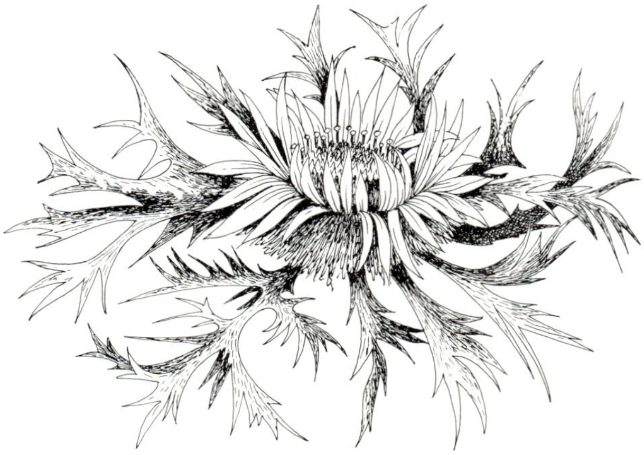

CARUM CARVI

CARAWAY

Apiaceae / Umbelliferae

46 Eur, C+N+W Asia
N Am

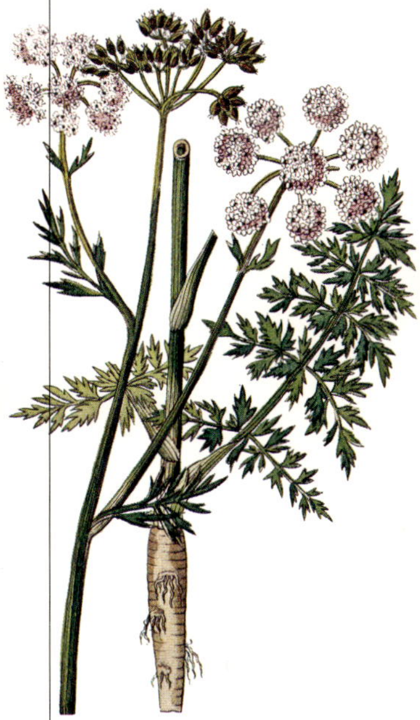

Sun, light, and warmth are most important if caraway is to thrive. It needs them particularly to develop the warming volatile oil it contains. Caraway grows wild in lean sunny uncultivated soil up to a height of 2000 m. It is cultivated for its seeds in many countries. The first year, only a ground rosette is formed, on a beet-like taproot. In the second year, the light green furrowed stems appear, bearing only a few small finely divided leaves. Each stem ends in a composite umbel of tiny white flowers. As the fruits ripen, they separate into 2 slightly curved parts, or half-fruits. These contain the warming essential oil, though the leaves if crushed also give off the characteristic scent by which the plant may be recognized. All plants producing essential oils need strong sunshine to do so.

CASSIA ANGUSTIFOLIA

SENNA, ALEXANDRIAN SENNA

Caesalpiniaceae / Leguminosae

47 C Af
Torrid Zones

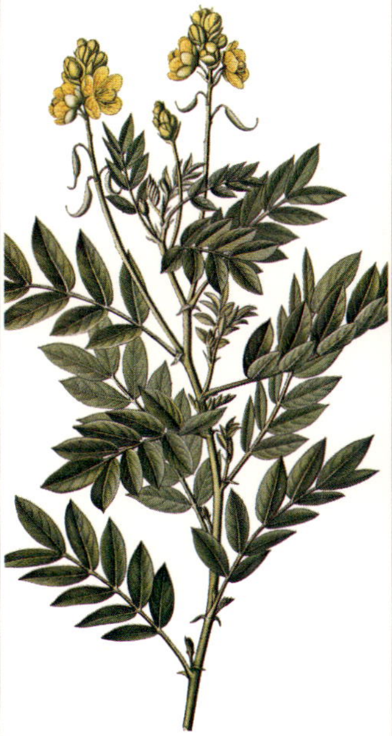

The genus *Cassia* comprises more than 400 species of subtropical plants. Apart from *Cassia angustifolia* and *Cassia senna* which provide senna leaves and pods, use is made of *Cassia fistula,* the false or purging cassia; the pulp of its pods also has laxative properties. *Cassia angustifolia* is a small shrub which, depending on the variety, grows to a height of 60 cm or may become a bush 1–2 m high. The stems are woody lower down and branch little at the top. The leaves are divided into pairs of narrow, lance-shaped, leathery green leaflets, 5–6 cm long and about 2 cm wide, ranged on either side of a main stalk which has a definite groove running down it. The stem terminates in a spike of yellow flowers. The flat, parchment-like pods are 3–5 cm long.

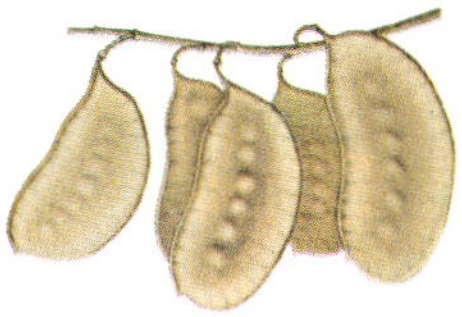

CASTANEA SATIVA

SPANISH CHESTNUT, EUROPEAN CHESTNUT

Fagaceae

48 SE Eur, SW Asia
S Eur

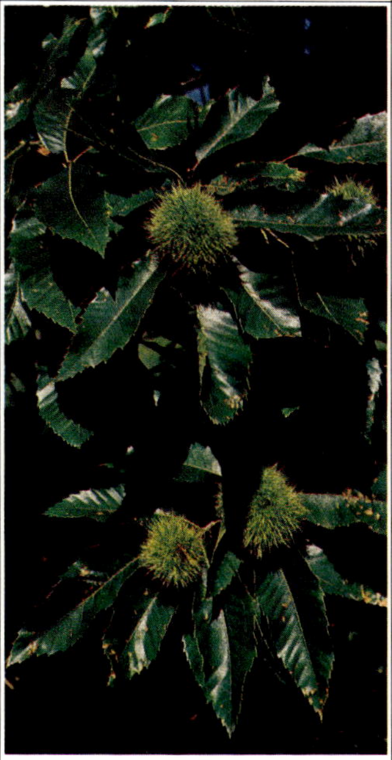

Spanish chestnut tends to form woods, often in company with the common oak. The stately tree may grow to a height of 35 m. The bark is smooth, olive brown, with lighter-colored lenticels, and becomes rugged and fissured with age. The large, firm leaves are short-stemmed, 10–20 cm in length, egg-shaped at the base, and pointed at the tip. They have prominent veins and are sharply toothed in the margins; the upper surface is a rich green and shiny like leather, while the underside is a paler green and slightly grayish and downy in spring. The male flowers grow in a number of small clusters on upright catkins approximately 20 cm in length; the female flowers in groups of 2–7 at the base of the male catkins, in the leaf axils. Two or 3 chestnuts are enclosed in a cup, soft on the outside but covered with spines. This is green at first and later becomes brownish, splitting into 4 when ripe.

CEANOTHUS AMERICANUS

NEW JERSEY TEA, REDROOT

Rhamnaceae

49 N Am

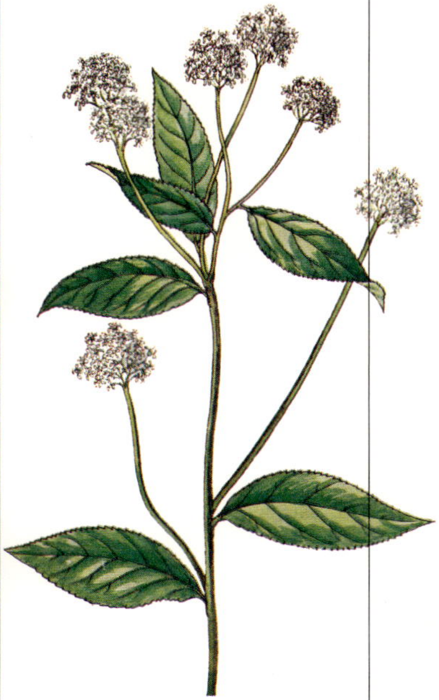

There are a number of varieties of Californian lilac, also known as wild snowball, and these are also grown as ornamental plants in Europe. The downy, later smooth, brownish-red or greenish branches form a shrub about 1 m in height. The alternate, short-stemmed leaves are egg-shaped, ending in a blunt point, pale green, smooth on the upper surface, with the veins and stalk on the underside covered with down. The leaf margins are bluntly toothed. From the upper leaf axils of this year's shoots grow spikes of white flowers. The bark of the root was traditionally used by the North American Indians to treat conditions affecting the mucous membranes and against fevers. The name "New Jersey tea" refers to the use of the leaves as a substitute for tea during the War of Independence. A number of active principles (tannins, alkaloids, saponins) have been found.

CENTAURIUM UMBELLATUM

CENTAURY

Gentianaceae

50 Eur, N Af, Asia
N Am

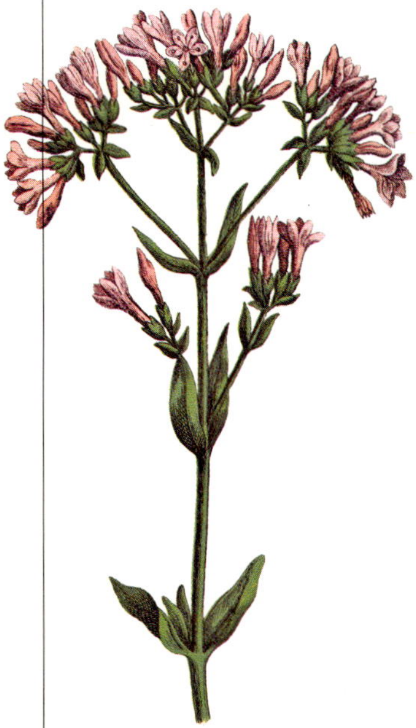

This annual or biennial herb was greatly esteemed by the Romans and during the Middle Ages in Europe. The name refers to Chiron the centaur, who was said to be a great healer. Centaury grows in chalky soil in sunny pastures, by waysides, and in forest glades. The root is light colored and produces a rosette of rich green inversely egg-shaped leaves. The square stems reach a height of 20–40 cm and bear alternate pairs of opposite lance-shaped leaves with prominent veins. They end in clusters of small pink tubular flowers opening into 5 widespread petals at the top. These are pollinated by insects only in the mornings. The seeds are carried by the wind. The bitters, which are typical of the gentian family, pervade the whole herb, a valuable remedy for overloaded stomachs. Compared to wormwood, centaury has the advantage that it contains no harmful substances in addition.

CEPHAELIS IPECACUANHA

IPECAC, IPECACUANHA

Rubiaceae

51 S Am
SE Asia, S-N Am

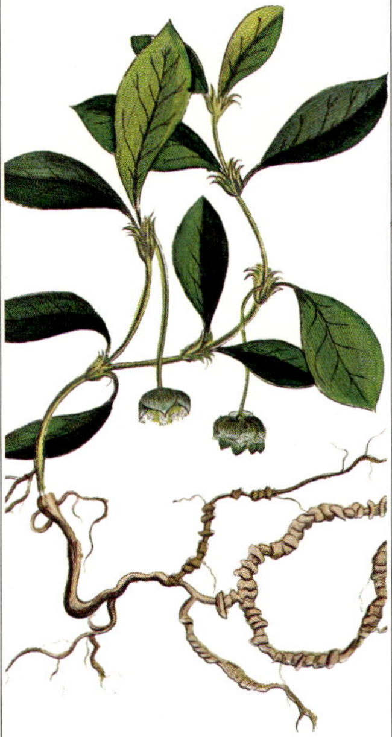

Ipecac, which is used to induce vomiting, is a small shrub growing to a height of 30–50 cm in the warm, humid rain forests of Central and South America. The elongated elliptical leaves are on short stalks and appear in 2–6 pairs. White floral corollas with 5-petal lobes form heads surrounded by 4–6 leaf-like bracts. The ovary develops into a fleshy stone fruit which is just about pea-size. To harvest the roots, the plant is dug up, the thickened rootlets are cut off, and then the whole shrub is replanted, to prevent its dying out (wild culture). Nowadays it is also cultivated in Asia (e.g., Malaysia). The active principles are widely used in cough mixtures. The major active principle, emetine, is still the standard remedy for amoebic dysentery.

CETRARIA ISLANDICA

ICELAND MOSS, ICELAND LICHEN

Parmeliaceae

52 C+N Eur, N Asia, N Am

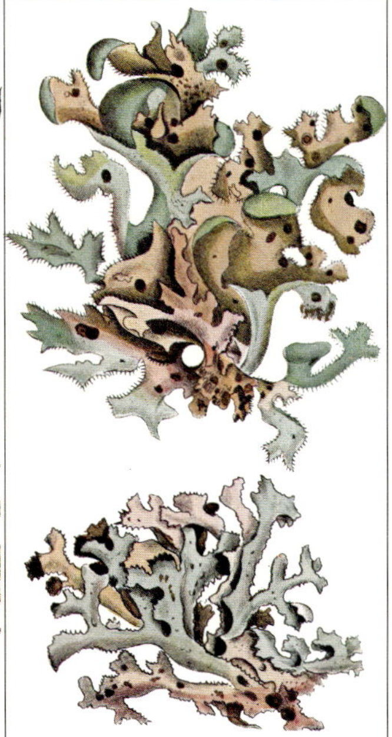

Iceland moss is not a moss, but a species of lichen made up of fungi and algae living in symbiosis. It grows among grass and mosses, mostly in the coniferous forests of misty mountains. The thallus is shrubby, deeply divided and smooth, and has stiff, broadly fringed edges. The rounded tips bear brownish scales and small warts. The lichen is olive-green or greenish-gray on the upper surface and lighter colored or whitish on the underside. As they die off, the thalluses turn rust-brown. The plant is rich in carbohydrates and provides food reserves for wild animals in northern countries. Modern research has shown that it contains vitamins and also antibiotic substances. It also contains some 70 percent of mucilage, which explains its traditional reputation as a soother of the irritated throat. There is also some evidence that it contains vitamins and has some antibiotic properties.

CHELIDONIUM MAJUS

CELANDINE, CELANDINE POPPY

Papaveraceae

53 Eur, N Af, Asia
N Am

In popular medicine, the greater celandine is known for the poisonous milky juice found in the flowering and underground stems. This produces bright orange stains and will remove warts; hence the plant is also called felonwort and tetterwort. Using the juice to remove warts may, however, cause ulceration. This undemanding herb grows in waste places, by walls and among stones, in the shade of bushes, and produces flow-

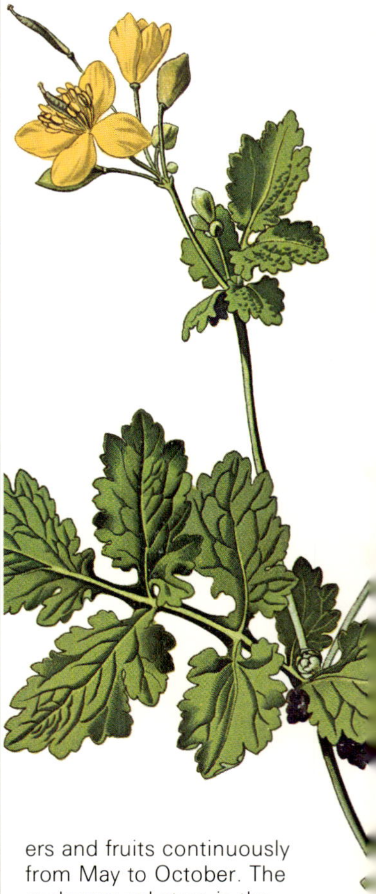

ers and fruits continuously from May to October. The underground stem is the thickness of a finger and reddish-yellow if cut. It produces upright hollow stems 40–80 cm high which have nodes and some stiff hairs.

The leaves in the ground rosette and those accompanying the stem are divided into 2–4 pairs, with softly rounded lobes, a rich pale green on the upper surface and gray-green on the underside. Four bright yellow petals form the flowers, which grow in long-stemmed clusters of 2–6. Green pods up to 5 cm long contain the small black seeds, which are distributed by ants. The greater celandine is poisonous.

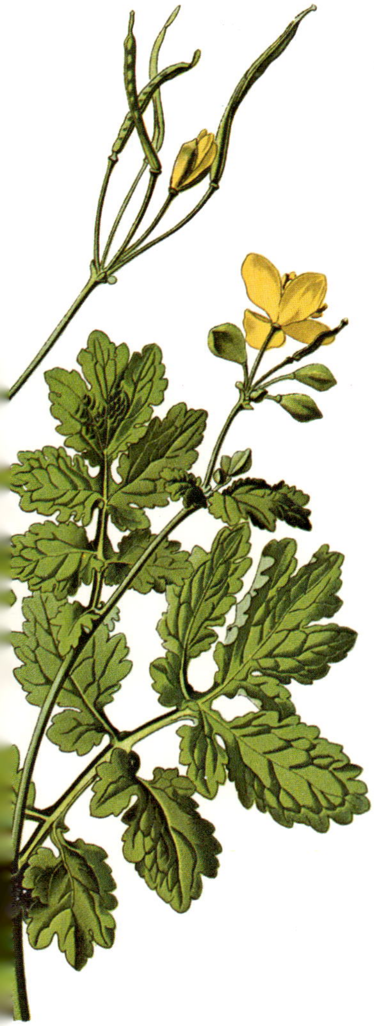

CHIONANTHUS VIRGINICUS

FRINGE TREE, OLD MAN'S BEARD

Oleaceae

54 N Am
Eur

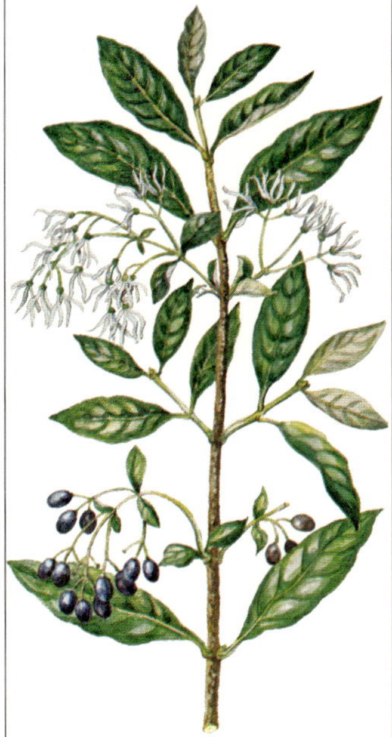

The most important representative of the *Oleaceae* is the olive tree, other members being the ash, lilac, and privet, and on the American continent, the fringe tree, also known as the snowdrop tree. This prefers to grow on river banks and in damp shrubberies. As a shrub, it grows to a height of about 3 m; as a tree, up to 10 m. The trunk is about 20 cm in diameter; its bark is grayish-brown. The branches are dark green and slightly hairy. The leaves are about 10–20 cm long, elliptical to egg-shaped; the upper surface is dark green and glossy and the underside is a lighter color, and downy when young. Buds on last year's branches develop into long flowering stems bearing spikes of white flowers. The 4 petals are narrow straps up to 3 cm in length. In autumn, the dark blue, elongated oval stonefruits ripen. Medicinal use is made of the root bark and the fresh bark of the branches, primarily in the United States.

CHONDRUS CRISPUS

IRISH MOSS, CARRAGHEEN

Gigartinaceae

55 N+W Eur, E-N Am

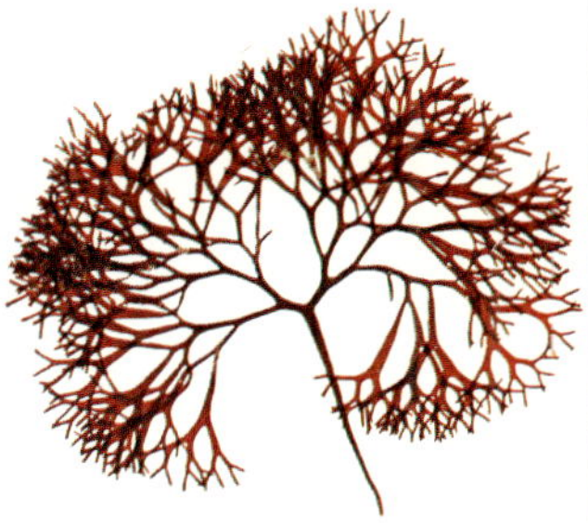

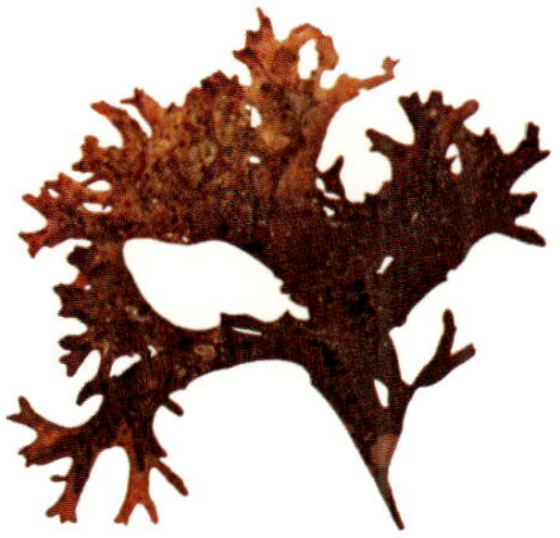

Neither Iceland moss *(Cetraria islandica)* nor Irish moss is botanically classified as a moss. *Cetraria* is a lichen and *chondrus* a red alga. They are found just below the water line along the Atlantic shores of Europe and North America, where they attach themselves to rocks and stones with fixing organs (hapterons). The thallus (plant body) consists of cartilaginous forked branches 15–20 cm in length which take the form of flat or grooved, broad or narrow ribbons. The cells contain chlorophyll, but also a special pigment which makes them appear red, purple, or brown, depending on the light intensity. At low tide, the fleshy, gelatinous algae are pulled off by hand or with rakes. Sometimes they also pile up on the shore after being torn from their hold by gales. They are washed repeatedly in fresh water and bleached in the sun or with bleaching agents. The cartilaginous ribbons turn a pale yellow.

CHRYSANTHEMUM VULGARE

TANSY, COMMON TANSY, BUTTONS

Asteraceae / Compositae

56 Eur, Asia
N Am

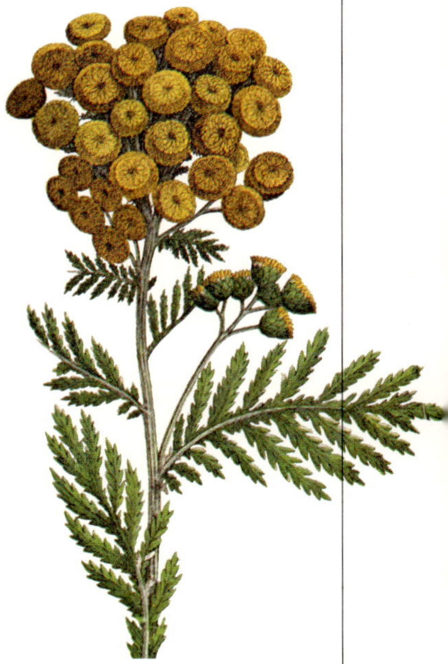

The older botanical name of this plant still used by some authors is *Tanacetum vulgare*. The name "tansy" is said to derive from the Greek word *athanasia*, immortality. A hardy perennial, it grows from a cylindrical root with numerous heads. The angular stems may be up to 1 m high and bear alternate, doubly divided feathery leaves with toothed margins which are a cheerful green, slightly downy, and dotted with glands. The stem ends in a loose umbel-like cluster of yellow flower heads with flattened tops (the "buttons") made up of short tubular florets. They give off a strong, camphor-like scent. In large doses, tansy is poisonous, but it is often grown as an ornamental plant. Its usefulness as a remedy for worms is in dispute, and getting the right dosage presents problems. Safer and equally effective worm remedies are now available.

CICHORIUM INTYBUS

CHICORY, SUCCORY

Asteraceae/Compositae

57 Eur, NW Af, W Asia
Temperate Zones

The wild chicory grows almost anywhere, an indestructible wayside companion in dry fields with clayey soil, and even among the broken stones on small field paths. Cultivated chicory is widely grown for the root, which is rich in carbohydrates (added to coffee). The tough angular stems stand stiffly upright, with spiky branches; they are hollow and contain milky juice. The narrow lobed leaves of a dull pale green clasping the stems are sparse, and the whole plant tends to be hairy. Short axillary stalks

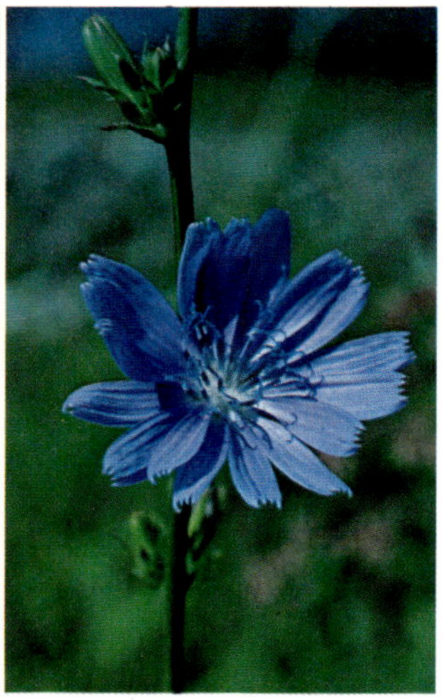

bear the clear blue disk-shaped flower heads (about 3–4 cm in diameter) with purple stamens at the center. Related species are grown for salads and as a vegetable (endive, chicory). Gently roasted and ground, the roots have long been used as a substitute for, or a diluent of, coffee.

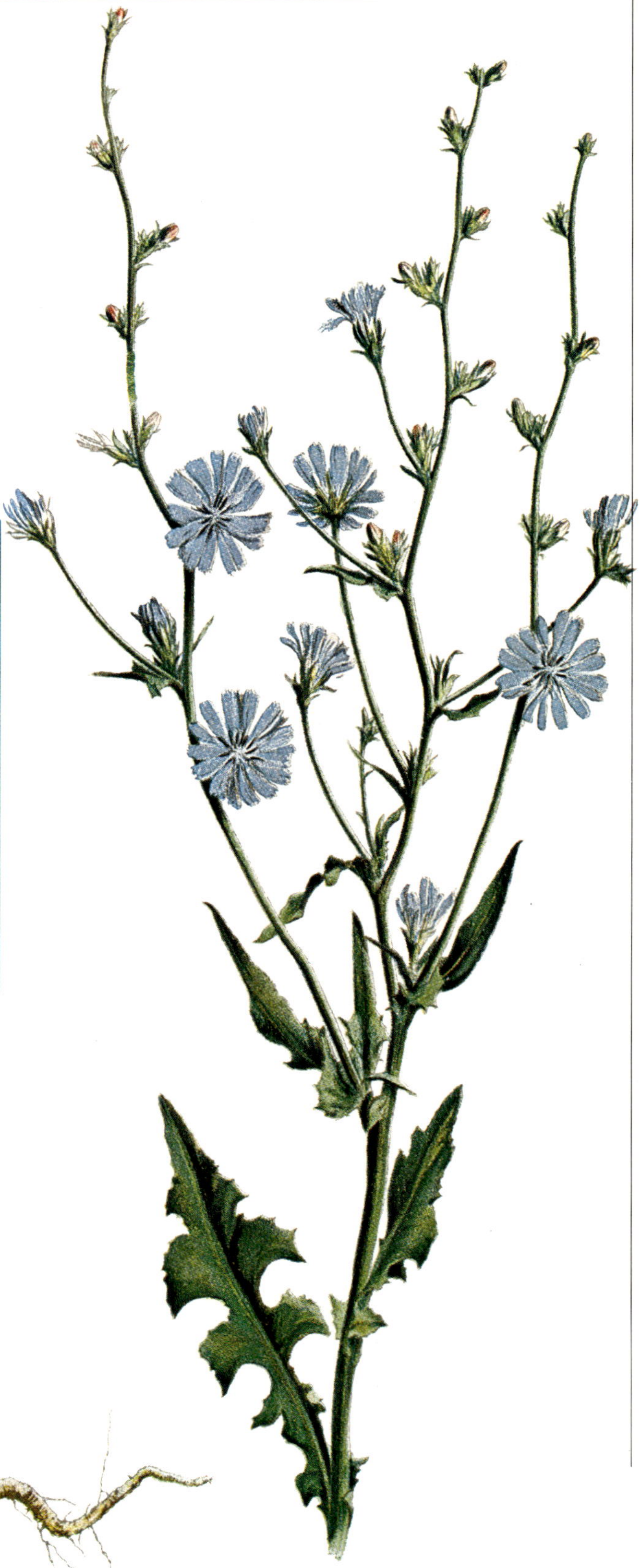

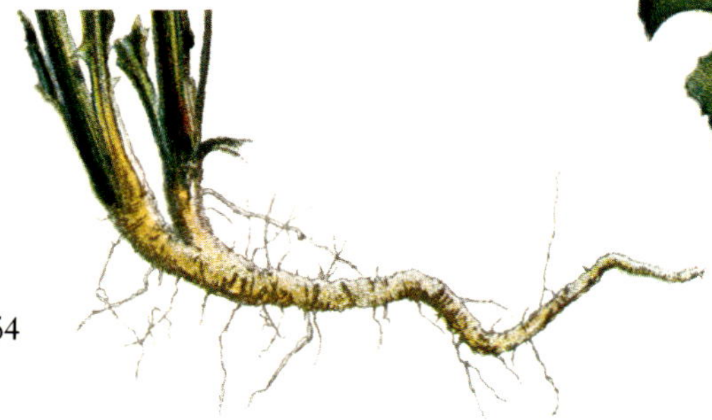

CIMICIFUGA RACEMOSA

BLACK COHOSH, BLACK SNAKEROOT, BUGBANE

Ranunculaceae

58 E-N Am

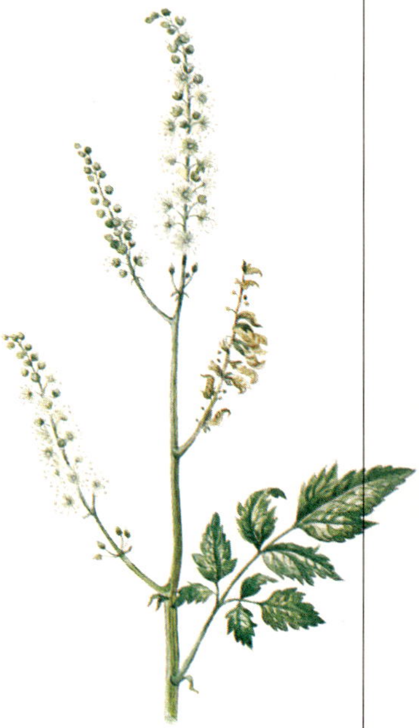

Perennial growing to a height of 1.5–2.5 m in damp or dry woods, hedgerows, and forest clearings. A creeping underground stem produces stout ascending herbaceous branches. The large, stalked leaves are up to 70 cm long and divided 3 times, their leaflets an elongated egg-shape, indented like a hand, and with strongly toothed margins. The leaves are dark green. The flowers grow in a rod-like terminal spike, white blossoms with 4 petaloids and numerous protruding stamens. The fruit is an egg-shaped capsule with numerous flat brown seeds (bug-like, hence bugbane). Medicinal use is made of the underground stem. This has dark reddish-brown fibers and a horny bark. It is collected after the fruit has ripened and is cut in pieces. It contains a large amount of resin, is bitter, and has mild expectorant properties. *Cimicifuga* is a major remedy in homeopathic medicine.

CINCHONA SUCCIRUBRA

YELLOWBARK CINCHONA, PERUVIAN BARK

Rubiaceae

59 S Am
Af

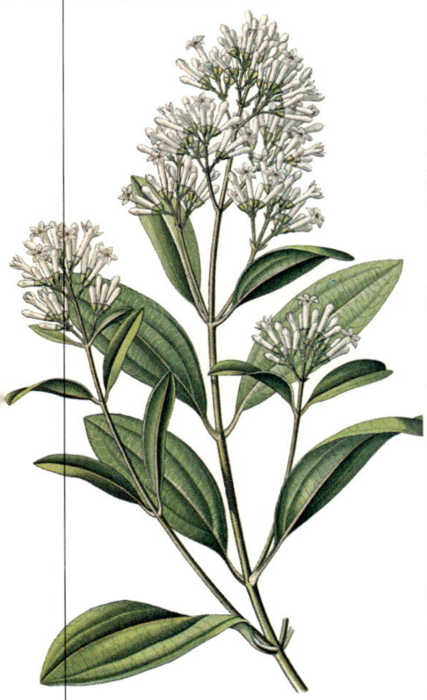

The bedstraw family *(Rubiaceae)* is very large. In northern parts, its members include many perennials *(Asperula, Galium, Rubia)*, and in the tropics it includes large trees, among them the Peruvian bark tree. The Latin name is thought to derive from the Peruvian word *kina* (bark). The bark has a long history as a drug introduced from overseas. Nowadays cinchona bark comes almost exclusively from plantations in the East Indies and Africa. The various species differ in their alkaloid content. The trunk reaches a height of 20–25 m. It has a reddish-brown bark and a beautifully leafy crown. The leaves are 25–40 cm in length, broadly elliptical, downy, and often red on the underside. They are opposite, on stalks 3–4 cm in length. From the leaf axils grow lateral branches with erect pyramid-shaped inflorescences of rose-red tubular flowers. The bark of the branches and roots is beaten and peeled off.

CINNAMONUM ZEYLANICUM

CINNAMON

Lauraceae

60 S Asia
S Am

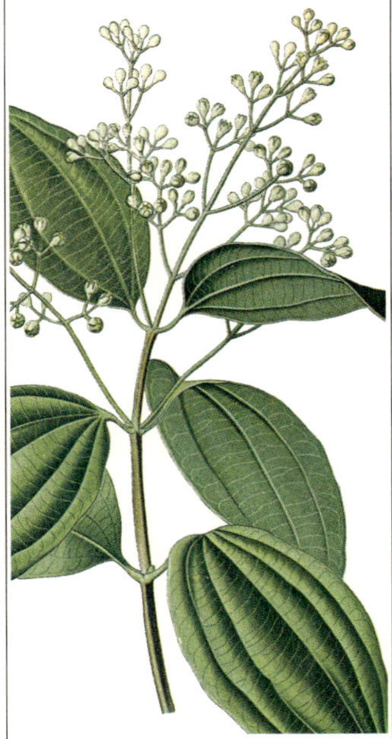

The evergreen cinnamon tree will normally grow to a height of about 10 m. In the plantations, the young trees are cut back to just above ground level, and the numerous unbranched stump-shoots are used to obtain the plant drug. The cylindrical woody core of these branches is covered with a smooth pale bark. Their large opposite leaves are 10–20 cm in length and broadly oval in shape, ending in a point. They are leathery, a glossy dark green, with the underside a paler color, and have prominent veins. The long-stemmed erect clusters of flowers grow from the upper leaf axils. The flowers are small, yellowish-white, and downy. The fruit, a club-shaped reddish brown berry about 15 mm in length, is enclosed in a bell-shaped calyx. The whole plant has a fragrant scent of cinnamic aldehyde and eugenol. The inner bark is used medicinally and as a spice.

CITRUS AURANTIUM

BITTER ORANGE, SOUR ORANGE

Rutaceae

61 S Asia
S Eur, S-N Am, S Am

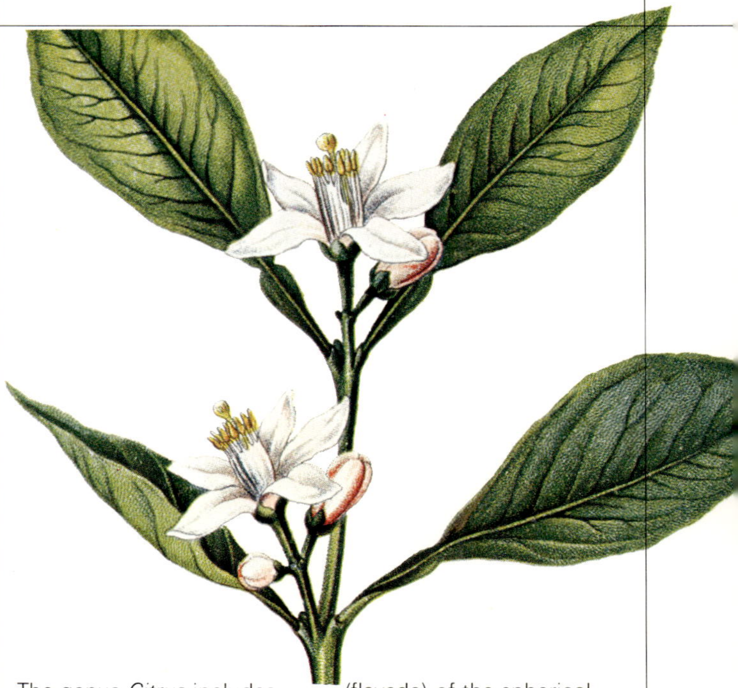

The genus *Citrus* includes many species and subspecies providing us with citrus fruits such as oranges, bitter oranges, Seville oranges, lemons, grapefruit, tangerines. Equally numerous are the medicinal principles obtainable from their leaves, flowers, fruit peel, fruit flesh, and so on. The bitter orange *(Citrus aurantium)* is of medicinal interest. In the plantations, the trees are headed to keep the trunk to a height of 4–5 m. They have numerous branches, with spines and pale green shoots. The dark evergreen leaves are pointed oval, 10–15 cm long, leathery, and have numerous oil glands. They are arranged in a spiral along the branches, often on winged stalks. The bisexual flowers are a brilliant white; they grow in the leaf axils or form small clusters at the tips of the branches. The 5 sepals form a tight bud and then spread wide as the flower opens, to reveal the 5 petals. The orange-red outer peel (flavedo) of the spherical fruit contains numerous glandular spaces filled with a volatile oil. Beneath it lies the yellowy white and slightly bitter pith (albedo), covering the actual fruit flesh. The leaves also contain aromatic bitters. Quite different constituents are found in oil of orange flowers, or orange flower water, obtained from the flower buds and blossom. Infants are given a tea of orange flowers as a gentle sleeping draught.

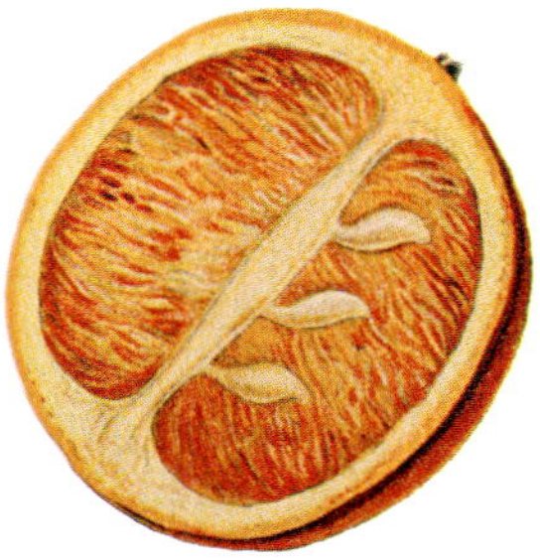

CLAVICEPS PURPUREA

ERGOT

Hypocreaceae

62 Eur, N Af, Asia, N Am
Temperate Zones

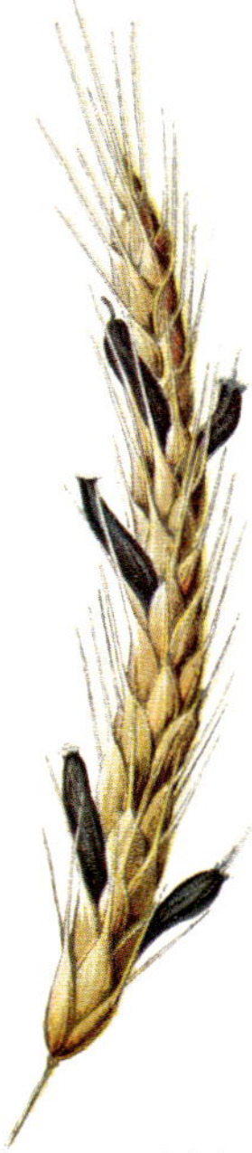

Ergot is a fungus which particularly attacks ears of rye. The wind carries the spores to the flowering host plant where they grow into a mycelium, a network of fungus growth, which secretes a yellow, unpleasantly sweet fluid to attract insects. As the corn grows, grains attacked by the fungus atrophy, and a hard, purplish-black sclerotium, a permanent mass of compacted cells develops. This forms the basis of quite a number of important medicinal products. If it drops to the ground at harvest time, it will germinate in spring and produce spore heads with new spores. Rye containing ergot has in earlier times led to episodes of mass poisoning (ergotism, or St. Anthony's Fire), even though the fatal effect of the black grain has been known since 600 B.C. Today, ergot rye *(Secale cornutum)* is cultivated on a large scale.

CNICUS BENEDICTUS

BLESSED THISTLE

Asteraceae / Compositae

63 S Eur, N Af, SW Asia
Warm Temperate Zones

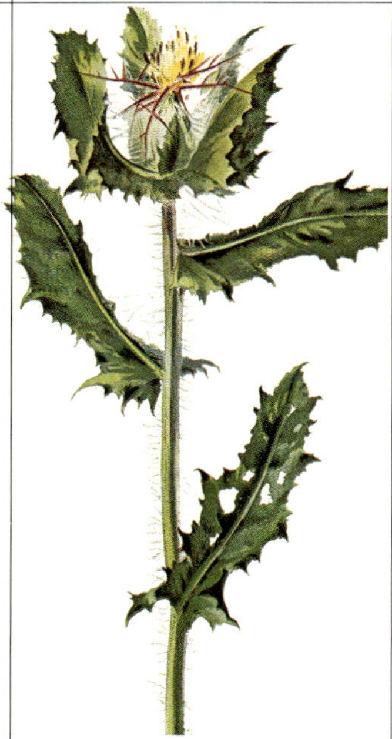

This herbaceous plant, a native of the Mediterranean, is cultivated for medicinal purposes in the north.
In the wild, the thick taproot likes to grow in sunny, stony waste places. The ground rosette consists of dark green narrow, lancet-like leaves, toothed and deeply incised, which are 5–30 cm in length. The 5-sided stems grow 40–60 cm high, with elongated pointed leaves held close. The leaves are toothed and wavy, with spiny margins. Both stem and leaves are hairy. The yellow composite flowers at the end of the stem are partly enveloped in a prickly calyx, with each bract ending in a downward-curving spine.
Also known as Holy Thistle, it has long enjoyed a popular reputation as an appetite stimulator. "Blessed herb" is an old name of the herb avens *(Geum urbanum)*.
It has long enjoyed a reputation as an appetite stimulator.

COCHLEARIA OFFICINALIS

SCURVY GRASS, SPOONWORT

Brassicaceae / Cruciferae

64 C+N Eur, Asia, NE-N Am

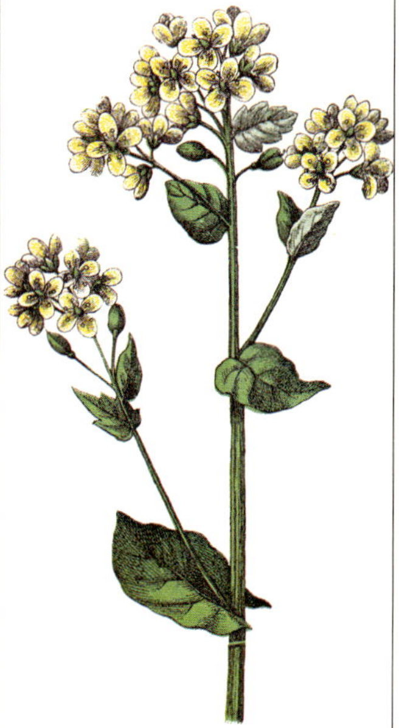

Scurvy grass grows in salty soil on seacoasts and riverbanks; an alpine species *(C. pyrenaica)* in ditches and swamps in mountain regions. It is similar to watercress and also has a similar salty, slightly sour taste. The basal leaves are long-stemmed, broad, and spoon-shaped, which is why the plant is also called spoonwort. The leaves clasping the angular stem higher up are a pale green, pointed oval and have bluntly toothed margins. The small white crucifer (petals forming a cross) flowers form dense clusters at the end of the stem. Small pods 1–2 cm in length contain the seeds, as is usual among the Cruciferae. The name scurvy grass points to the earlier use of the plant to prevent this vitamin C deficiency disease. The fresh plant is still popular for its vitamin content. Unfortunately, pollution is causing it to become quite rare, and the plant now has to be cultivated to obtain the juice.

COFFEA ARABICA

COFFEE

Rubiaceae

65 E Af, Arabia
Torrid Zones

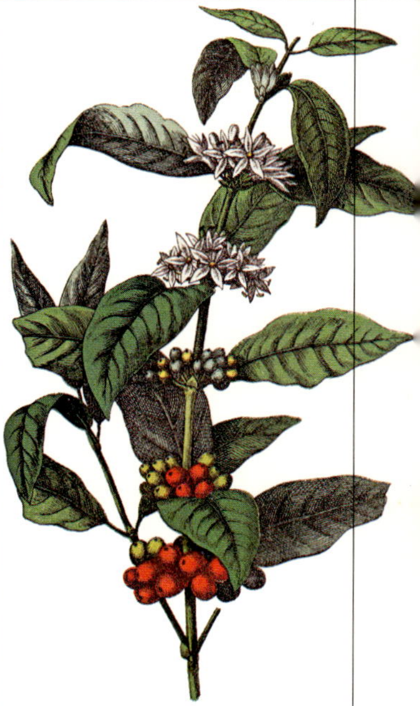

Coffee beans are usually marketed under the name of their country of origin, or port of exportation (Mocha, Brazil, Puerto Rico). In the plantations, the shrubs are kept to a height of about 2.5 m. The branches bear leathery, laurel-like leaves, up to 20 cm in length, which are a pointed oval, dark green and wavy, with prominent veins. From the upper leaf axils grow rich clusters of 5–15 snowy white star-shaped flowers with a scent similar to that of jessamine. The fruit is cherry-like, about 1.5 cm in diameter; it is an elongated oval, green, then red, and finally a dark purple. The pulp contains two seeds covered with a tough, parchment-like skin. These are the actual coffee beans. Various methods are used to remove the pulp and parchment. In the unprocessed beans, the caffeine is bound to an organic acid and requires roasting in order to be liberated.

COLA ACUMINATA

COLA

Sterculiaceae

66 C Af
S Am, Jamaica

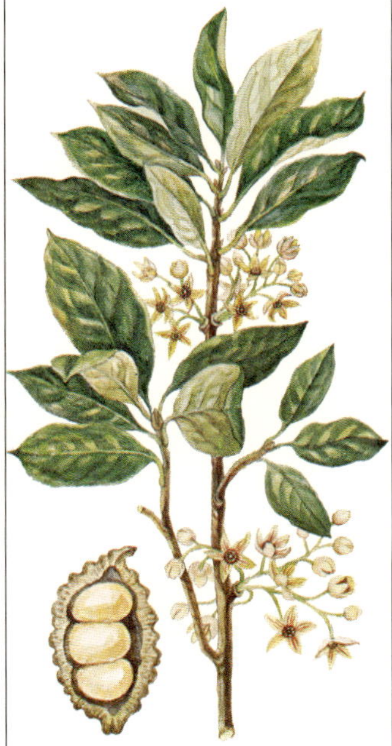

Long before the soft-drink industry discovered the stimulant principles of the cola nut, the plant drug was known for its high content of caffeine and other stimulants. The natives have always used cola as a general stimulant. The tree grows to a height of 15–18 m. In appearance it is similar to the horse chestnut. The long-stemmed leaves, up to 25 cm in length, are entire simple or in 3 lobes, tough, and elliptical with pointed tips. The bisexual flowers grow in spikes on the trunk and older branches. The fruit consists of 4–6 follicles arranged in a star shape; these are about 15 cm in length and each contains 5–9 irregularly shaped seeds. Freed from their dark brown wrinkled leathery or woody coat, the seed kernels consist of a white or brown embryo and its cotyledons. These kernels are the actual cola drug. They are reddish-brown seeds, convex on one side, 2–4 cm long and about 3 cm wide.

COLCHICUM AUTUMNALE

AUTUMN CROCUS, MEADOW SAFFRON

Liliaceae

67 Eur
C+N N Am

Flowering in autumn, the meadow saffron forms large colonies adorning damp meadows in both lowlands and mountain regions. The corm, sitting 10–20 cm below ground, produces a leafless white flower stem, 10–15 cm high, which bears the pale mauve 6-pointed flower. At the base this ends in a thread-like tube extending down to the corm. The ovary overwinters in the ground and is raised above it in spring, together with the green parallel-veined leaves. At this time the plant reaches a height of 25–40 cm. The fruit develops into a capsule which breaks open in early summer. This is when the small brown seeds are harvested, or borne away by the wind and by ants. A new corm then develops in the ground, at the end of the stem. The meadow saffron is poisonous and should be used only in pharmaceutical preparations.

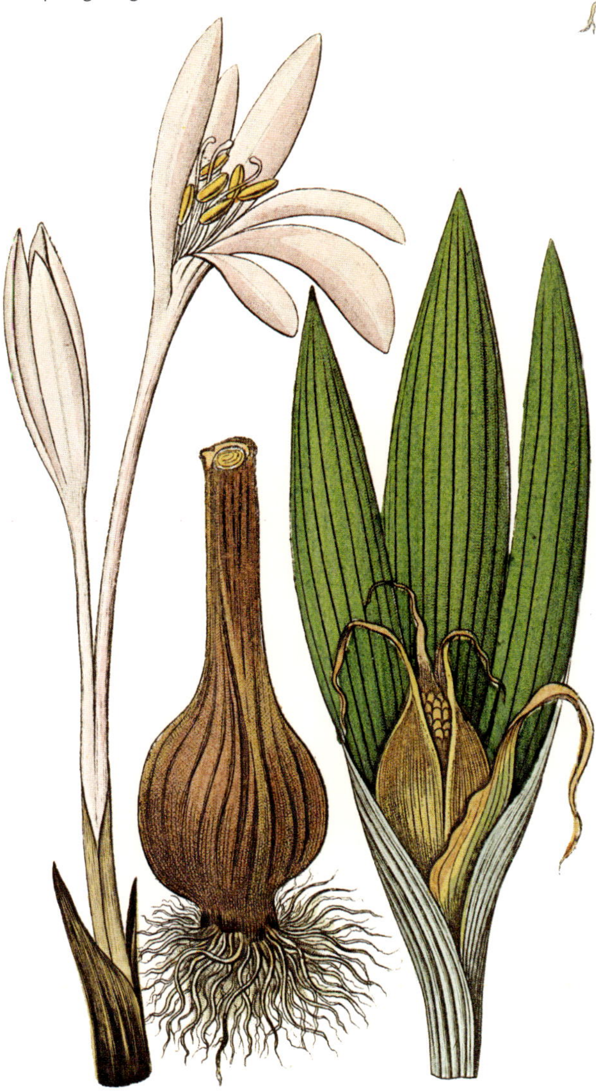

CONVALLARIA MAJALIS

LILY-OF-THE-VALLEY

Liliaceae

68 Eur, Asia
N Am

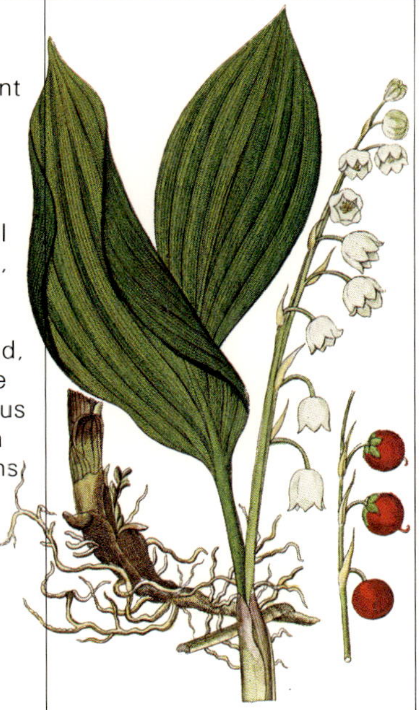

The lily-of-the-valley, popular as a garden flower, also grows wild on slightly moist clayey soil in deciduous forests and mountain meadows, often in large patches. The creeping underground stem increases greatly in length during the summer. It bears buds which wait until spring to produce 2 long-stemmed, upright, deep green elliptical pointed leaves 10–25 cm in length. Then the leafless flowering stem appears, with a one-sided spike of 5–10 white bell-shaped flowers. By autumn these have turned into bright red globular berries. The scent of the flowers is enchanting. All parts of the plant are poisonous and contain powerful medicinal substances. Tinctures and extracts of *Convallaria* are active constituents in drugs used to treat heart disease. Correct dosage as prescribed by the physician is important, to avoid possible ill effects.

CORYDALIS CAVA

CORYDALIS

Papaveraceae

69 C+S Eur

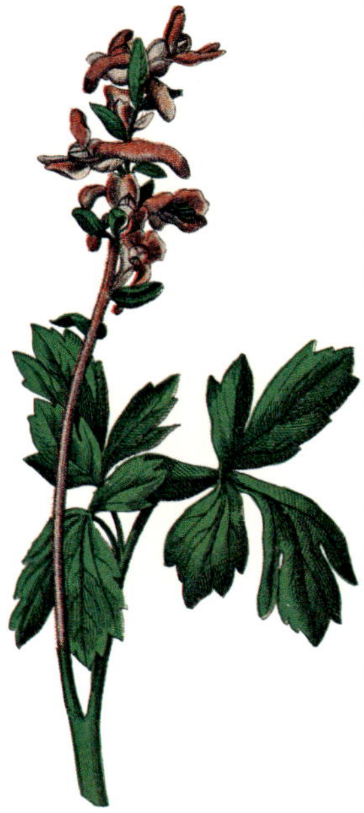

Corydalis grows in deciduous forests, shrubberies, grass, gardens, and hedges. The herbaceous plant overwinters with a hollow *(cava)* tuber with thread-like rootlets. The stem bears 2 alternate stalked leaves, bright green on the upper surface, and bluish-green on the underside. They are divided, with leaflets forming groups of 3, incised, tender, and fade easily. Every 3 or 4 years, the terminal spike of flowers appears. One of the reddish-purple or blue-violet petals is drawn out into a slim spur which contains nectar. Each flower is borne on a small, green egg-shaped bract. Small green pods contain the tiny dry seeds. When ripe, these are borne off by the wind and by ants. Corydalis grows 20–30 cm high. The active principles are used in neurotherapy. Experimental research suggests that their action may be superior to that of isolated chemical compounds.

CRATAEGUS OXYACANTHA

HAWTHORN

Rosaceae

70 Eur, NW Af, W Asia

The hawthorn was already known to the ancient Greeks, but went out of medicinal use until rediscovered in the nineteenth century by an Irish physician. The spiky bush or tree reaches a height of up to 4 m and grows on the edge of woods and forests; it is frequently planted as a hedge. It is not found at altitudes above 1500 m. All along the twiggy branches grow sharp thorns and small stalked deeply lobed leaves which are a shiny fresh green. In May to June, a snow-white blossom appears among the green; the flowers are about 1.5 cm across, with 5 petals and numerous reddish stamens surrounding 1 or 2 styles

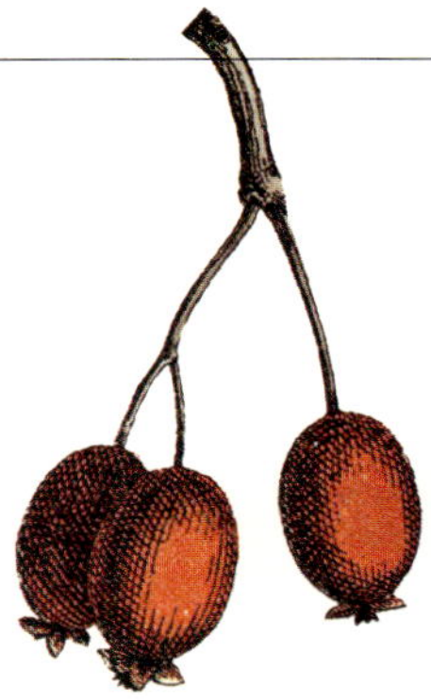

(depending on the species). The fruits are brilliant red, round to oval pseudo-fruits 8–10 mm in diameter hanging down in clusters. The leaves, flowers, and fruit contain medicinally active principles and are widely used in heart remedies, particularly on the Continent.

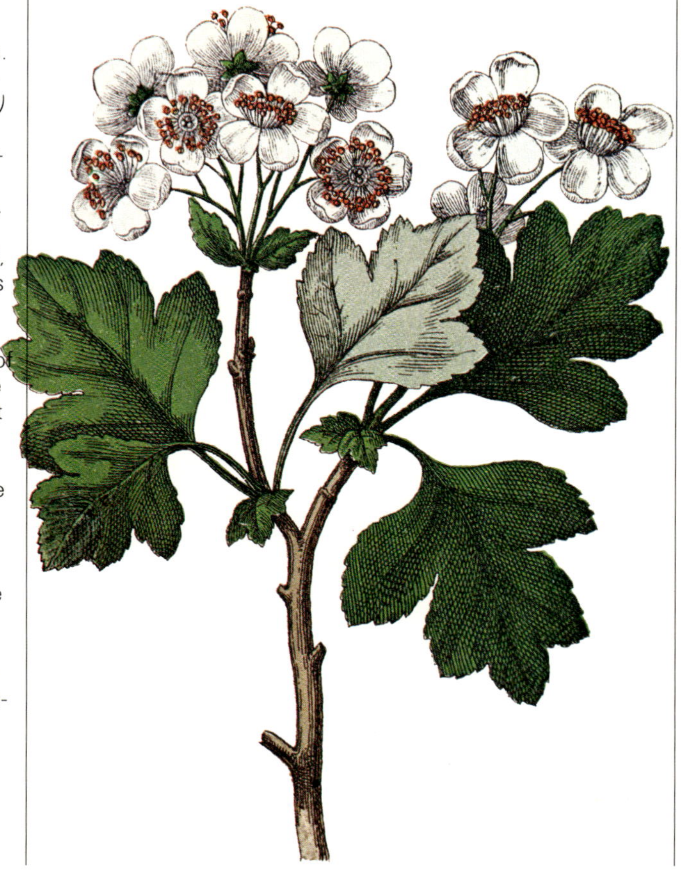

CUCURBITA PEPO

PUMPKIN, SQUASH

Cucurbitaceae

71 C Af, S Asia *Torrid+ Warm Temperate Zones*

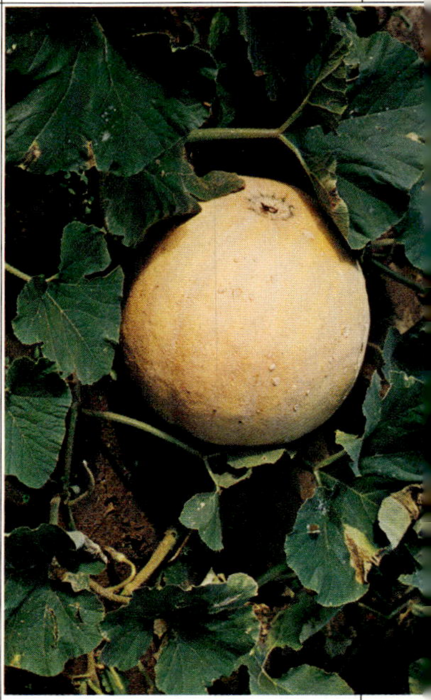

Pumpkins like a very rich soil and flourish on compost heaps, often growing wild after they have been cultivated. The creeping stem reaches a length of several meters, and lateral stems bear large dark green lobular leaves which have prominent veins and are very hairy. Branching tendrils help the plant to hold on to its surroundings. The bright yellow star-shaped flowers have short stems. Their ovaries develop into large yellow pumpkins, with flattened oval white seeds in the watery fruit flesh. With the hard shell removed, the seeds are chewed, or they may be pounded before they are taken. There has not been much research on the active principles so far. It is improbable that the fatty oil is really useful as a treatment of tapeworms, as has been claimed.

CUCURMA LONGA

TURMERIC

Zingiberaceae

72 S Asia
Torrid Zones

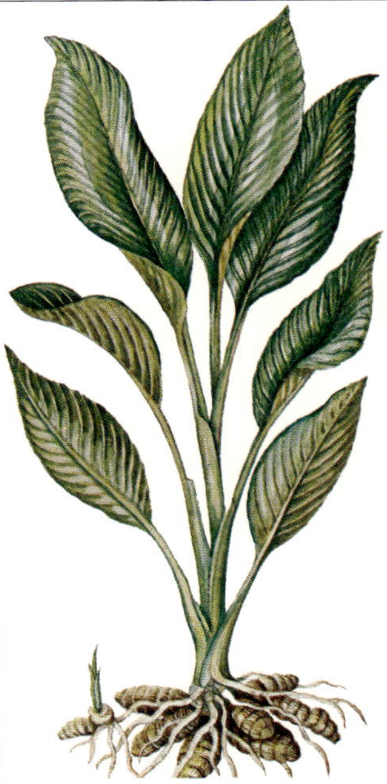

Cucurma root is one of the spices used to flavor and color curries, and also serves as a textile dye in East Asia. Recent researches have brought it back into favor for its property of stimulating biliary function. The tuberous principal root produces a considerable number of lateral roots, some of them bearing root leaves and showing transverse ring markings when those leaves have died. The lateral roots will sometimes separate from the main root and develop into separate plants. Short axial shoots produce long green stems with erect leaves 1 m long, thin and narrow like lily leaves, with margins entire, sheathing the stem at the base. The large yellow flowers are funnel-shaped and usually grow in pairs in the axils of greenish-white leaf structures. The root is marketed in lengths of 3–4 cm; it shows transverse ring markings and is horny on the outside.

CYDONIA OBLONGA

QUINCE

Rosaceae

73 W Asia
Eur, N Am

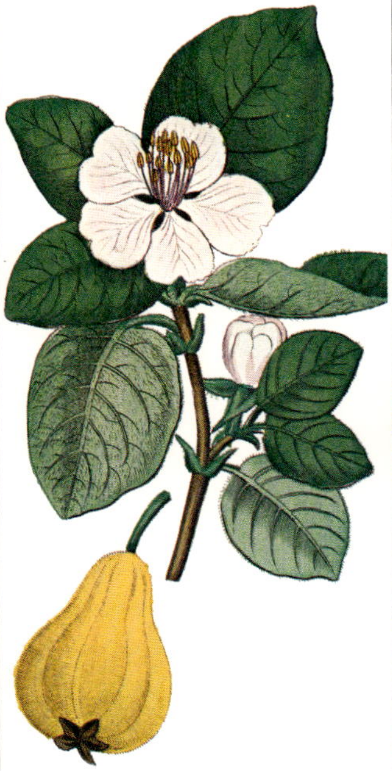

The quince, quite common in the gardens around our houses, grows to a height of 4–6 m. In northern parts, it is more usual to train it. The stiff branches bear short-stemmed egg-shaped leaves covered with matted down. There are no thorns. The flowers are pink or white stars of 5 petals and larger than apple blossom. The ovary and the floral base form a pome, the pear-shaped quince, with a rough yellow skin covered with a woolly pelt which rubs off easily. The flesh is firm, not very juicy, and rather sour. It is made into preserves. The cores with the pips which contain mucilage are used for their aperient properties.

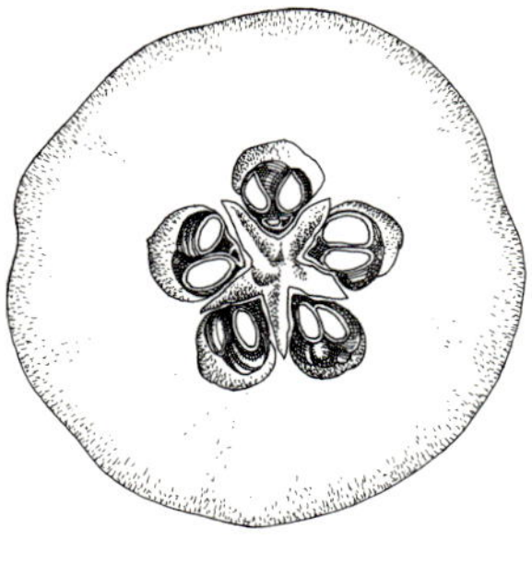

CYNARA SCOLYMUS

ARTICHOKE,
GLOBE ARTICHOKE

Asteraceae/Compositae

74 S Eur
Warm Temperate Zones

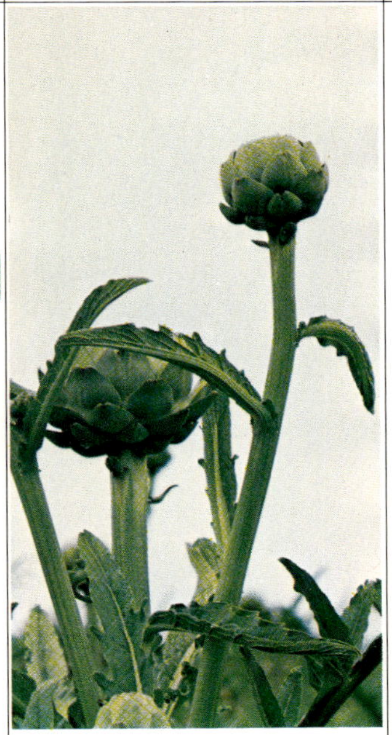

The artichoke is related to the thistles. It produces a sturdy, fleshy upright stem which grows from a basal rosette of leaves. These are 20–30 cm in length, doubly divided and toothed, gray-green and downy on the underside. The leaves borne on the stem are similar in shape but narrower and more elongated. The flower heads are prickly, with fleshy scale leaves. The soft inner tips of these and the flower base (the "bottom") are eaten as a vegetable before the violet ray florets open. The bitter substances obtained from the leaves, the stem, and the root are a useful dietary aid for those with poor liver function and high cholesterol levels. The use of artichoke extracts in aperitifs is sound practice, as is their use in teas for preventive treatment after liver diseases. The leaves contain an enzyme which even in high dilutions will coagulate milk.

CYNOGLOSSUM
OFFICINALE

HOUND'S TONGUE

Boraginaceae

75 Eur, W Af, Asia
Temperate Zones

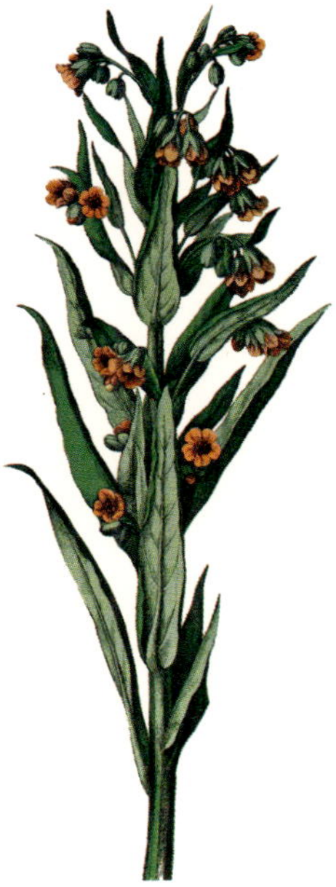

The name derives from the softly downy, pointed leaves which are similar to a dog's tongue. The plant grows to a height of 40–80 cm, on roadsides, in forest glades, hedges, and stony slopes. The spindle-shaped root produces an angular stem with numerous alternate leaves in the second year. Stem and leaves are covered with a grayish pelt of hairs. Small coiled spikes of short-stemmed maroon flowers grow from the upper leaf axils. The fruits are in 4 parts and have small hooked spines at the top, by which they become attached to animals brushing past. The whole plant smells rather unpleasantly of mice, especially if the leaves are rubbed between the fingers. The active principles are contained in the root and in the herb. They are similar to those of comfrey *(Symphytum officinale)*, which belongs to the same family, and are used in a similar way.

CYTISUS SCOPARIUS

BROOM, SCOTCH BROOM

Papilionaceae

76 S+W Eur

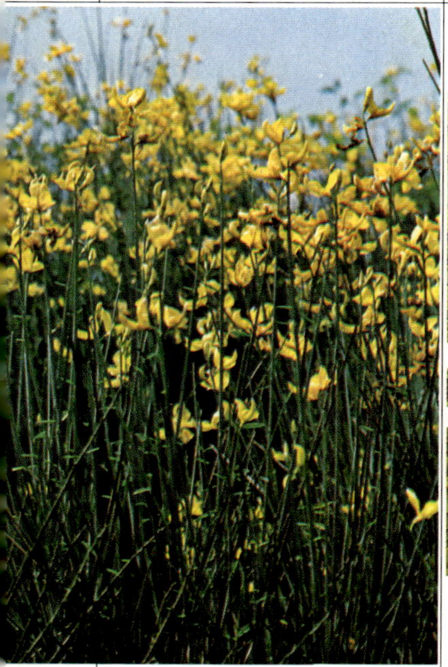

The long slender branches are strongly ridged and woody and are used to make brooms; hence the English name. The branches bear numerous golden-yellow flowers which cheer up sunny slopes, forest glades, and heaths in early spring. The shrub grows to a height of up to 2 m and is deeply rooted. The dark green branches bear small leaves that have 3 leaflets lower down and are single higher up, barely visible among the flowers. The large yellow peaflowers are the most outstanding feature of the broom. The fruits are flat brownish-black pods containing a number of brown seeds. The young tips of the branches and the seeds contain substances with useful medicinal properties. The flowers of a relative, the dyer's greenweed *(Genista tinctoria)* are used to dye fabrics. Another species in Mediterranean countries is the Spanish broom *(Spartium junceum)*.

DATURA STRAMONIUM

THORNAPPLE, JIMSONWEED

Solanaceae

77 C Am
Warm Temperate Zones

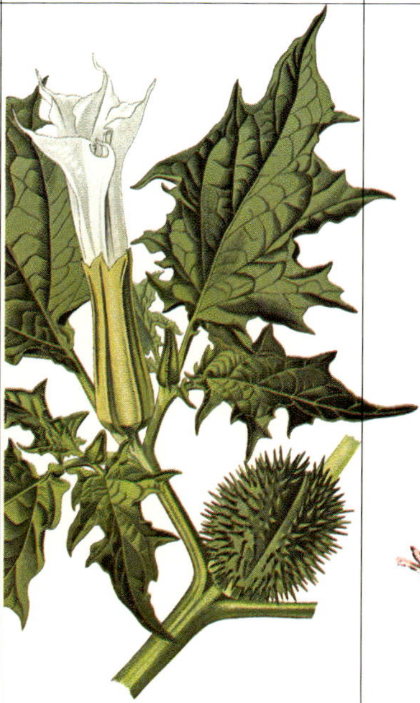

The thornapple, a member of the nightshade family closely related to belladonna, sometimes grows wild also in more northern areas – in fields, waste places, and sunny spots at the edges of woods. The tap root produces a freely branching, firm round stem 40–100 cm in height. The dark green leaves are oval, often triangular and quite large, with deeply incurving toothed margins. From the leaf axils grow the single flowers, white trumpets 6–10 cm in length, opening above a green calyx. They are pleasantly scented, in contrast to the rather repellent smell of the leaves. The fruit is a spiny capsule, similar to that of the horse chestnut. When ripe it opens to reveal small black seeds. The seeds and particularly also the leaves contain poisonous principles which are used in cigarettes and smoke candles for asthmatics. The thornapple is cultivated to obtain these active principles.

DIGITALIS PURPUREA

FOXGLOVE

Scrophulariaceae

78 W Eur, NW Af
Eur, N Asia, N-N A

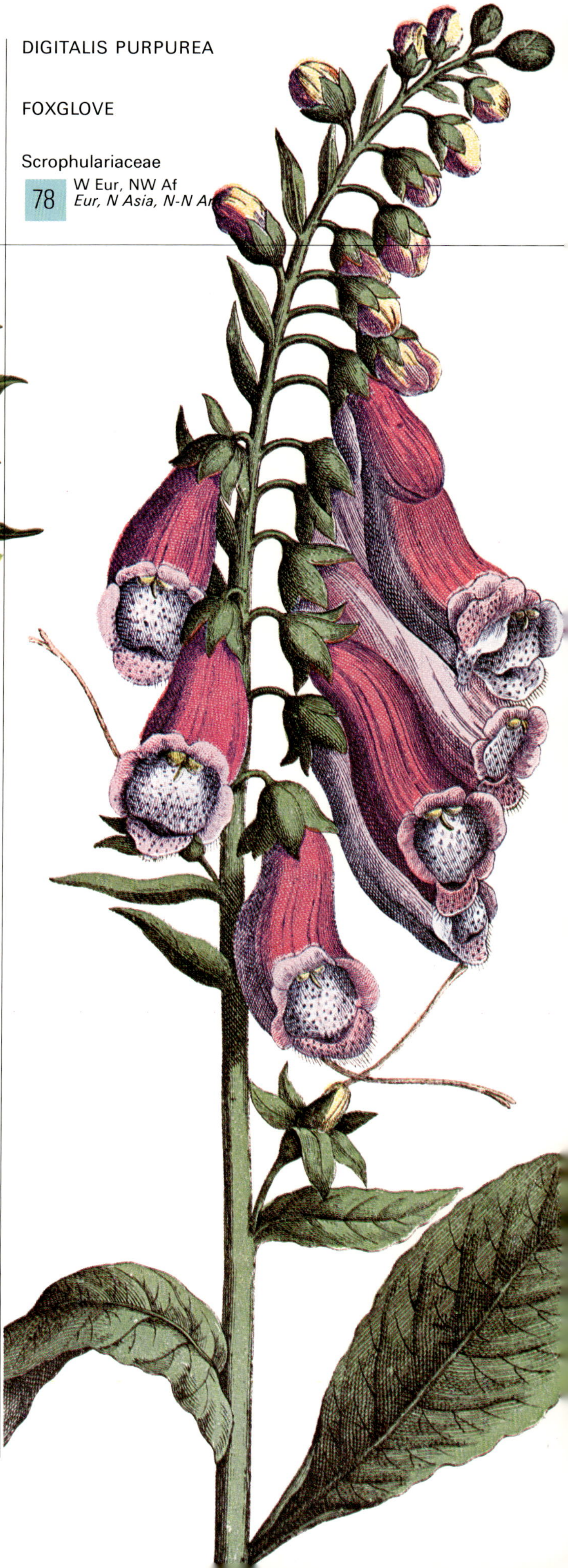

This is one of the medicinal plants which have been very fully analyzed. Even today, there are no synthetic drugs to take the place of its cardiac glycosides in the treatment of the failing heart, and digitalis continues to hold its place in modern drug therapy. Most industrial countries therefore cultivate the foxglove, sometimes in varieties more adapted to the climate, such as the woolly foxglove *(Digitalis lanata)* in the Mediterranean region. In the eighteenth century Dr. William Withering, an English physician, published *An Account of the Foxglove* in which he described the cultivation, collecting, drying, preparation, and use of the plant. The foxglove does not like much lime. In the wild, it may be found in open woodland and among the bushes growing on slopes. Other varieties grow on lime and in gardens. The common foxglove is cultivated for its leaves. During the first year, it forms a basal rosette of large, elliptical, very downy leaves. The following year, a strong unbranched stem, hairy but with only few leaves, grows to a height of 70–150 cm. It terminates in a long, slender flowering spike, with the pendant tubular flowers growing from the leaf axils. The deep pink to purple flowers are 4–5 cm in length and hairless on the outside, while the inside is hairy and paler in color, with numerous dark crimson spots. The fruit, in autumn, is a hairy sphere containing tiny seeds which are distributed by the wind. The active principles are contained in egg-shaped leaves which are covered with a gray pelt of hairs on the underside.

DIOSCOREA VILLOSA

YAM

Discoreaceae

79 E-N Am

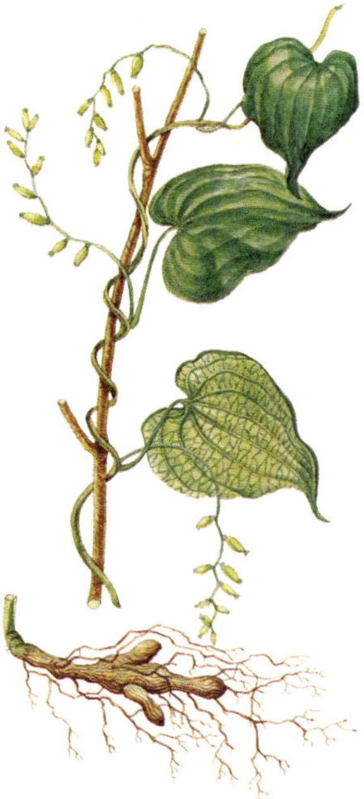

This is a major food plant with potato-like tubers. It is cultivated in many southern countries, and grows wild in damp woodlands and thickets. Other species of *Dioscorea* are attractive ornamental shrubs *(Dioscorea bulbifera)*. A knotty, woody rootstock with long, creeping runners produces thin, smooth twining stems which grow to a length of 5 m. The long-stemmed leaves are heart-shaped and pointed, green and smooth on the upper surface, and a matt green on the underside, with 9–11 prominent longitudinal veins. From the upper leaf axils grow long, pendant loose clusters of small greenish-white single flowers that are almost sessile. The fruit is a 3-celled winged yellowish-green capsule. Medicinal use is made of the tubers of *Dioscorea villosa*, for the saponin they contain. This principle is also found in other species from Guatemala and Mexico *(D. spiculiflora* and *D. floribunda)*.

DROSERA ROTUNDIFOLIA

SUNDEW

Droseraceae

80 Eur, Asia, N Am

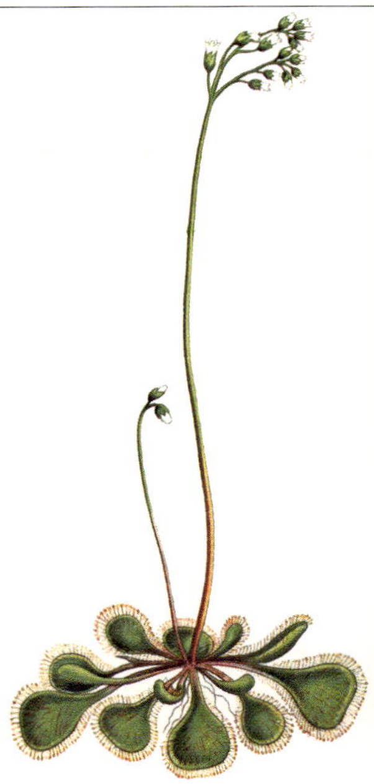

This small but most interesting plant likes to grow in moors, sphagnum bogs, and swamps, mostly in northern latitudes, from the lowlands up to altitudes of 1800 m. The root is supported by lateral rootlets and bears a rosette of long-stemmed circular dish-shaped leaves (oval in other species). The leaves are covered with small, upright glandular hairs bearing small droplets at the tip which glitter in the sun like dewdrops. It is to these that the plant owes the name "sundew" (*drosos* in Greek). The sticky drops attract insects that are held fast on the glandular hairs and literally digested by the fluid. Delicate slender flowering stems about 10–20 cm high grow from the rosette of leaves; they bear a short coiled spike of tiny white flowers. When the small seed capsule opens, the wind distributes the tiny seeds. Useful medicinal principles are derived from its juices.

DRYOPTERIS FILIX-MAS

MALE FERN

Polypodiaceae

81 Eur, N Af, Asia, N Am

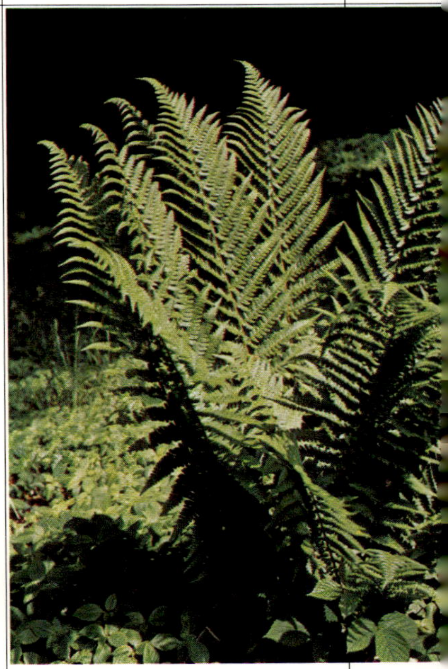

The ferns are classified among the vascular cryptogams (plants not bearing obvious flowers). There are more than 7000 species, found in open woodlands on soil rich in humus, but also to some extent in heathland and shady forest glades. The underground stem of the male fern is large, up to 30 cm in length, and often branched. It has fibrous roots 1–2 mm in thickness. The stem is surrounded with the angular leaf bases of earlier leaves. The rosette of leaves forms a funnel. The leaves are curled up like a crozier to begin with, and unfold into pale green fronds up to 1 m long, each frond divided into alternate divided leaflets growing smaller toward the tip. The underground stem and leaf stalks are covered with thin brown scales. In summer, light green sori (collections of spore-bearing structures) develop on the undersides of the leaflets. They turn brown as they ripen in autumn.

ECHINACEA ANGUSTIFOLIA

PURPLE CONEFLOWER, RUDBECKIA

Asteraceae/Compositae

82 C+SW-N Am

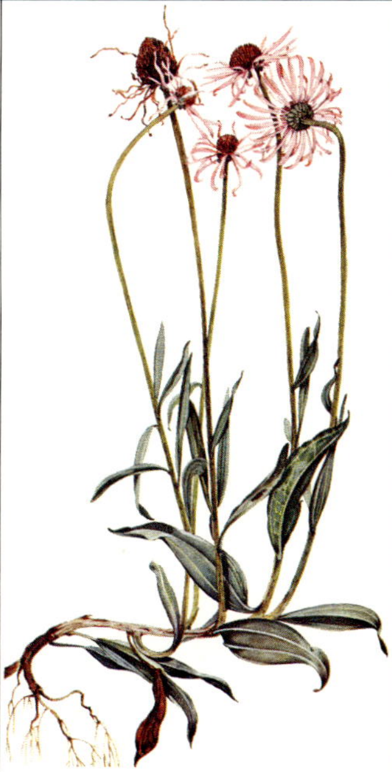

The purple coneflower or Rudbeckia is found in prairies and on sandy banks; the red variety, also in open deciduous forests and on sunny slopes. In Europe the purple coneflower is grown as an ornamental plant. It is a perennial, with a fairly large tap root surviving through winter. This produces simple rough stems, 60–90 cm long, hollow near the base, and thickening slightly close to the flower head. The leaves are elongated, narrow or slightly elliptical, dark green, with margins entire. They are coarsely hairy and covered with protuberances. The ground leaves are long-stemmed, while the few leaves growing on the stem are almost sessile. The base of the flower forms a high cone, with narrow, roughly hairy bract leaves with margins entire. The ray florets are generally down-turned. The tubular florets are greenish, 5-toothed, with the dark red style divided at the top.

EPHEDRA SINICA, EPHEDRA DISTACHYA

EPHEDRA, SEA GRAPE

Ephedraceae

83 a) E Asia
b) S Eur, M+W Asia

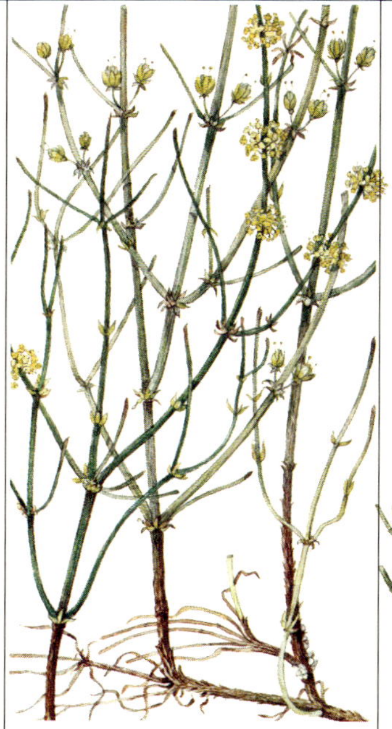

The seemingly leafless Ephedra species grow on dunes, in the tundra, and on rocky slopes. Known for thousands of years in Chinese medicine, as a remedy for asthma and as a circulatory stimulant, the plant drug made its appearance in the *materia medicas* of the rest of the world from the sixteenth century onward. Its principal alkaloid, ephedrine, is nowadays also synthesized as a medicament used in a variety of conditions. The pale green, grooved stems are erect or prostrate, and 30–90 cm in height. They are articulated, the length of the internodes being 3–5 cm. The scale-like leaves growing at the nodes are 2–4 mm long and toothed at the tip. The inconspicuous yellowish-green flowers appear in terminal catkins; male and female flowers are separate. In August the female develop into fleshy red cones 5–6 mm long, the ephedra or seagrapes. These are poisonous.

EQUISETUM ARVENSE

HORSETAIL, SCOURING RUSH

Equisetaceae

84 Eur, N Af, N Asia, N Am

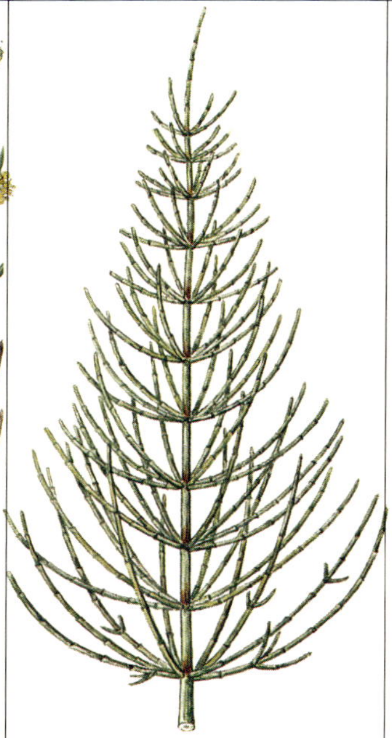

Horsetails are very common on clayey, sandy soil on roadsides, along embankments, and in fields. They derive from a primeval plant which 400 million years ago (in the Paleozoic period) formed whole forests. The horsetail is a nonflowering plant; it increases through spores. Early in spring, a yellowish-brown, pencil-slim stem rises 15–20 cm above the ground. It bears scaly whorls and at the tip a scaly head of spores which are borne away on the wind. The fruiting stem withers and its place is taken by a pale green brush, 20–35 cm high, of regular whorls. Crystals of silica (in the form of opal) are formed on the cell walls of the grooved stems and branches as they dry. These cause scratches when the plant is ground and formerly were used to scour pewter (pewterwort). The marsh horsetail, a relative, contains additional substances which are poisonous.

ERIGERON CANADENSIS

FLEABANE, HORSEWEED

Asteraceae/Compositae

85 N-N Am
Temperate Zones

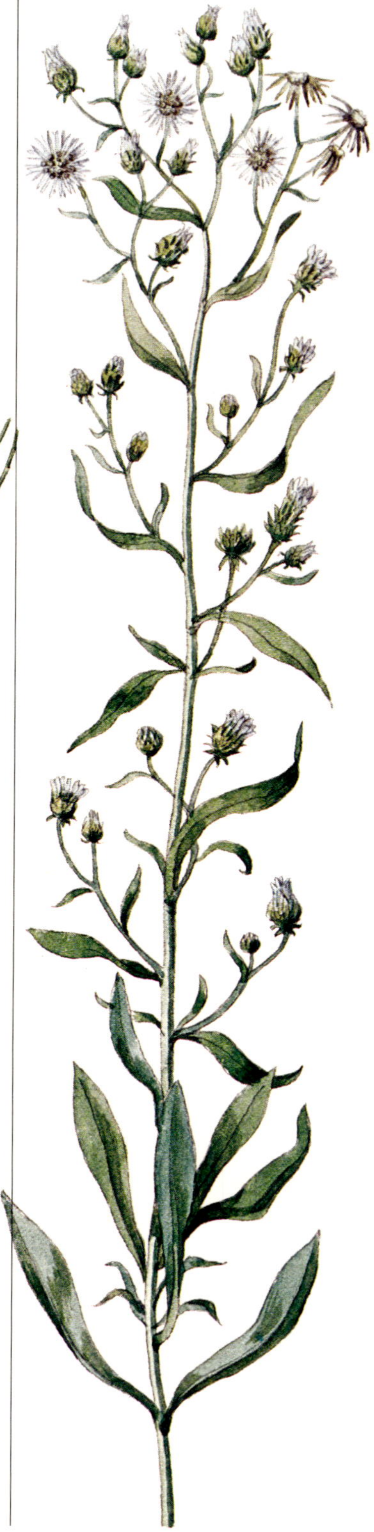

If a piece of land is left uncultivated anywhere, the fleabane soon makes luxuriant growth there. Herbal lore has it that fleabane bound to the forehead is "a great helpe to cure one of the frensie" (Parkinson). On sandy hills and in cut-down forests, the plant often forms large colonies, displacing the flora usually found there. No wonder it is called a weed, though botanists do not care for the term. In the spring the underground stem produces leaf shoots with unbranched, leafy angular stems that are 40–100 cm in height. The leaves are a rich green, narrow and lance-shaped, and slightly hairy. The stem

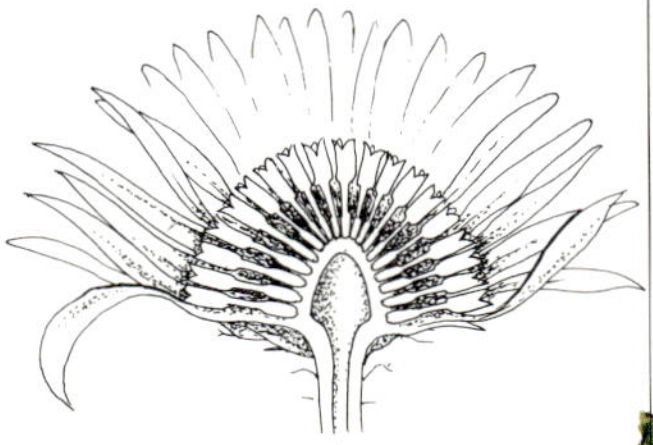

ends in much branched clusters of small flower heads with whitish ray florets. These fade quickly, and fruiting heads with silky white hairs develop. This is why the plant bears its Greek name *Erigeron* (*eri*=early, and *geron*=aged person) – growing old early. To make up for it, the leaves of this active weed contain principles with diuretic and styptic properties which are quite frequently used in the United States.

ERYTHOXYLUM COCA

COCA

Erythroxylaceae

86 Peru, Bolivia
E Af, E Asia, NE-S Am

This shrub 2–3 m high is hardly known in its wild state today, as the plant has been cultivated for centuries, in a number of varieties. The straight erect woody branches bear opposite pairs of short-stemmed pale or grayish-green leaves. These are 5–8 cm long and 2.5–4 cm wide, their shape a pointed oval. The central vein on the underside is accompanied on either side by a line of thickened cells which strengthen the leaf. The small stipules in the leaf axils become horny later. The greenish-white flowers also grow in the axils, in small clusters. The red stone fruits are barely 1 cm in diameter, like small cherries, each containing 1 seed. The most important active principle, cocaine, is found in the leaves. It is a narcotic and is also addictive. In their countries of origin, coca leaves are chewed to relieve hunger, thirst, and physical fatigue. After removing the veins, the leaves are prepared with lime or ashes and made into bite-sized parcels which are chewed for a long time. The natives only rarely become addicted from chewing coca.

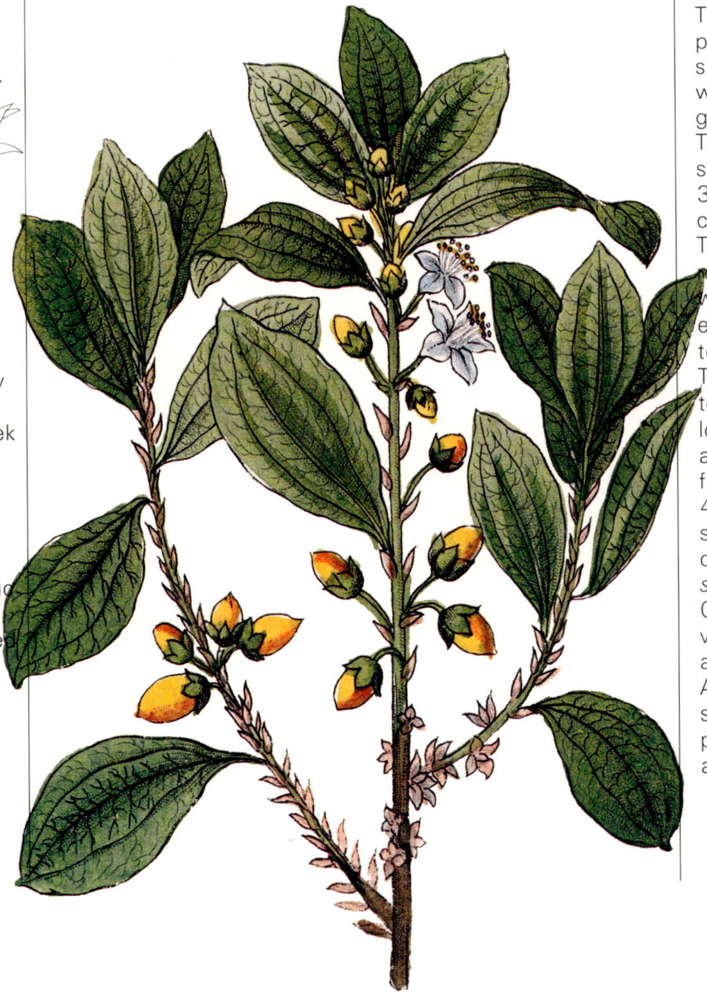

ESCHSCHOLZIA CALIFORNIA

CALIFORNIAN POPPY

Papaveraceae

87 W-N Am
Warm Temperate Zones

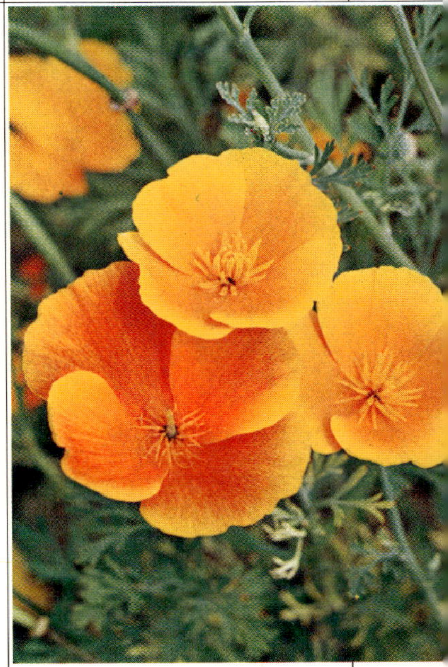

This annual or perennial plant likes a sheltered, sunny site and prefers a sandy soil, where it will continue to grow after it has flowered. The thin, smooth round stems are gray-green, 30–60 cm in height, and contain a colorless juice. The leaves are few and much divided, ending in thin wisps. The color of the flowers ranges from pale yellow to orange in the wild state. The 4 petals have crinkled top edges. They form a shallow bowl, with numerous anthers at the center. The fruit is an elongated capsule 4–6 cm in length; in other species it is a pod. Many different varieties of *Eschscholzia* (named after the German physician Dr J. F. von Eschscholtz) are grown as ornamental plants. The American Indians used the slightly narcotic juice of this plant as a remedy for toothache.

EUCALYPTUS GLOBULUS

EUCALYPTUS,
BLUE GUM TREE

Myrtaceae

88 Aus
Warm Temperate Zones

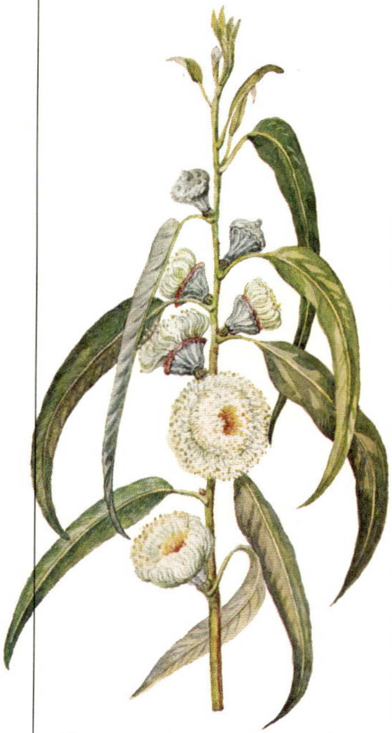

The eucalyptus tree makes rapid growth, reaching a height of 20 m in 6–8 years. In Australia, certain species grow to a height of more than 100 m. It is popular as an ornamental tree in temperate regions. The bark of the straight trunk is smooth and ash gray, and studded with glands. The wood is reddish. The first leaves growing on the young branches are thin, oval to heart-shaped, opposite and without stalks. Their place is later taken by others, about 20 cm in length, which are sickle-shaped, their tips at a slant, and narrow down into a stalk up to 2 cm in length. Stiff and leathery, these are bluish-green in color, with a strong central vein, and dotted with oil glands. The flowers grow in erect terminal clusters. Their petals are joined in a firm capsule, with whitish stamen filaments emerging when the flowering is over. The bluish capsules are often used in floral arrangements and wreaths.

EUPATORIUM
CANNABINUM

HEMP AGRIMONY

Asteraceae/Compositae

89 Eur, Asia

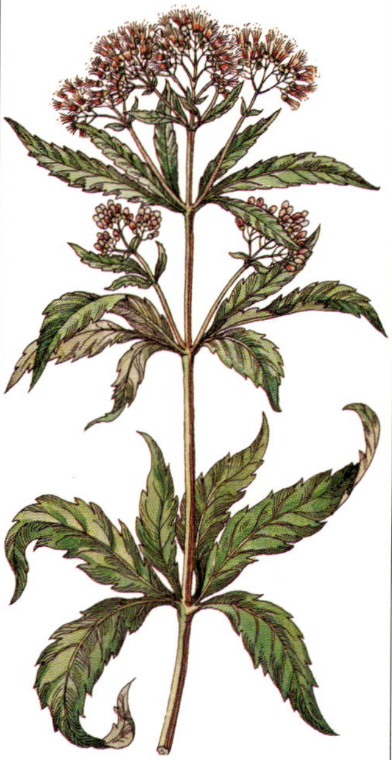

On the edge of damp woodlands and on river banks, the hemp agrimony may form large colonies. The upright, bluntly angular stem may grow as high as 150 cm; coarsely hairy, it is often tinged with red, and branches at the top. The leaves show some variation of form, being elongated and pointed, lance-shaped, and generally toothed. The tiny flowering heads are a muddy pink; they grow in dense flat-topped terminal clusters and may be confused with those of valerian. The small fruits are carried on the wind by their crown of hairs. The whole herb and the root contain bitter aromatic principles. The frequency and ready availability of hemp agrimony should ensure a plentiful supply of its active principles. Extracts from the plant are already being used to good effect in some preparations for the treatment of the common cold and flu.

EUPHRASIA
ROSTKOVIANA

EYEBRIGHT,
DRUG EYEBRIGHT

Scrophulariaceae

90 Eur

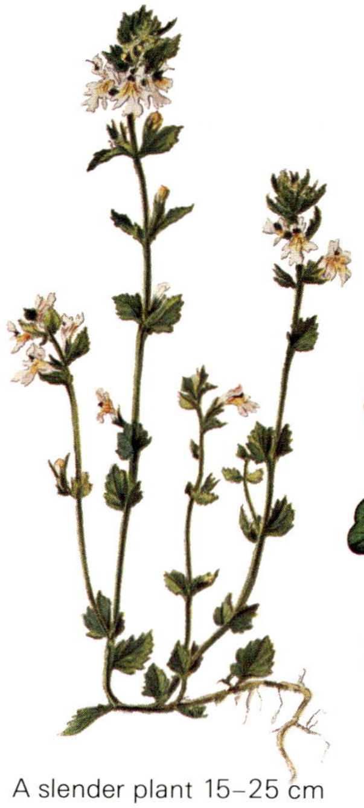

A slender plant 15–25 cm high, eyebright likes sunny places among sparse bushes, on the edge of woods, and in heathlands, from the lowlands up to high mountain regions. It is semiparasitic, attaching itself by suckers to the roots of neighboring grasses. Eyebright is an annual, producing small branching stems with opposite broadly egg-shaped leaves with toothed margins; both stem and leaves are covered with downy hair. Higher up the stem, smaller leaves are followed by the small, beautifully marked flowers. These sit in the leaf axils. The upper lips are about 1 cm in length and have purple veins. The lower lip has 3 lobes and a bright yellow spot where it enters the throat of the flower. Eyebright flowers from May until autumn. A subspecies appears in pastures cropped by animals or cut for hay in midsummer and flowers in autumn. The Greek prefix *eu-* means "good" or "well."

FICUS CARICA

FIG

Moraceae

91 S Eur, SW Asia
Warm Temperate Zones

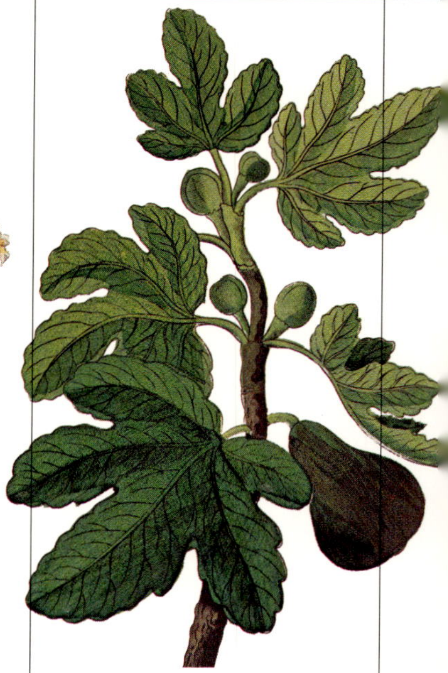

Like the olive and the almond, the fig tree is one of the major food-producing plants in southern regions of the world. Containing about 50 percent of invert sugar, figs preserve themselves and are a valuable food reserve when dried. The edible true figs are, without exception, produced in large plantations. Fig trees have broad, open-structured crowns, their branches being horizontal and sometimes climbing. They reach a height of 5–8 m. The olive-green branches bear stalked, dark green leaves in a variety of shapes. Basically round, they are usually lobed to give a shape like a hand, with the individual lobes widening near the tip. The dark green upper surface is covered with small bristles; the underside and the stalk, with downy hairs. A soft, fleshy, pear-shaped receptacle encloses the flowers growing on female trees—the only ones to be cultivated.

FILIPENDULA ULMARIA

QUEEN-OF-THE-MEADOW, MEADOWSWEET

Rosaceae

92 Eur, Asia
N Am

Meadowsweet, on stems 80–150 cm high, waves above damp meadows, on the banks of brooks, and in ditches to altitudes of 1500 m. The creeping underground stem with its thickened nodules persists through winter, and in spring produces a ground rosette of leaves and then tough erect furrowed stems which branch at the top. The foliage leaves are divided into larger leaflets, with smaller ones in between; they have silvery hairs on the underside and prominent reddish veins. The tiny, creamy white flowers cluster at the top. They attract insects with their strong, sweet scent.

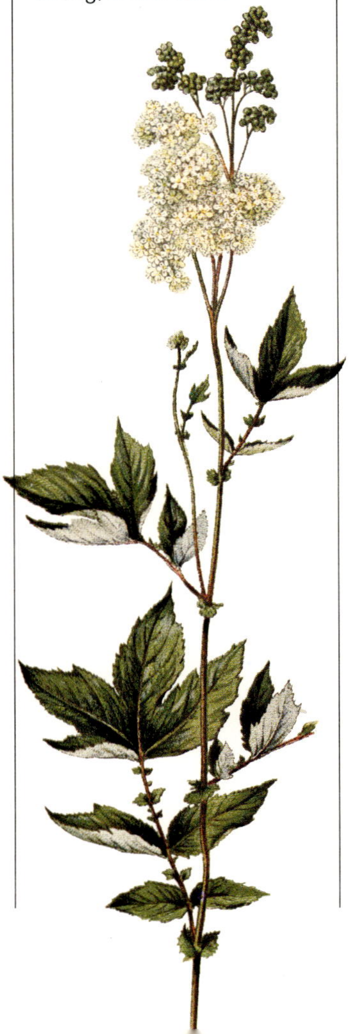

FOENICULUM VULGARE

FENNEL

Apiaceae / Umbelliferae

93 S Eur, N Af, W Asia
Temperate Zones

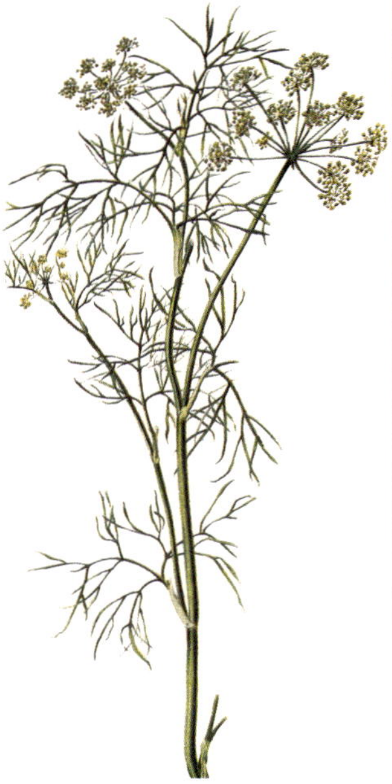

Fennel is one of the most attractive Umbelliferae (carrot family). In gardens and in southern lands, the branching herb can reach a height of 2 m. The round, finely fluted tubular stem grows from a thick, solid root. The leaves are divided 3 or 4 times, ending in almost thread-like structures of a tender blue-green, their stems emerging from fleshy leaf sheaths. A large umbel, again branching into rays, bears the small insignificant yellow flowers that are frequently visited by bees and other insects. The elongated round seeds are ridged and blue-green to begin with, turning a greenish-brown as they ripen. The whole plant gives off a characteristic scent similar to aniseed. The highest concentration of the volatile oil is found in the seeds. Vegetable fennel, the bulbous sheaf of thickened leaf stalks from a cultivated variety, provides a delicious aromatic winter vegetable. In southern regions it is also eaten raw.

FRAGARIA VESCA

STRAWBERRY, WOODLAND STRAWBERRY

Rosaceae

94 Eur, Asia, NW-N Am

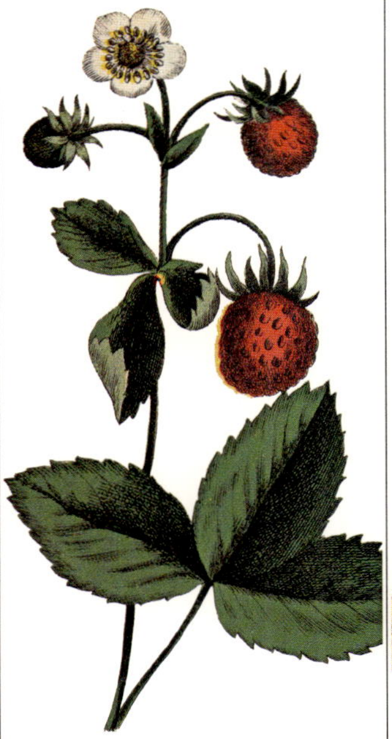

All summer long, the red berries gleam among the thin undergrowth where the sun reaches the humus-rich soil. One of the smallest members of the rose family, the strawberry buries its woody rootstock in the ground. Numerous creeping runners produce the upright leaf stems that are densely hairy near the ground and only slightly hairy higher up. The leaves, with pointed teeth, are divided in three, green and glossy on the upper surface and covered with silky hairs on the underside. The tall flowering stems are also hairy, with flowers of a clear white which have 5 petals and 5 sepals on a greenish receptacle. This develops into the strawberry which is an aggregate of tiny nutlets ("seeds") sitting on the enlarged fleshy receptacle. The wild strawberry flowers and fruits through summer and into autumn. The leaves contain substances that stimulate the liver.

FRAXINUS EXCELSIOR

ASH

Oleaceae

95 C Eur

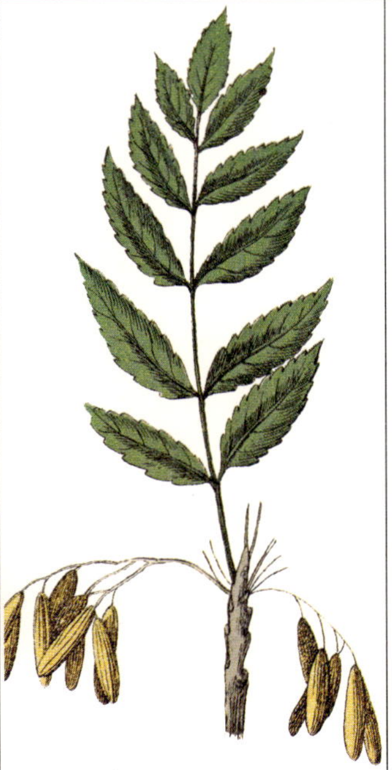

Ash trees with their rich foliage may reach a height of up to 30 m. They prefer a damp soil and plenty of light on low ground, in river valleys and meads. The cylindrical trunk is protected by a smooth, gray-green bark which later becomes brownish-black and fissured. Stout branches bear opposite pairs of leaves, at right angles to the preceding pair, each leaf divided into pairs of leaflets with an odd one at the tip. The leaflets are dark green on the upper surface and lighter in color beneath, an elongated pointed egg-shaped, with irregularly toothed margins. The flowers appear before the leaves and are small clusters of purple stamens. The fruits, the "keys," are elongated, flat, and hairless, usually with a single seed, and prolonged into a wing, several fruits hanging together in a short-stemmed bunch. Medicinal use is made of the dried leaflets. The bark of the branches contains a sugar, mannitol.

FUCUS VESICULOSUS

ROCKWEED, BLADDERWRACK

Fucaceae

96 N+W Eur, E+W-N Am

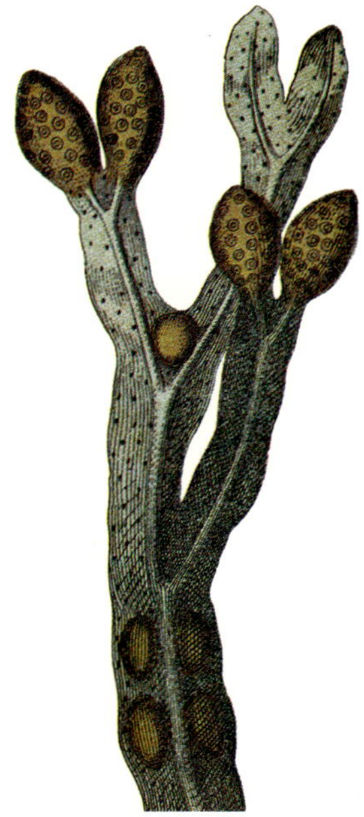

This seaweed is a brown alga which is gathered along the Atlantic coast, by the North Sea, the Baltic, and along the Irish coasts. Prior to the discovery of natural iodine salts, rockweed was one of the chief sources of iodine. The fresh thallus is a slimy, slippery ribbon up to 1 m in length and 2–4 cm wide. On either side of the midrib are oval bladders filled with air that give the thallus buoyancy. The alga attaches itself to stones in the tidal region with a suction disk, piling up on the shore when torn away by gales. Dried rockweed, which comes in brittle brownish-black strips or flakes, contains not only iodine, but also other trace elements dissolved in seawater, and mucilage. Other sea algae and marine sponges also have a high iodine content, but this tends to vary considerably so that pharmaceutical utilization is difficult, particularly as people vary in their sensitivity to iodine.

FUMARIA OFFICINALIS

FUMITORY, EARTH SMOKE

Papaveraceae, Fumarioideae

97 Eur, N Af, W Asia
Temperate Zones

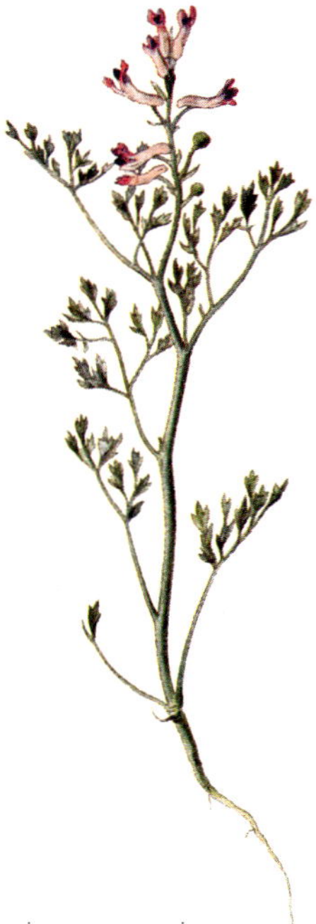

Fumitory owes its name to the appearance of the gray-green leaves that often look a little browned, as if smoked. The fumitory grows in friable, rather moist soil on rubbish heaps, in fields, orchards and gardens, and by the roadside. It is an annual, with erect ridged stems 20–30 cm in height. The stalked alternate leaves are several times divided, with pointed lobes to their gray-green leaflets. From the axils of small bracts grow flowering shoots bearing an extended spike of tubular purple flowers. The 4 petals with their dark red tips are arranged in 2 circles. The pointed, toothed sepals are very short, and narrower than the tube of petals. The fumitory produces nectar and is pollinated by insects. The fruits are small nutlets containing oil. They are carried off by ants. The active principles (alkaloids and other compounds) have not been fully analyzed so far; they have been used in skin conditions.

GALEGA OFFICINALIS

GOAT'S RUE, EUROPEAN GOAT'S RUE

Fabaceae, Papilionaceae

98 C+SE Eur, W Asia

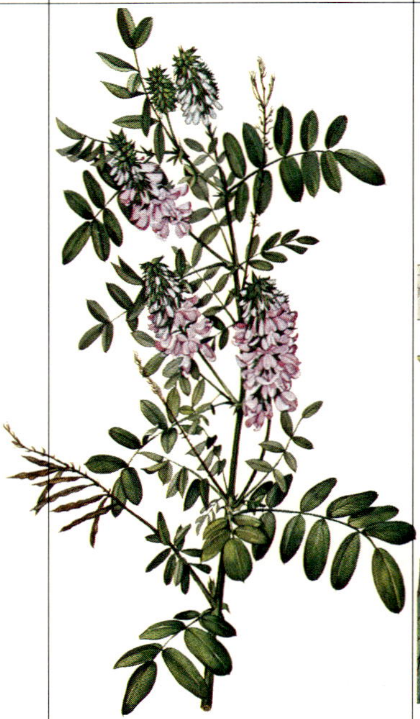

Goat's rue, a handsome perennial up to 1 m high, is often cultivated as an ornamental plant. It also grows wild in sunny, damp meadows, on the banks of brooks, and in river valley woods. The beet-like root produces erect hollow stems with only a few branches. The leaves consist of up to 17 blue-green lance-shaped leaflets growing in pairs with an odd one at the tip of the stalk, each ending in a small spine. Long-stemmed flower spikes grow from the leaf axils; the pale blue or bluish-white flowers with their broad "standards" at the top make these stand out clearly against the rich foliage. Flowering continues from summer into autumn. The whole of the dried herb is used medicinally, formerly to stimulate lactation (*gala*=milk, *agere*=to promote), and today as a tea which slightly reduces blood sugar levels.

GALEOPSIS OCHROLEUCA

HEMPNETTLE

Lamiaceae/Labiatae

99 W Eur
C Eur

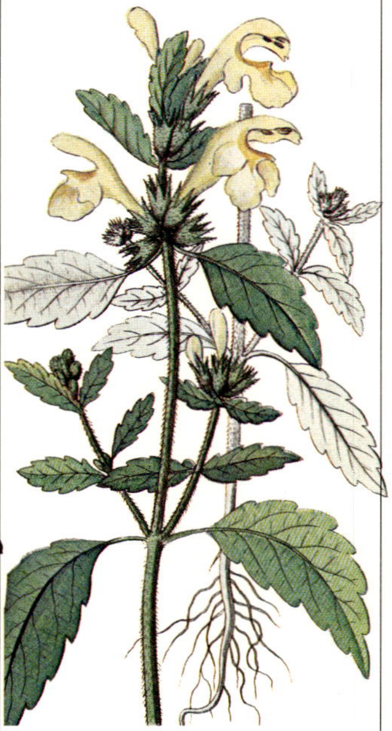

There are a number of species of hempnettle, which show an unmistakable relationship to the white deadnettle. They grow in fields, in waste places, among bushes, and on sunny slopes. A thin tap root produces a square, softly downy stem, often with a tinge of red, which grows to a height of 15–30 cm. The elongated egg-shaped opposite leaves are also hairy, with coarsely toothed (only rarely untoothed) margins. They grow from the swollen stem nodes. In the upper leaf axils, 3–5 two-lipped flowers grow in apparent whorls. The convex, 3-lobed lower lip has a small pointed hollow tooth on either side. The color of the flowers differs with the species, ranging from a deep pink to white or yellow. The hempnettles all contain a high proportion of silica (up to 18 percent in the ash) which inhibits inflammation. Teas of silica-containing plants are useful in the treatment of bronchitis.

GALIUM ODORATUM

SWEET WOODRUFF

Rubiaceae

100 Eur, Asia
N-N Am

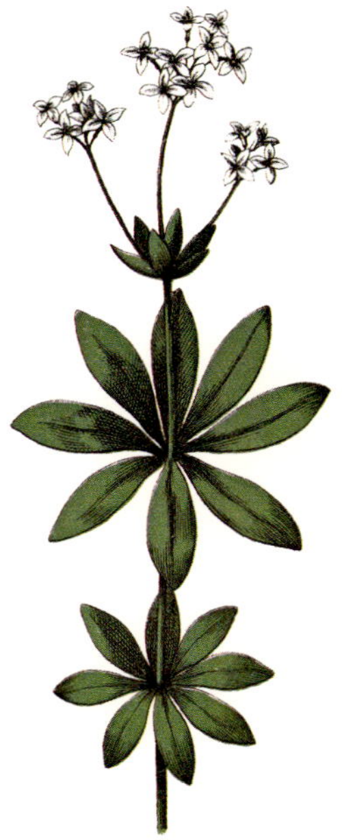

A pleasing small plant, growing about 20 cm high, this carpets shady deciduous forests where the soil is rich in humus. With its regular whorls of leaves it has something of the appearance of a technical drawing. The creeping underground shoots produce thin angular stalks with whorls of 6, and higher up 8, narrow lance-shaped leaves of a rich green. The stalks terminate in graceful loose heads of tiny white star-shaped flowers. Pollination is by flies and other insects. The fruit has small hooked hairs that catch on to the fur of animals brushing past, and this is how the seed is dispersed. The whole plant has a pleasant aromatic scent (coumarin), which develops more fully as the plant dries. This scent has won woodruff popularity since pre-Christian days. It has been used to flavor wine, and to give a sweet odor to linen closets.

GALIUM VERUM

BEDSTRAW, OUR LADY'S BEDSTRAW

Rubiaceae

101 Eur, N Asia
N Am

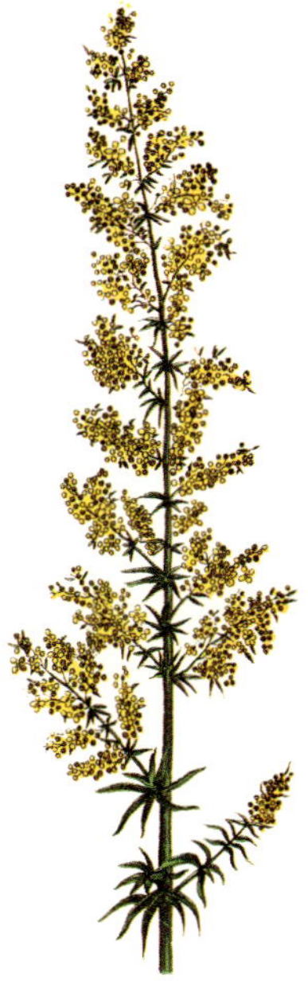

Bedstraw was formerly used in many countries to curdle milk for cheese-making (*gala*=milk). It grows in dry meadows, open woodlands, and on sunny slopes, from the lowlands up to altitudes of 1800 m. The nodular underground stem produces a round or occasionally angular stem 30–80 cm in height. Small branches stand well away, bearing whorls of 4–8 small lance-shaped leaves circling the stalk, their undersides covered with a downy pelt. The whorls of leaves resemble those of the sweet woodruff *(Asperula odorata)*, which is a relative. The stems terminate in elongated clusters of numerous golden-yellow star-shaped flowers, shining like golden bushes among nature's summer greenery. Although the dairy industry no longer has need of it, lady's bedstraw is still used as a metabolic stimulant. Other bedstraw species *(Galium silvaticum* or *Galium mollugo)* have white flowers.

GAULTHERIA PROCUMBENS

WINTERGREEN, TEABERRY, CHECKERBERRY

Ericaceae

102 E-N Am

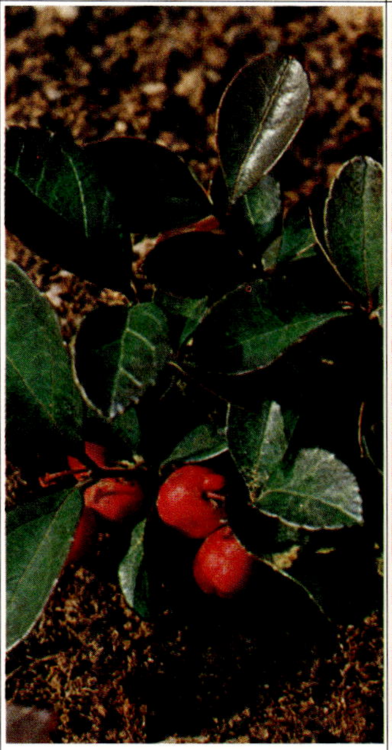

This is a small dwarf shrub, 10–15 cm high, commonly found in the cool, damp woodlands of North America. From the thin underground roots grow erect stems covered with glandular hairs, bearing a few leaves close to the summit. These are 2–4 cm long, a pointed egg shape, stiff and leathery, a glossy dark green on the upper surface and paler beneath, the margins bristly and toothed. As the name suggests, the plant is evergreen. The small bell-shaped pendant flowers at the top of the stem are withe or rose pink. In autumn, the plant bears small glossy red berries. The leaves and berries are pleasantly aromatic. The young leaves are chewed when they are a tender pale green, and the berries may be gathered throughout winter and eaten. The dark green leaves are used for "mountain tea." The plant contains a volatile oil with a high proportion of methyl salicylate which is of medicinal value.

GELIDIUM AMANSII

AGAR AGAR

Gelidiaceae

103 E Asia, W-N Am

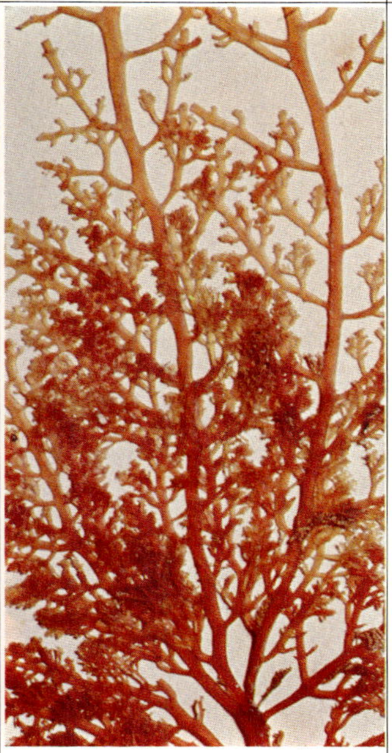

Various kinds of red algae (particularly *Gelidium* species) are gathered by hand or with rakes on underwater sandbanks and rock shelves along the seashore, down to a depth of 30 m. These algae do not have a stiff body, but merely a flexible skeleton of cellulose-type carbohydrates containing a great deal of mucilage. The soft, much branched ribbons and fronds are about 1 m in length, slightly reddish, and almost transparent. They are first of all dried, washed in fresh water, and cleaned. Later the algae are boiled in water to dissolve out the agar which sets to a stiff jelly when cold. Industrial processes are used to purify it by filtration and precipitation with acids to remove impurities and algal residues, and finally the water is removed by freezing and the agar is dried. The finished product consists of horny flakes or strips without smell or taste. It contains up to 90 percent of agaropectin and agarose.

GELSEMIUM SEMPERVIRENS

YELLOW JESSAMINE

Loganiaceae

104 SE-N Am

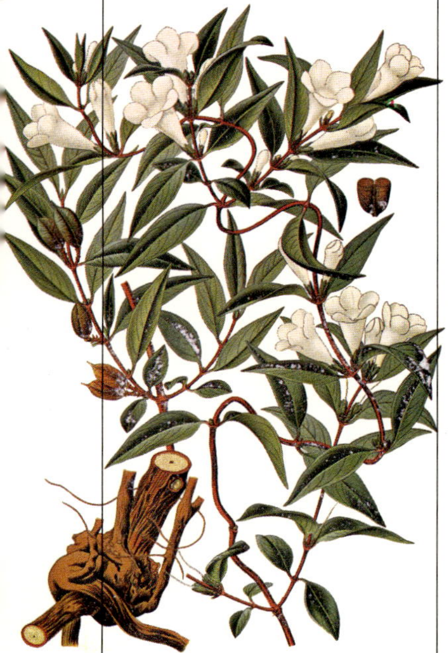

This is a climbing plant with slender branches up to 5 m long. Its natural habitat are the forests and thickets of the southern states of North America. A stout nodular underground stem produces partly woody shoots, branching freely. These bear narrow lance-shaped opposite leaves of a glossy dark green. From the leaf axils of the upper shoots grow the brilliant yellow tubular flowers, 4–5 cm in length, their 5 petal lobes forming a trumpet-like rim. The plant produces its highly fragrant blossoms all through the summer. All parts of the yellow jessamine *(Gelsemium)* contain powerful alkaloids and are poisonous. Medicinal use is made of extracts and tinctures obtained from the underground stem and roots. Jessamine or jasmine tea consists of the nonpoisonous white flowers of *Jasminum odoratissimum,* a shrub cultivated in the Mediterranean region and also in Formosa.

GENTIANA LUTEA

YELLOW GENTIAN, DRUG GENTIAN

Gentianaceae

105 C+S Eur

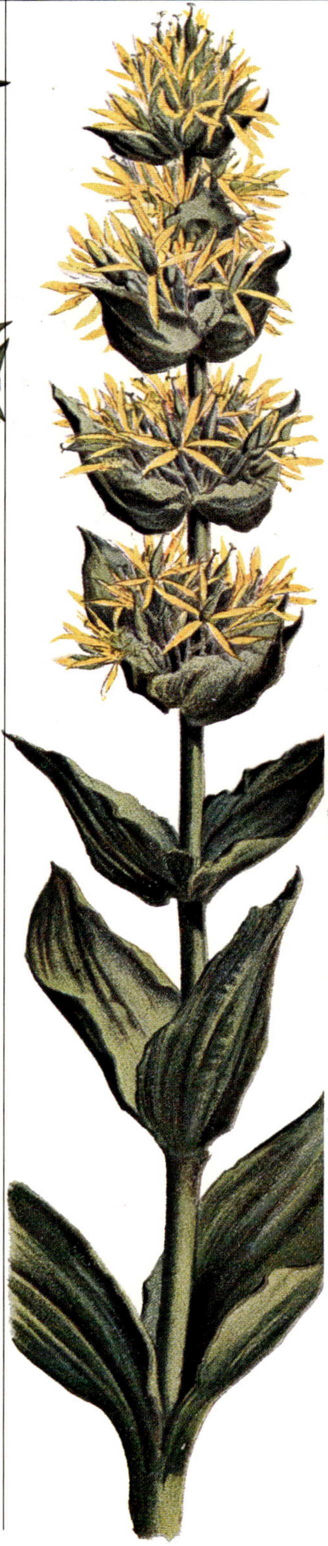

The yellow gentian, the largest member of this richly diverse family, likes soils rich in lime, at altitudes of 700–2400 m. For several years, the powerful tap root produces only a ground rosette of large, elliptical leaves with prominent veins on the underside. Then a sturdy unbranched flowering stem grows 70–120 cm high. This bears gray-green, oval, pointed opposite leaves, like two small hands protectively cupped around the numerous, long-stemmed, golden-yellow star-shaped flowers. The purple gentian *(G. purpurea)* is similar in structure. The roots of both species are used in an alcoholic beverage (gentian brandy),

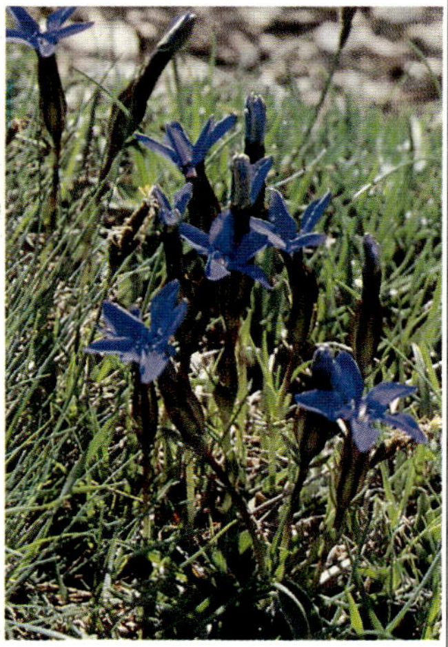

and because of this the plants have disappeared from many areas. The bitters contained in the roots are of medicinal value, and the plant is cultivated to obtain them. Alpine meadows are made glorious with various species of blue and purple flowering gentians.

GERANIUM ROBERTIANUM

HERB ROBERT

Geraniaceae

106 Eur, N Af, Asia, E-N Am

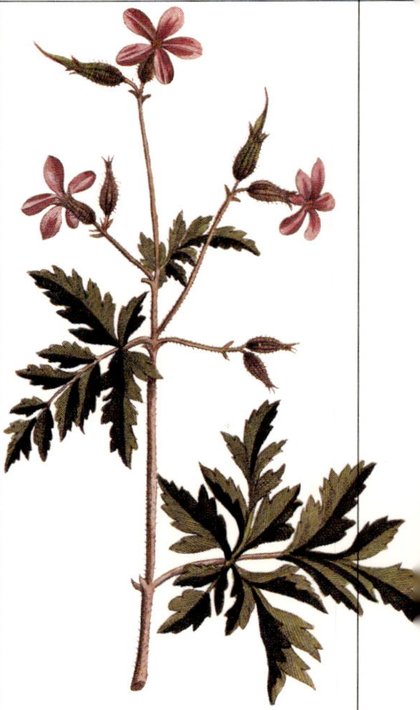

The herb robert likes to grow in hedges and open woodlands, in cracks in walls and rocks, in fields and dry waste places anywhere from the lowlands up to altitudes of 1800 m. Branched fibrous roots produce thin reddish stems, branching stiffly, 20–50 cm in height. The long-stemmed leaves are symmetrical and divided into 3–5 lobes which in turn are divided twice over. The leaves and stems are softly downy, as are the reddish sepals of the flower. The short-stemmed flowers are grouped in twos or fours and have 5 rose-pink petals striped with red. The fruit is about 2 cm long, ending in a pointed beak. This has given other Geranium species the name cranesbill. Rubbed between the fingers, the herb gives off a strong, somewhat harsh scent. Different herb robert and cranesbill species develop in different habitats. *Geranium robertianum* is the only one of medicinal value.

GEUM URBANUM

AVENS, CLOVE ROOT, HERB BENNET

Rosaceae

107 Eur, N Af, Asia
N Am, Aus

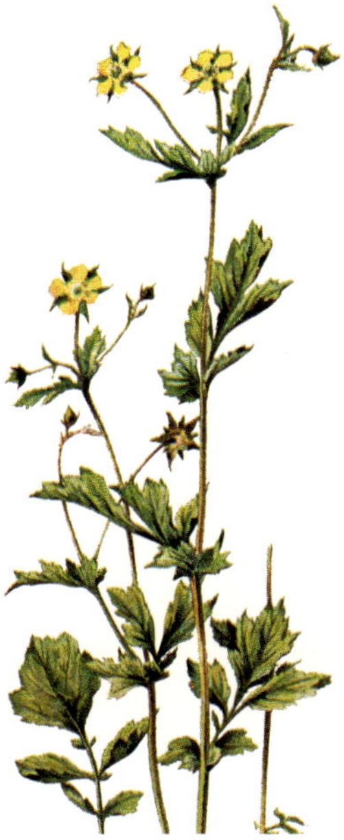

This graceful plant, 30–70 cm in height, adorns shrubberies, hedges, open woods, and waste places. With its pendent of brownish-pink flowers it grows in damp places and near streams. In spring, the beet-like underground stem which smells of cloves (hence the name "clove root"), produces large stalked basal leaves that are divided, with toothed margins. Later, the branching flowering stems arise. These bear smaller leaves divided in three. The stems are slightly hairy and have a reddish-brown tinge; the leaves also have a few hairs, and toothed margins. The 5 roundish-oval petals of the terminal flowers are a golden yellow, with the green tips of the sepals visible between them. A small brown tassel contains the fruits, which are caught up in the pelts of animals passing by and distributed in this manner. The herb and the root contain active principles valued in phytotherapy.

GINKGO BILOBA

GINKGO, MAIDENHAIR

Ginkgoaceae

108 China, Japan

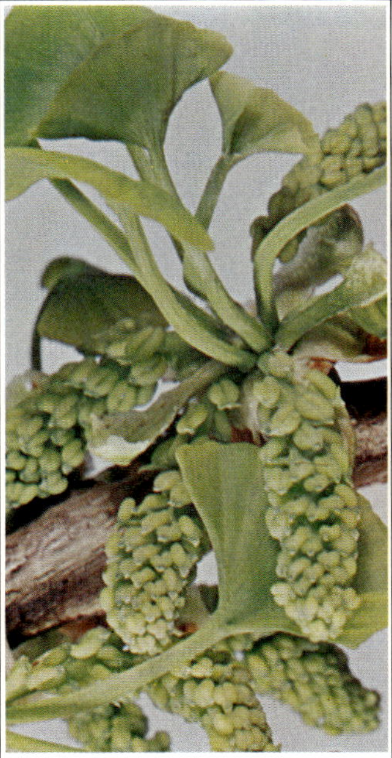

Gingko or maidenhair tree is the last representative of a class of plants which formed part of the flora in Mesozoic times. Cultivated for centuries in the temple precincts of the Far East, it is also widely found as an ornamental or avenue-forming tree in other countries. In the countries of its origin the tree grows to a height of 30–40 m, its branches forming a broad crown. The wide fan-shaped leaves, pale green and hairless, are most decorative. They are borne on long stalks arising from a leaf sheath on the stem, and their veins fork repeatedly. The flowers, male and female on separate trees, grow singly from the leaf axils. The male spore-carrying bodies grow in short, loose catkins. The fruits are yellow, plum-shaped, and contain a woody stone. They are pleasant to eat when fresh, but develop a disagreeable smell if they become overripe.

GLYCYRRHIZA GLABRA

LICORICE

Fabaceae

109 SE Eur, SW Asia
SW Eur, N Af, C Am

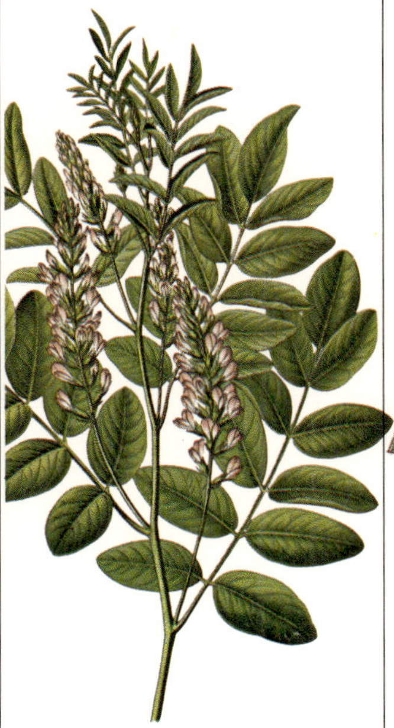

Licorice is one of the most widely used medicinal plants. Pencil-like pieces of the dried runners consisting of yellow fibrous wood are chewed for their sweetness. The plant is perennial, reaching 2 m in height from a root system of taproots, branch roots, and meter-long runners. It often covers large areas in southern Italy, Spain, and Russia and other countries east of the Mediterranean. The woody stems bear a graceful foliage of dark green leaves, with pairs of narrow, lance-shaped leaflets on a stalk terminating in one odd leaflet. From the leaf axils grow long-stemmed spikes of numerous bluish-purple to blue-violet butterfly-type flowers. An important principle found in the root is glycyrrhizin, which has a cortisone-like action. In the areas where it is cultivated and harvested, pieces of root are finely ground, mixed with water, and boiled to obtain the licorice extract.

GOSSYPIUM HERBACEUM

COTTON

Malvaceae

110 S Asia
Torrid and Warm Temperate Zones

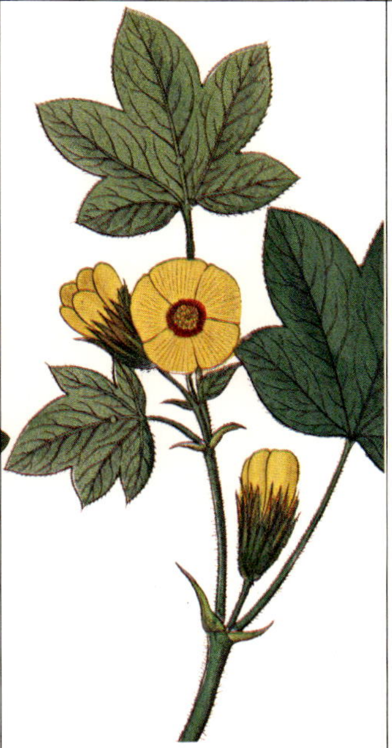

Numerous varieties of cotton have been cultivated in various countries, to achieve the best production for the climate. New varieties are now being developed in the search for a long-stapled cotton resistant to insect pests. Cotton plants are shrubs about 0.5–1.5 m high. The branches are slightly hairy and bear leathery, broadly heart-shaped and short-tipped leaves with a network of veins. The small leaves surrounding the floral structure are lobed and have toothed margins; they show some variation according to the species and variety. The short-stemmed flowers have yellow petals and a purple spot in the center. The fruits are beak-shaped capsules with 3–4 compartments. These split open when ripe, letting the downy seed hairs, the cotton, burst forth. Cotton seeds give an oil containing a high proportion of unsaturated fatty acids. Medicinal principles have been found in the root bark.

GRATIOLA OFFICINALIS

HEDGE HYSSOP, GRATIOLA

Scrophulariaceae

111 Eur, C+N Asia

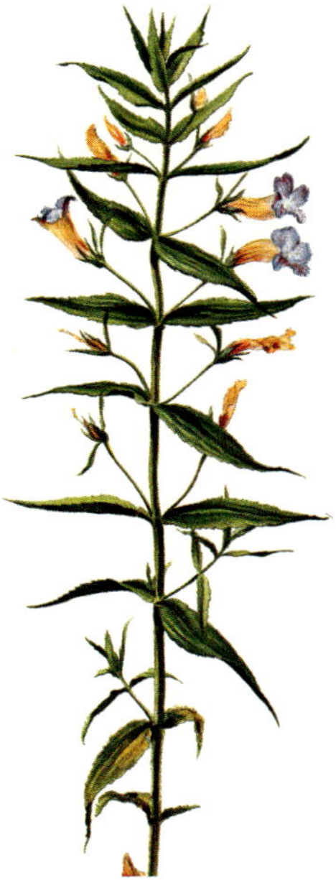

In swampy meadows, on the banks of streams and rivers, and in peat bogs, this perennial spreads its thin, creeping white underground stems. It reaches a height of 20–35 cm and prefers a warm site. The erect hollow flowering stem is square in the upper part. It bears opposite lance-shaped leaves of a richgreen, with slightly toothed margins. The flowers grow from the upper leaf axils, with stalked calyces of 5 sepals holding the tubular, creamy white corolla, which often has reddish stripes. The fruits are pointed, egg-shaped capsules. The flowering herb is gathered in July–Aufust. It contains a number of principles, some of them poisonous, which have not yet been fully analyzed and produce unpleasant side effects. The plant was formerly known as Gratia Dei (grace of the Lord), which suggests that it was greatly valued as a medicinal herb. Pharmaceutical preparations are necessary for accurate dosage.

GUAIACUM OFFICINALE

LIGNUM VITAE, GUAIACUM

Zygophyllaceae

112 C Am, N-S Am

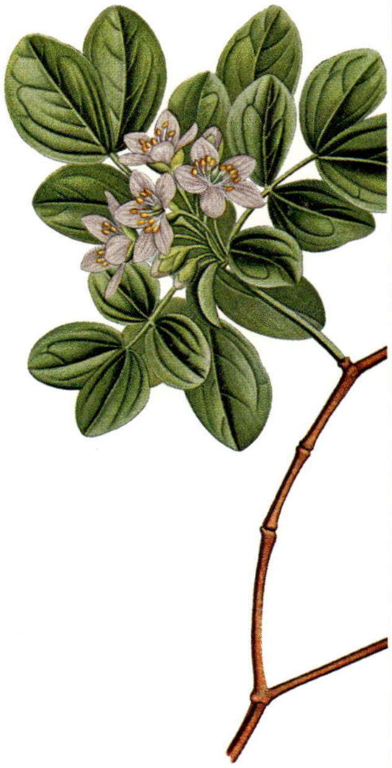

During the sixteenth century, in the days of the great Paracelsus, *Lignum vitae,* or Guaiacum wood, enjoyed a great reputation in the treatment of syphilis. It was later found that this action was due to a resin produced in special cells in the wood. Today the resin is mainly used in the treatment of rheumatism and as a laxative. Lignum vitae is an evergreen tree growing up to 10 m high. Its greenish-brown wood is extremely heavy and resinous. Woody branches bear leaves divided into 2–3 pairs of leaflets. These are 3–5 cm long, light green, and a pointed egg shape. The blue flowers grow in terminal clusters. The fruit is an egg-shaped, dark brown capsule 2 cm in length. To obtain the resin, the trees are felled, and after stripping the bark the fibrous wood is rasped or cut up into small brownish-green pieces which darken when stored, because of oxidation. The resin is sold in rounded tears the size of a hazelnut.

HAMAMELIS VIRGINIANA

WITCH HAZEL

Hamamelidaceae

113 E-N Am

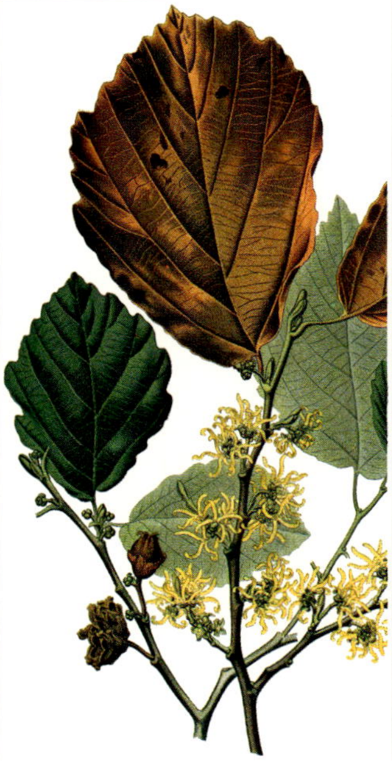

The witch hazel from the woodlands of the eastern United States has much in common with the European hazel *(Corylus avellana).* It is a shrub about 6 m in height, with straight woody branches and a gray-brown bark. The elongated ovate leaves are green, smooth or slightly hairy on both sides, with marked veins along the margins with their shallow, rounded teeth. The flowers grow in the leaf axils of the upper branches, their bright yellow petals taking the shape of narrow, often twisted straps. They appear only after the leaves have dropped off. The fruits, woody capsules of a rounded egg shape similar to hazelnuts, ripen in the following spring or summer. Then the capsules burst and the seeds are ejected with some violence. Because of this peculiarity, as well as the late flowering of the shrub, the American Indians considered the plant bewitched and gave it the name witch hazel.

HARONGA MADAGASCARIENSIS

HARONGA TREE

Hypericaceae

114 Madagascar *Torrid Zones*

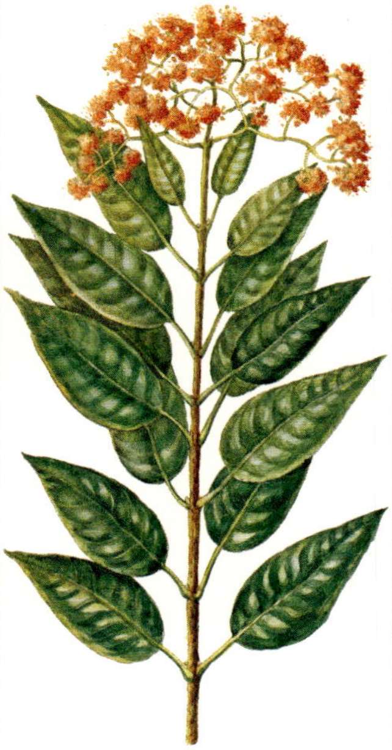

The haronga tree or shrub grows to a height of 6–8 m. The short-stemmed opposite leaves are evergreen, 10–15 cm in length, with margins entire, thin and membranous. They have prominent veins. The upper surface is dark green, the underside covered with rust-red stellate hairs. These may also be noted on the stems. Looking at the leaf against the light, one sees black dots and the transparent veins. The terminal flowers are small and rust-colored; they grow in a compound cluster. Numerous erect stamens emerge above the star shape formed by the 5 petals. The small spherical fruits have a thin outer coat and contain 2 elongated flat seeds. The whole plant is filled with a resinous juice the color of carrots which contains harunganin (an orange-red principle) and other anthraquinone derivatives. The bark, roots, and resin are used as natural dyes.

HARPAGOPHYTUM PROCUMBENS

GRAPPLE PLANT

Pedaliaceae

115 S Af

This plant owes its common name to the branching woody fruit equipped with barbs suggestive of a devil's claw (German name) or of a grapple—whichever way one's imagination may tend. The plant prefers a good depth of clayey sandy soil by the roadside, around watery places and waste ground, where natural vegetation has been checked. The shoots growing from the large, tuberous main root are 100–150 cm in length and lie flat on the ground. They produce erect, stalked, fleshy, lobed leaves. From the leaf axils grow single flowers, 4–6 cm in length and bright purple, similar to those of the foxglove. The woody fruits already mentioned are 10–20 cm long and lie flat on the ground. Along their longitudinal edges are anchor-like outgrowths 5–8 cm in length, and barbs like burs. These catch in the feet of passing animals and are thus distributed. The lateral roots form storage tubers, up to 60 mm wide and 20 cm long, which may be found at a depth of 40–90 cm in the friable soil, and from which interesting principles have recently been isolated.

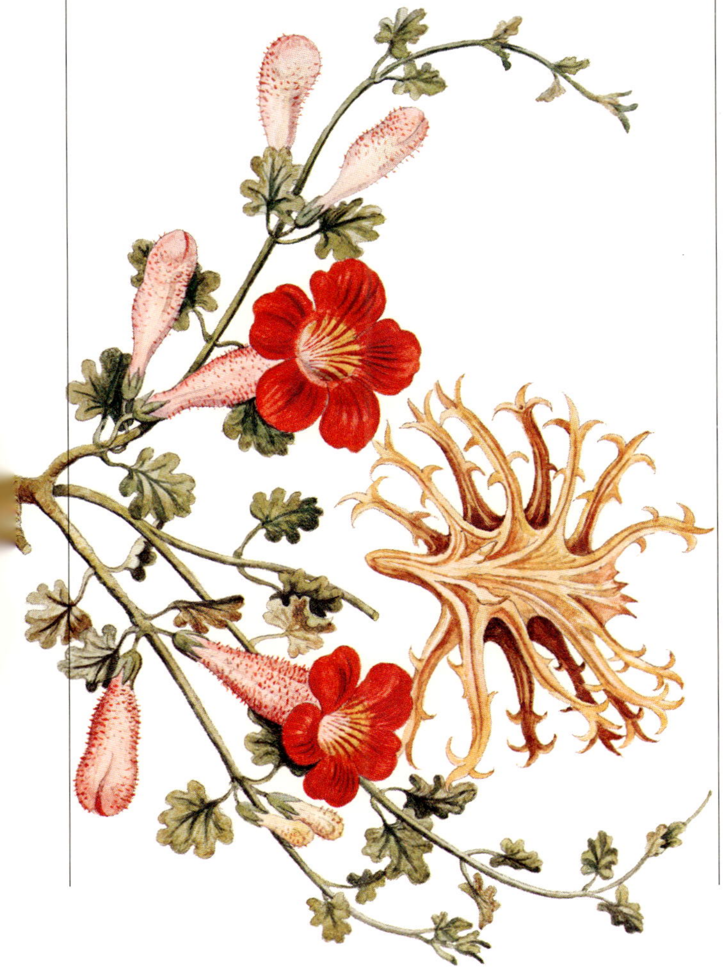

HEDEOMA PULEGIOIDES

AMERICAN PENNYROYAL

Lamiaceae/Labiatae

116 E-N Am

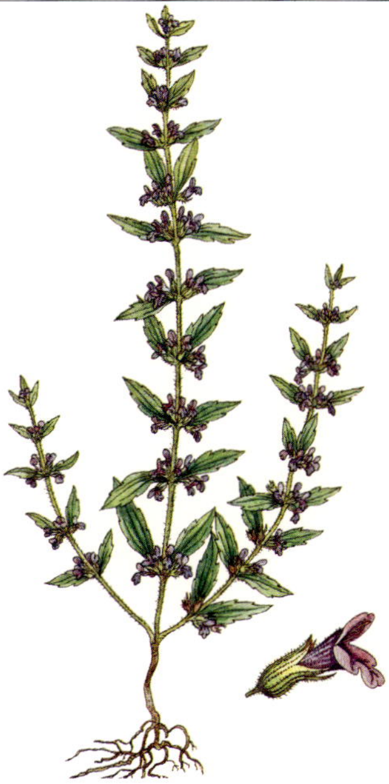

The American pennyroyal is similar to the pennyroyal widely distributed in Europe. It is an annual, with a much branched root system producing slim, erect, somewhat angular stems 30–50 cm in height. The short-stemmed opposite leaves are a pointed oval or elliptical, 1–3 cm long, and have toothed margins. They have small leaf-like stipules in the leaf axils. The flowers are small, barely 5 mm in length, and consist of a hairy calyx with a whitish-purple to pale blue labiate corolla. They grow in whorls of a few flowers in the leaf axils. The stem and leaves are gray-green with glandular hairs. The leaves have a strong minty scent and a pungent aromatic flavor. The volatile oil found in them contains a small amount of menthol, but other principles could produce undesirable side effects. The herb was formerly used as an insect repellent, and its fragrant volatile oil in perfumes and soaps.

HEDERA HELIX

ENGLISH IVY

Araliaceae

117 Eur, NW Af, SW Asia *N Am*

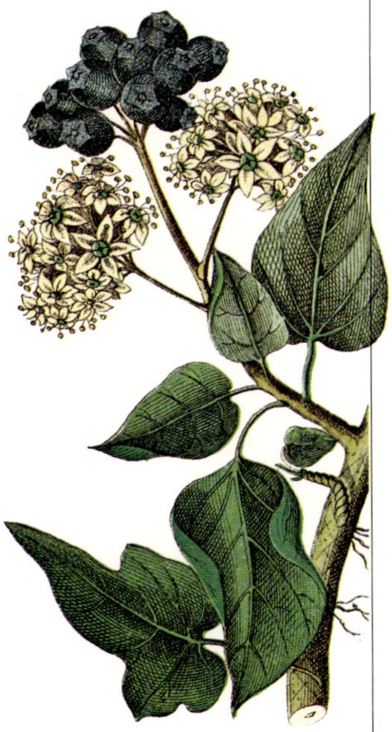

For a long time this evergreen climber went unrecognized as a medicinal plant. More recently, French pharmacologists have found it to contain active principles effective against spasmodic coughs. Its round, woody, branching stems grow from a woody underground stem. The stems grow up trees and walls, wherever their small roots can find a hold, but do not live off the supporting plant the way parasites do. The upper surface of the dark green leaves with 3–5 lobes is glossy and marked with light-colored veins. The leaves are leathery and persist through winter. If the stems do not find an upright support, they often cover large areas of the ground in forests. The upper ends of the branches bear insignificant umbels of green flowers that in autumn turn into small blue-black berries. These are poisonous. The young leaves contain a number of saponins and other principles.

HELICHRYSUM ARENARIUM

EVERLASTING FLOWER

Asteraceae

118 Eur, W Asia

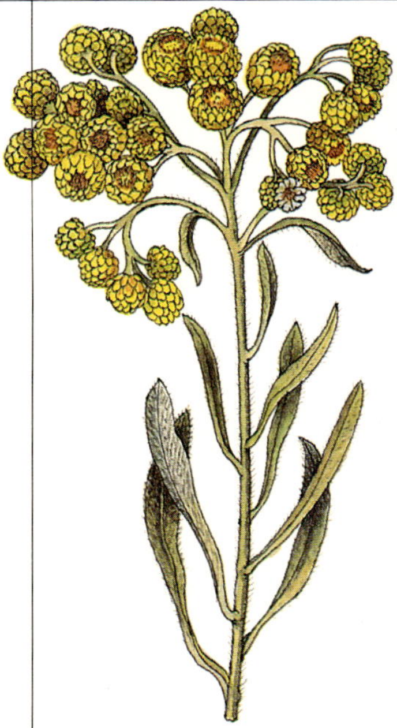

This perennial likes a sandy soil on roadsides and the edges of forests, in dunes and waste places. There it establishes itself with multi-headed, partly wooded roots. It hates wet soil and lime, being entirely designed for a dry environment. In the spring, erect nonflowering stems 10–30 cm in height appear, as well as the densely foliar, very woolly flowering shoots. The narrow, lance-shaped leaves are alternate, merging into the stem lower down, but erect and sessile higher up. The stem terminates in small, dense heads of tiny yellow flowers, their calyces covered with dry membranous scales. Like the immortelles grown as garden perennials, the flowers retain their shape and color when dried. They have a slightly aromatic odor. The flower heads are widely used to improve the appearance of herbal tea mixtures. More recently, they have been shown to promote biliary function and relieve spasms.

HELLEBORUS NIGER

BLACK HELLEBORE

Ranunculaceae

119 C+S Eur

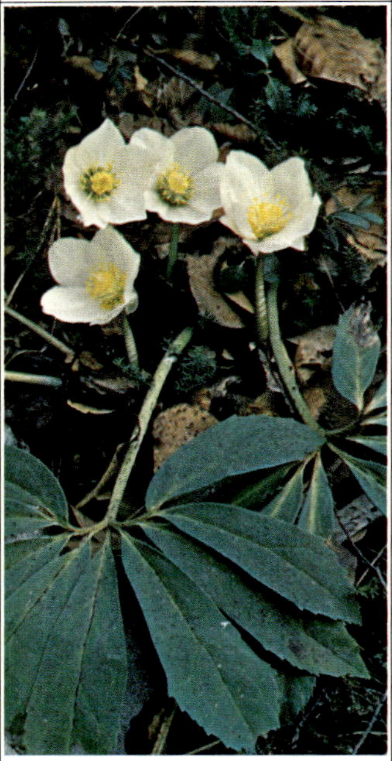

This plant of the woods and mountains has a preference for lime soil, on stony or bushy slopes. It is sometimes called Christmas rose because it flowers in winter. It is often found as an ornamental plant in gardens and cemeteries. A short underground stem produces long-stemmed, leathery basal leaves that are dark green, glossy or dull, each divided into 7–9 leaflets with toothed margins. The stems often have a reddish tinge. The hairless, round, flowering stems bear 1–3 light green bracts, with margins entire, and a terminal flower, white or tinged with red and 4–7 cm in diameter, with 5 ovate, petal-like sepals arranged in a star around the numerous stamens and the ovary. The whole plant is poisonous. Medicinal use is made of the black or brownish-black dried roots of this and other species of *Helleborus*. Preparations of *Helleborus* should be taken only on a doctor's prescription.

HERNIARIA GLABRA

RUPTUREWORT

Caryophyllaceae

120 Eur, N Af, SW Asia *N Am*

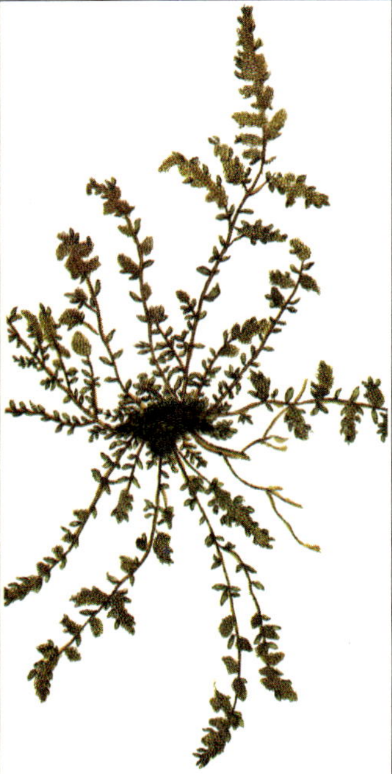

This graceful small herb covers dry sandy soil, heathland, and waysides with delicate branching stems 15–20 cm in length. It will probably never become famous, though it does contain some very useful principles. Cultivation would not be worth the trouble, and gathering it wild would yield little to show for much effort. Chemists and pharmacists have tried, however, to isolate its saponin-like principles and use them as the model for a synthetic drug, a method that has often proved useful. The rupturewort spreads its thread-like branches to cover a circular area. The tiny lance-shaped leaves, barely 1 cm in length, have entire margins and are accompanied by small membranous leafy appendages (stipules). Small clusters of yellowish-green flowers grow in the outer leaf axils. When dry, the whole herb smells of coumarin, but rapidly loses its medicinal powers on storing. Another species *(Herniaria hirsuta)* is hairy.

HIBISCUS SABDARIFFA

ROSELLE, JAMAICA SORREL

Malvaceae

121 Af, S Asia *Torrid Zones*

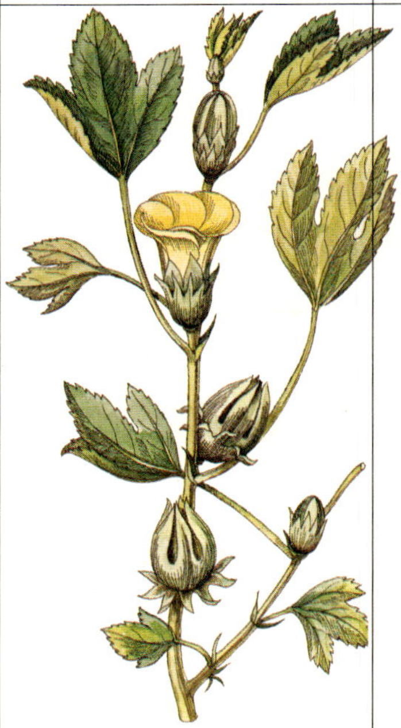

The genus *Hibiscus* comprises around 200 species of annuals, perennials, shrubs, and trees forming part of the subtropical and tropical flora. Some are cultivated as ornamental plants in northern countries. *Hibiscus sabdariffa* is generally annual, reaching a height of 2 m or more. Its erect hairless stems branch little. The egg-shaped undivided lower leaves are soft and downy. Higher up the stem the leaf shape changes to a stalked, 3–5 lobed form. The stem terminates in a loose cluster of bright, pale yellow flowers. The 5-lobed inner cup fuses with the stiffly bristly leaflets of the outer cup, and when the flowering is over these form a fleshy red calyx. This calyx contains a number of plant acids and pigments and is used to make a popular refreshing drink. In the countries of origin, roselle fiber is obtained from the reddish stems. Pharmacologically the plant is of minor interest.

HIPPOPHAË RHAMNOIDES

SEA BUCKTHORN

Elaeagnaceae

122 Eur, Asia

The sea buckthorn is one of the pioneering plants. It takes root in sand containing primitive rock and gradually produces the humus in which other plants are able to grow. It needs plenty of light to do well, and disappears as soon as shade-giving shrubs grow anywhere near it. The woody shrub has spreading roots to give it a hold in the loose sand. The rigid stems branch stiffly, and slow growth produces branches with gray-brown bark and sharp thorns.
In spring, the young shoots produce inconspicuous brown flower buds. The wind carries the pollen from the tiny male flowers to the female flowers growing on another plant. Then at last the shrub seems to come to life. Elongated narrow silvery-green leaves weave an open, airy tissue around the young shoots, letting light penetrate freely to all parts of the plant. On the branches of the female plant, orange-yellow berry fruits grow close to the stem. These contain vitamin C, carotene, and other active principles. No description of the sea buckthorn will be found in the old herbals, for this odd-man-out in the small family of oleasters used to be of interest only to botanists. Sea buckthorn from southern mountain valleys has high vitamin C content.

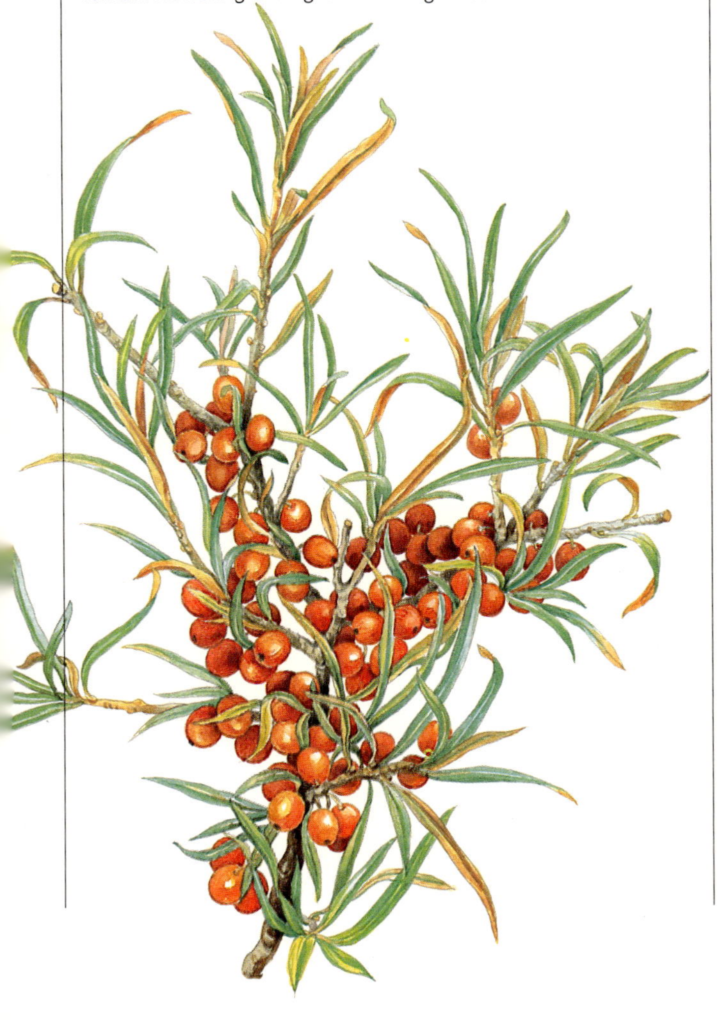

HUMULUS LUPULUS

HOP, COMMON HOP

Moraceae

123 Eur, Asia, N Am *Temperate Zones*

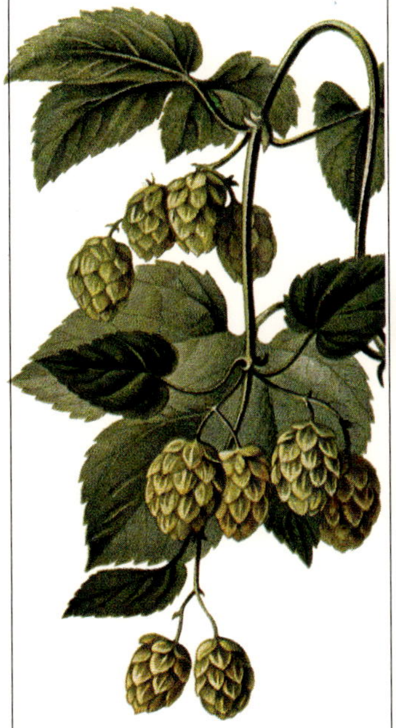

Hop is related to the hemp family. The plant climbs up hedges, fences, and copses, reaching a height of 2–3 m. Cultivated hops are grown on poles 4–6 m high. In the spring, the branching rootstock produces thin, roughly hairy vines that hold on to twigs, branches, and wires with anchor-like climbing hooks. The long-stemmed opposite leaves are similar to those of the vine, but are deeply lobed and hand-like, with sharply toothed margins. Male and female flowers grow on separate plants. The female flowers are cone-like catkins ripening into small egg-shaped fruiting cones, with browny scales covering small granular yellow glands. These contain the most important active principles, the hop bitters. Brewers use the whole cones, as they give beer its pleasantly bitter aroma, improve its keeping qualities, and give it certain sedative qualities. Hop pillows have a reputation as a safe sedative.

HYDNOCARPUS KURZII

CHAULMOOGRA

Flacourtiaceae

124 S Asia

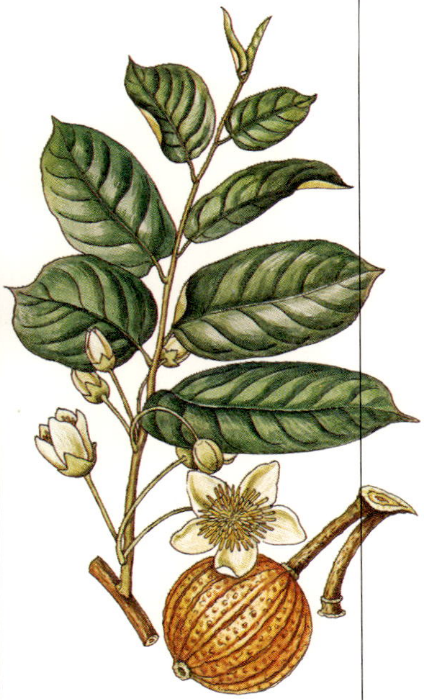

Chaulmoogra oil is obtained from a number of *Hydnocarpus* species growing in dense jungle country. It is a yellowish or brownish oil or soft fat containing fatty acids and other principles, and was for long the standard treatment for leprosy. The oil is not suitable for culinary purposes. *Hydnocarpus* trees have thick trunks and long, pendant branches. They reach a height of about 15 m. As it is difficult to harvest the seeds from the wild plant, the trees are frequently cultivated. The leaves are elongated, about 20 cm in length, with margins entire, and terminate in a short point. Male and female flowers grow on separate plants. The flowers growing in clusters in the leaf axils are a pale yellow. The fruits are round and brown and quite large. They contain numerous egg-shaped seeds, each about 2 cm long. The bark contains principles capable of reducing fevers.

HYDRASTIS CANADENSIS

GOLDENSEAL

Ranunculaceae

125 E-N Am
NE Eur, N Asia

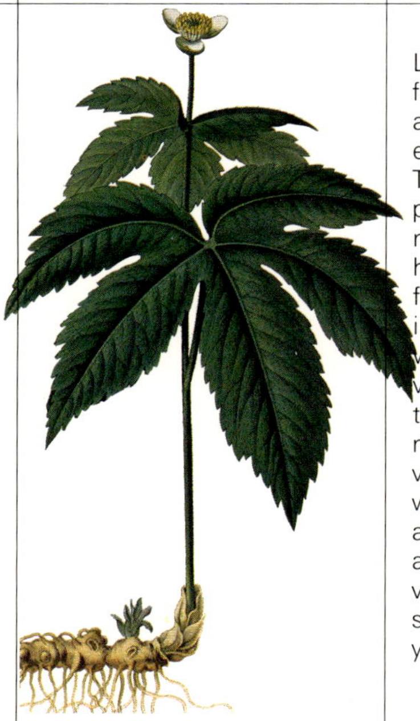

This is very much a woodland plant with a preference for the damp mountain forests of North America and for soils covered to a good depth with dead leaves. A creeping underground stem (rhizome) with numerous roots produces flowering shoots 30–40 cm high. These bear 2 hand-shaped, deeply lobed dark green leaves near the top, which are 5–10 cm wide and 20–25 cm long. The insignificant short-stemmed greenish-white flowers form a spherical head. The fruit is a head of a dozen small juicy red berries. The knotted rhizome, a dark gray-brown on the outside and greenish-yellow inside, is cut up and dried. As the plant is no longer very plentiful in its natural habitat, efforts have been made to cultivate the goldenseal, but this succeeds only if the conditions under which it grows in the wild state can be maintained. The root tastes very bitter if chewed and colors the saliva yellow.

HYOSCYAMUS NIGER

HENBANE,
BLACK HENBANE

Solanaceae

126 C+S Eur, N Af, Asia
N Am, Aus

Like many of the nightshade family, henbane presents an appearance likely to evoke fear and suspicion. The herb has hallucinatory properties and was used in magic; witches are said to have brewed love potions from it. Henbane grows in waste places and by the wayside and prefers the vicinity of human habitations. The spindle-shaped root produces an angular, very hairy flowering stem which is 50–80 cm in height and often much branched at the top. The biennial variety only produces a rosette of leaves in the first year. The leaves are elongated and oval, and incised to give a few large teeth with pointed tips. Their color is a striking gray-green, and they are covered with a velvety down. The funnel-shaped flowers all turn to one side on the upper stem, forming a loose cluster somewhat like an ear of grain. They are a dirty yellow with brown or purple veins. The seeds are enclosed in a bell-shaped lidded capsule, which opens when ripe. The active principles found in the leaves are similar to those of belladonna. The whole plant is very poisonous, and great caution is indicated in its use.

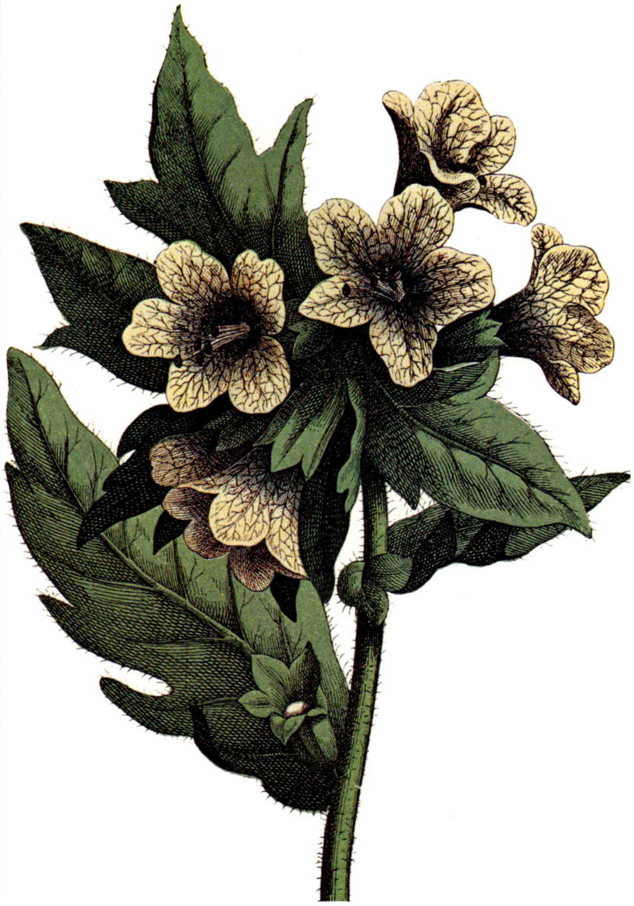

HYPERICUM
PERFORATUM

SAINT JOHN'S WORT

Hypericaceae

127 Eur, NW Af, N Asia
Temperate Zones

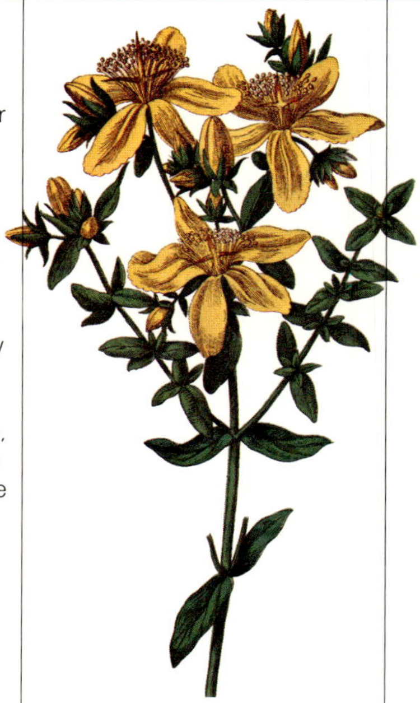

Saint John's wort likes a dry, sunny position on the edge of meadows, on railway embankments, the edge of woods, and in bushy places. The byname, *perforatum,* refers to the tiny oil glands dotting the leaves, which give them a perforated appearance. This herb contains a number of important principles. In spring, the much branched rootstock produces several hard smooth stems, 50–80 cm in height and often with a reddish tinge. These branch widely at the top, so that the terminal flowers get a maximum of sun. The opposite leaves, elongated oval and with margins entire, are dotted with tiny black glands in the margins. Like small golden-yellow suns, the numerous 5-petaled flowers sit on pointed green calyces covered with tiny reddish-black glands. A cluster of brownish stamens emerges at the center. If the flower is squeezed a red oil runs from them.

ILEX AQUIFOLIUM

EUROPEAN HOLLY

Aquifoliaceae

128 C+S Eur, NW Af, SW Asia

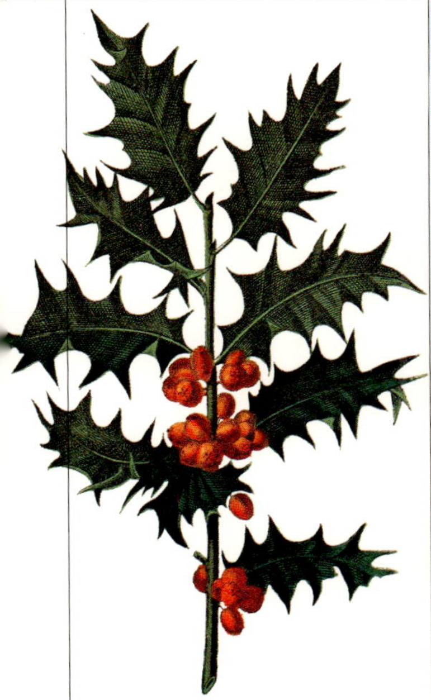

This shrub grows to a height of 2–5 m and may under favorable conditions develop into a tree. It forms part of the undergrowth, mostly in beech woods, but also adorns the edge of forests, parks, and gardens. The dark evergreen foliage with the red berries in autumn is highly decorative. The stem with its smooth bark and woody branches bears green shoots with leathery elongated oval leaves, shiny on the upper surface and pale green on the underside. These have wavy margins with prickly tips. On older bushes some of the leaves may have smooth margins. In spring, small waxy white flowers on short stems grow from the leaf axils, male and female flowers on different plants. In the autumn the fruits ripen to become scarlet berries the size of a pea. The berries are poisonous, though not to birds, and it is through them that the seeds are distributed. The active principles are found in the young leaves.

ILEX PARAGUARIENSIS

PARAGUAY TEA, MATÉ

Aquifoliaceae

129 C-S Am

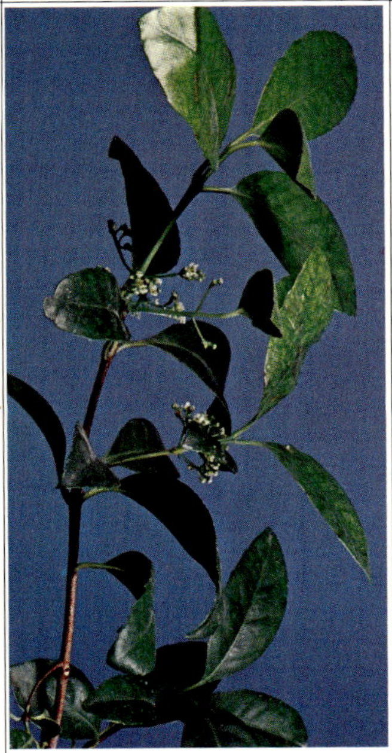

Most of the Ilex species of the holly family are native to tropical countries. There they grow as trees, 6–12 m in height, unless cultivated to a lower height for easier harvesting of the leafy twigs. In the extensive *Ilex* forests, these are cut off with a knife. The leathery leaves of the maté tree are 6–12 cm long, an elongated oval, and pale green in color. When harvested, they need to be dried quickly to prevent fermentation and black discoloration, and this is done over open wood fires. In the collecting depots they are dried further by modern methods. The leaves are then chopped up finely. Maté contains caffeine and is something of a national drink in many parts of South America. Jesuit missionaries cultivated it in Indian settlements in the seventeenth century, and it was formerly known as Jesuit's or missionary tea. The leaves contain stimulants (such as caffeine) and make a refreshing, reviving drink.

INULA HELENIUM

ELECAMPANE, SCABWORT

Asteraceae / Compositae

130 SE Eur, W Asia
Eur, C+E Asia, N Am

This handsome, luxuriant plant concentrates all its active principles in the thick, branching rootstock. In spring it produces large elliptical basal leaves up to 25 cm long, and at their center a stiff robust stem that branches at the top and is covered with matted hairs. The upper leaves are elongated and pointed and sit directly on the stem. The flowers growing at the end of the stem and from the leaf axils are striking – large yellow disks, 6–8 cm in diameter, on a hemisphere of green bract leaves arranged like overlapping tiles. The golden-yellow tubular florets at the center are surrounded by narrow ray florets of a paler yellow. The elecampane likes a moist position on the banks of streams and ditches, where it grows singly. It was formerly cultivated for use as a dyeing agent and for medicinal purposes. Apart from a pigment dyeing blue, the root contains inulin (a sugar similar to fructose) and a bitter aromatic volatile oil.

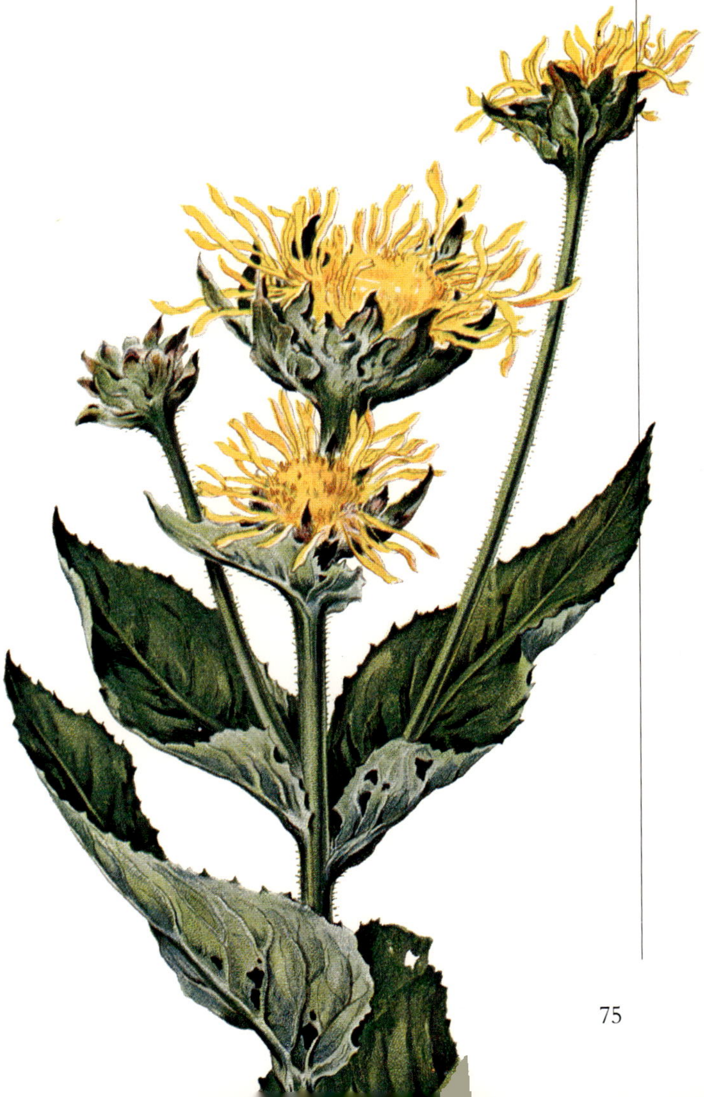

JUGLANS REGIA

ENGLISH WALNUT

Juglandaceae

131 SE Eur, SW Asia
Temperate Zones

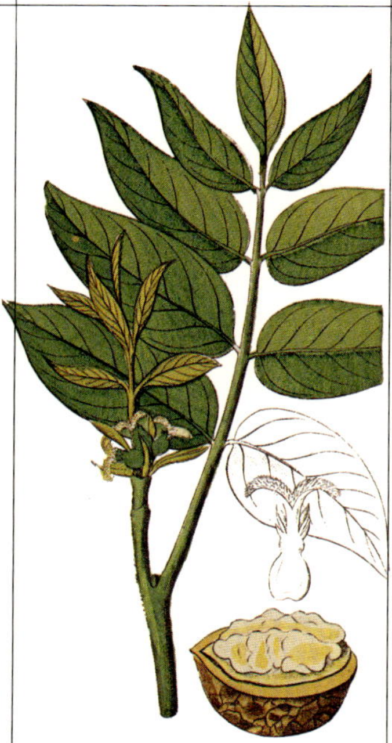

This stately, well-formed tree, up to 30 m high, tends to grow singly. The slowly increasing heart wood is protected by fissured gray bark. The stalked leaves are up to 40 cm long and divided into pairs; the 7–11 oval leaflets are about 15 cm in length, with margins entire and a raised midrib on the underside. The male flowers are in solid hanging catkins. The female flowers appear at the tips of the branches. In autumn, a pale green, tough, fleshy husk holds the single-seed fruit in its hard woody shell. A whole range of active principles are utilized: tannins from the leaves, vitamin C and pigments from the husk or pericarp, the oily kernels, and concentrated tannins in the membranes dividing the nut.

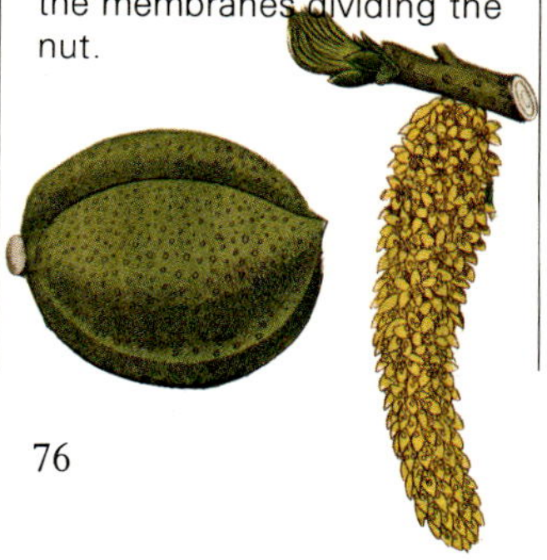

JUNIPERUS COMMUNIS

JUNIPER, COMMON JUNIPER

Cupressaceae

132 Eur, NW Af, Asia, N Am

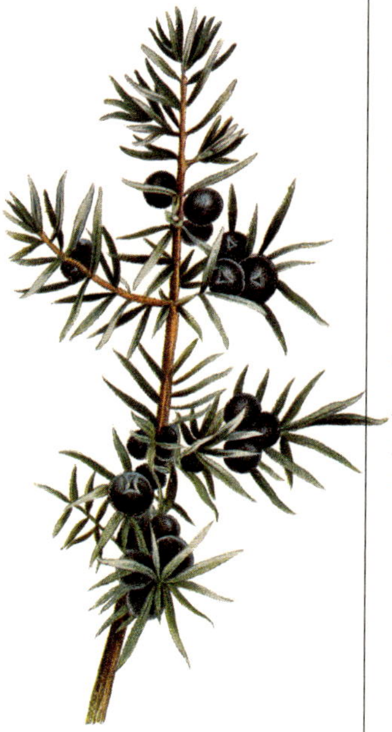

The juniper adapts its shape to the climate of the site. In the south, it produces a columnar shape 10 m high. In the mountains, well above the tree line, it grows as a dwarf juniper, resisting the harsh climate, a low shrub giving shelter to other plants. In the north, the dark shapes of junipers loom large in heath and moorlands. The spiky shrub with its woody branches bears thin, spine-tipped leaves in whorls of 3 needles, each with a central band of bluish-white on the upper surface. The insignificant male and female flowers grow on separate plants, with the pollen carried by the wind. The berries, green to begin with, ripen to become blue-black in 2 or 3 years. The brown flesh of the fruit contains the seeds and a highly aromatic volatile oil in which the most important active principles are found, and the plant also contains much invert sugar. The branches contain only a little of the volatile oil.

KRAMERIA TRIANDRA

PERUVIAN KRAMERIA, RHATANY

Krameriaceae

133 W-S Am
S Am

A low shrub about 60 cm in height, with a knotted and woody rootstock. The prostrate branches are covered with a silky down when young and later become gnarled and woody. The leaves are alternate and sit close together on the branches. They are egg-shaped, 1–2 cm long, and covered with silky hairs. Red flowers, each with 4 sepals and 4 petals, grow from the upper leaf axils. Medicinal use is made of rhatany root, which usually comes in cylindrical pieces of varying length and 1–3 cm in diameter. These have a reddish-brown, wrinkled, fissured or smooth surface and a brown woody core. The women of Lima formerly used pieces of the fibrous root to clean their teeth. The root is used in medicine for its powerful astringent properties.

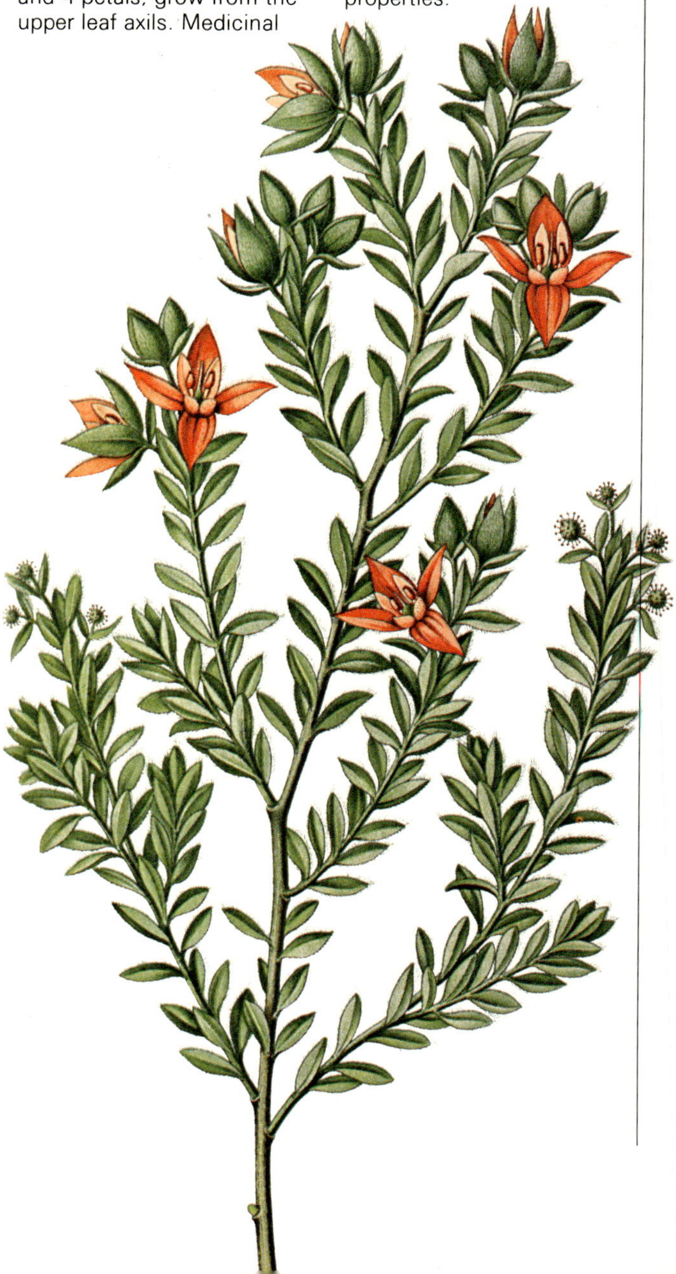

LAMIUM ALBUM

WHITE DEADNETTLE

Lamiaceae, Labiatae

134 Eur, Asia
Temperate Zones

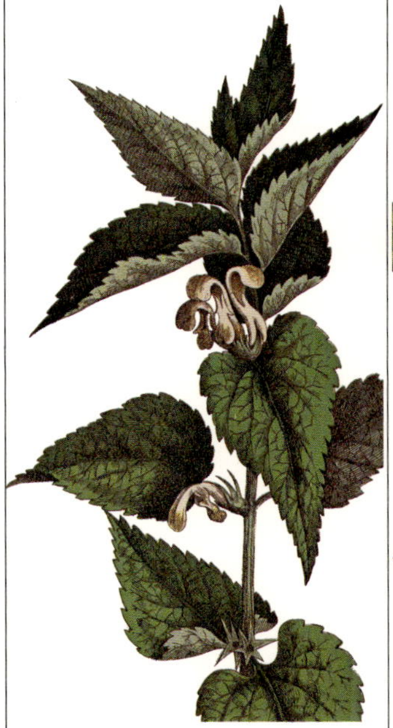

The name *Lamium* (Greek *lamos*=gullet) refers to the throat-shaped flower. The graceful herb, 20–30 cm in height, grows among the undergrowth, between grasses and shrubs, along hedges and fences, by waysides, and on rubbish heaps. The much branched underground stem produces numerous runners that in spring give rise to several flowering shoots. The erect, square, hollow stems are hairy and usually colored red near the ground. They bear downy, elongated heart-shaped dark green leaves ending in a point, similar to those of the stinging nettle. These are coarsely toothed and grow in opposite pairs set at right angles to each other. At the base of the leaves, the numerous flowers cluster in apparent whorls. Their white corollas, sometimes a muddy pink, are covered by a curving upper lip. Bees and bumblebees find abundant nectar in them, and children like to suck the flowers.

LAURUS NOBILIS

BAY, LAUREL

Lauraceae

135 S Eur, NW Af, SW Asia

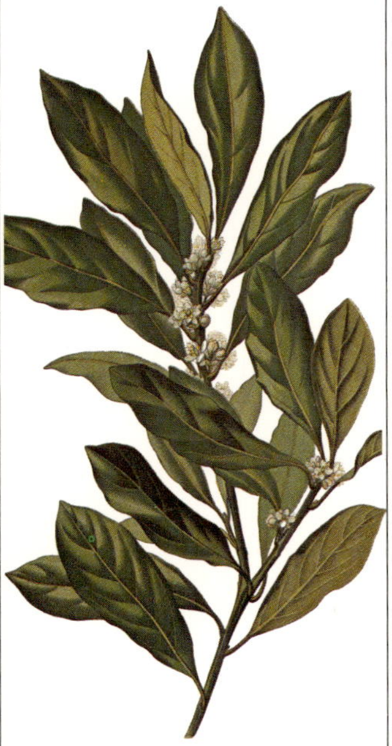

The sweet bay tree, favorite of the gods in ancient Greece, and the laurel branch, symbol of victory, have spread halfway round the world. Yet all that remains of the former glory of those leaves is the bayleaf in the casserole, a condiment prized by every good cook. The small tree or shrub has a smooth gray bark. The evergreen leaves are an elongated oval in shape, with margins entire, dark green and leathery, their upper surface glossy, and the underside a matt pale green. The sweet bay is able to adapt to many climates, but it is not hardy. Male and female flowers grow on different plants, small yellowish-white clusters appearing in the upper leaf axils. The fruits are cherry-sized berries, green at first and then a glossy black, and contain a single seed. The leaves have a spicy, aromatic scent. The fatty oil obtained from fresh laurel berries is pale green and ointment-like in consistency.

LAVANDULA ANGUSTIFOLIA

LAVENDER

Lamiaceae, Labiatae

136 S Eur, NW Af

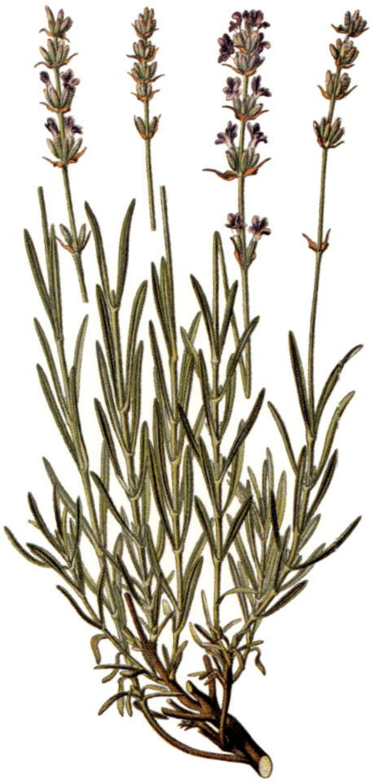

In northern areas, lavender grows as an ornamental plant in gardens, liking a dry, sunny position. It grows wild in southern France and Spain. There and in England it is widely cultivated for its oil, an important product used in the perfume industry. The broad rootstock produces branches, usually woody, with square green shoots 50–70 cm in length. These bear the gray-green narrow leaves with rolled-in sides that are covered with a silvery down. The whorls of small blue-violet labiate flowers stand out in extended spikes above the foliage. These contain most of the fragrant volatile oil and are cut off in their entirety, for its distillation. Other species, such as the spike lavender *(Lavandula latifolia)*, are larger, with broader leaves, but their oil is less sweet and more like camphor. The young shoots are occasionally used as a bitter aromatic herb. More recently, the plant has been analyzec for its tranquilizing effect.

LEONURUS CARDIACA

MOTHERWORT, COMMON MOTHERWORT

Lamiaceae, Labiatae

137 Eur, Asia
N Am

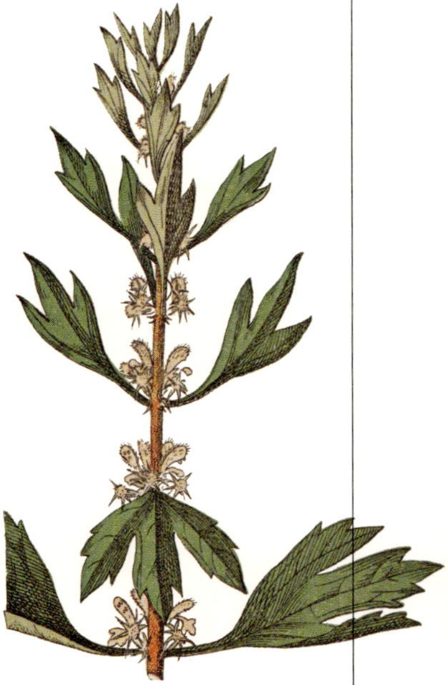

The ancient Greeks must have known of the strengthening effect on the heart of this plant, as the byname *cardiaca* (relating to the heart) indicates. The motherwort grows singly at the wayside, in hedges, and by old walls, perferring a dry position. The horizontal underground stem with its many roots produces erect square stems with hairs standing out stiffly. These often have a reddish-purple hue and grow to a height of 60–100 cm. The stalked leaves are in opposite pairs at right angles and deeply divided, hand-like, into 3–5 lobes. They are slightly downy, their upper surface dark and the underside light green. The leaf axils bear whorls of numerous flowers. The petals sit on a funnel-shaped calyx; they are flesh pink with red-brown markings and widen at the top. The whole plant has an unpleasant smell. More recent researches have confirmed its sedative and regulatory action.

LEVISTICUM OFFICINALE

LOVAGE

Apiaceae, Umbelliferae

138 SW Asia
Temperate Zones

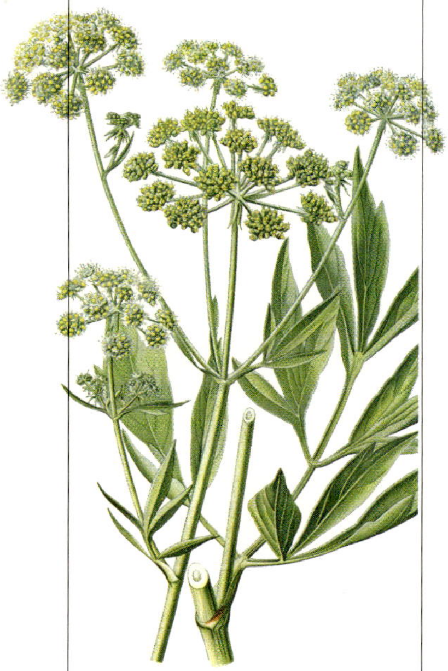

Popular as a kitchen herb in many countries, lovage is also cultivated for medicinal use. The large root does best in friable, moderately moist soil, in semishade. It produces erect tubular stems 1–2 m in height and branching at the top. The basal leaves are very large and tough, a glossy green on the upper surface, and divided 2–3 times. The stem leaves are less divided, their stalks getting shorter higher up on the stem. These are used to season soups and stews, but in small quantities only. The stems end in convex umbels of close rays bearing pale yellow flowers which are much visited by bees. The ribbed, often curved seeds ensure further distribution, though lovage may also be propagated by root division. The whole plant is strongly aromatic. The highest concentration of the volatile oil and other active principles is found in the root, which in some countries is still listed as an official drug.

LINUM USITATISSIMUM

FLAX, LINSEED

Linaceae

139 S Eur, SW Asia
Temperate Zones

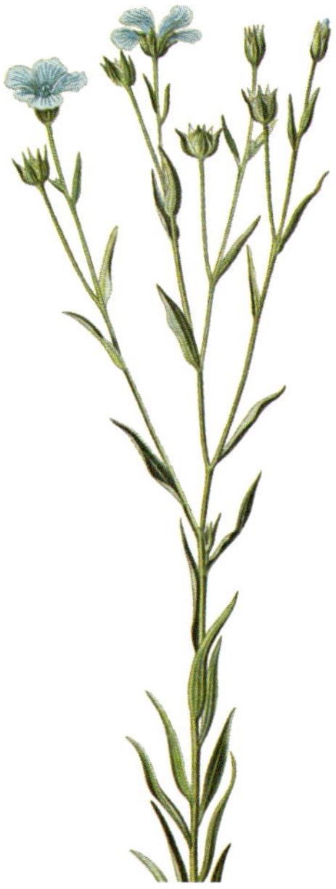

In the wild, flax is found only rarely. The annual plant has a whitish spindle-shaped root producing thin stems branching at the top. The small, veined alternate leaves are narrow and lance-shaped. Their color is a rich green. The delicate terminal flowers are blue, or more rarely white or pink. They have 5 petals arranged in a wheel, and usually last only a few hours. The fruit is a spherical capsule (boll) from which the seeds are obtained by thrashing. Each capsule holds 4–6 long, smooth glossy-brown seeds, their husks rich in mucilage and the kernel containing the fatty linseed oil. Both the mucilage and the oil are used medicinally, and linseed meal made from the cake remaining after expressing the oil is used for poultices. Other species of flax provide the fiber for linen (*linum*=thread=linen). The oil cake is very good for fattening cattle. The large seeds of a cultivated species serve as a diet food.

LOBELIA INFLATA

INDIAN TOBACCO, LOBELIA

Lobeliaceae

140 E-N Am

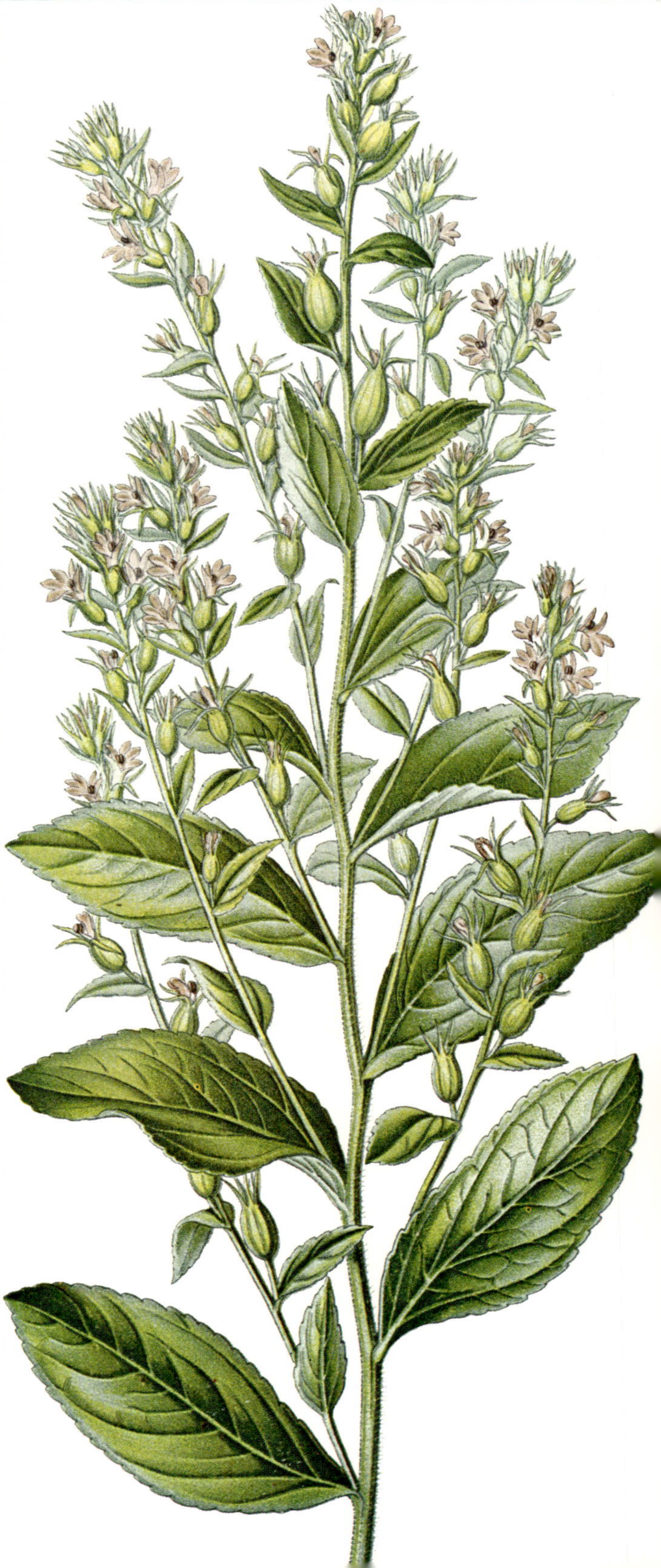

The species of *Lobelia* which is used medicinally belongs to the flora of northeast America, where it is also cultivated. The Indians used it as a medicinal herb, and because of its acrid taste it was called Indian tobacco. The Indians used decoctions of the root to treat syphilis and smoked the leaves to cure asthmatic complaints. Other species of *Lobelia* (e.g., *L. dortmanna*) grow in northern Europe. These are not used medicinally. The angular, roughly hairy stem of this annual is about 50 cm high, green or with a tinge of violet. The leaves are 4–7 cm long and a somewhat pale green; they are narrow, lance-shaped and pointed, short-stemmed, and have irregularly toothed margins. The tips of the teeth bear small whitish warts (water stomata). The leaf is hairy, particularly along the veins. The sparse, pale blue flowers are 2-lipped and grow in a terminal spike. The seed capsule is inflated *(L. inflata)* and contains numerous small seeds. The leaves have an acrid, burning taste. *Lobelia* contains a number of interesting alkaloids as active principles. These include lobeline, which has an action like that of nicotine.

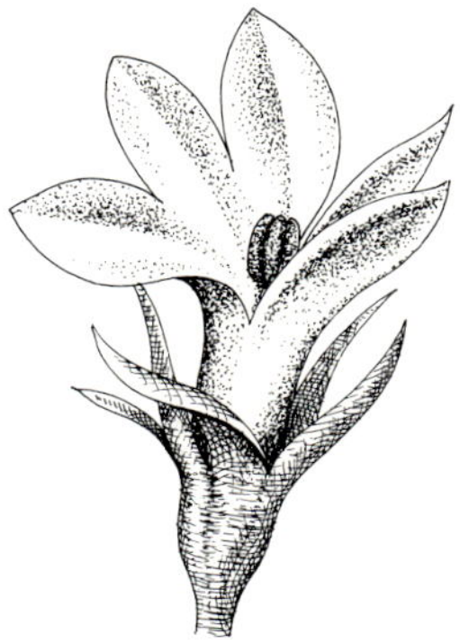

LYCOPUS VIRGINICUS

BUGLEWEED

Lamiaceae / Labiatae

141 E-N Am

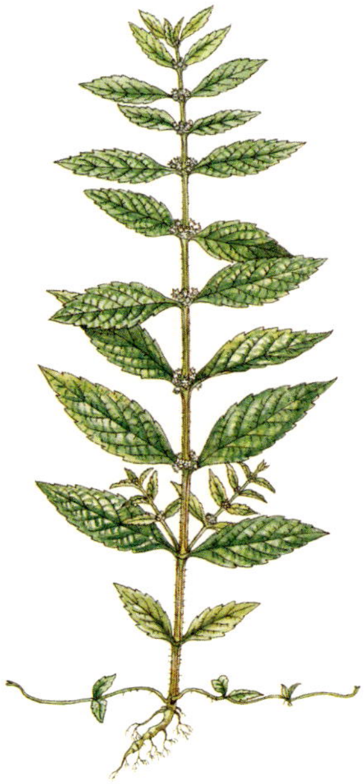

The bugleweed likes to grow in damp meadows, on riverbanks, in ditches, and in open woodlands. The perennial creeping underground stem is square, with a circle of long fibrous roots spreading from each node. The erect flowering stems grow to a height of 30–60 cm. They are bluntly quadrangular and downy, branching usually only near the top. The leaves are opposite, each pair at right angles to the preceding one; they are 6–15 cm long, in an elongated egg-shape ending in a point, and narrow down into the short stalk. The margins are toothed, and the underside of the leaf is dotted with glands. The small whitish labiate flowers grow in whorls at the base of the upper leaves. The fresh plant has been found to contain a volatile oil and also hormone-type substances which have not yet been fully analyzed. The gipsy wort, *Lycopus europaeus*, with incised leaves, also grows in North America.

LYTHRUM SALICARIA

PURPLE LOOSESTRIFE, SPIKED LOOSESTRIFE

Lythraceae

142 Eur, Asia *N Am*

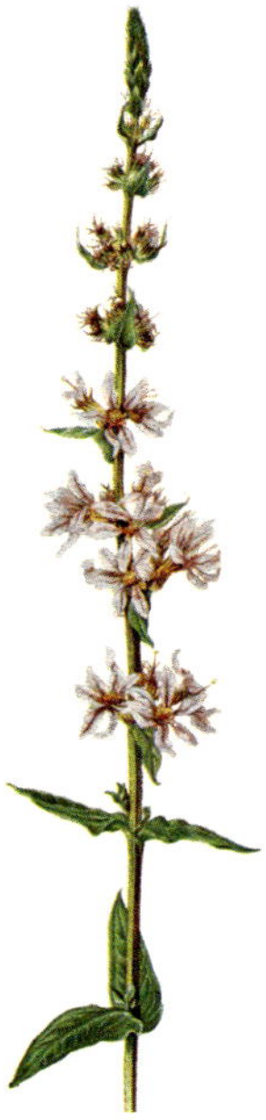

The purple loosestrife is one of our most common marsh ornamenting plains and river banks with its blood-red spikes of flowers. The thick, woody root produces simple angular stems 70–120 cm in height that do not branch much. The heart or lance-shaped, opposite pointed leaves on these stems are up to 12 cm in length, a rich green with prominent veins and fringed with short hairs in the margin. Numerous star-shaped flowers with 6 petals on a cup-shaped calyx form the purple-red terminal spikes. The plant flowers from July to August. The fruits are small capsules containing seeds covered with mucus-secreting hairs. These become attached to the beaks and feet of aquatic birds and are thus distributed. The byname *salicaria* is supposed to refer to the willow-like shape of the leaves (*Salix* = willow). The herb was formerly recommended for severe, dysentery-like diarrhea.

MALVA SYLVESTRIS

HIGH MALLOW, COMMON MALLOW

Malvaceae

143 S Eur, W Asia *Temperate Zones*

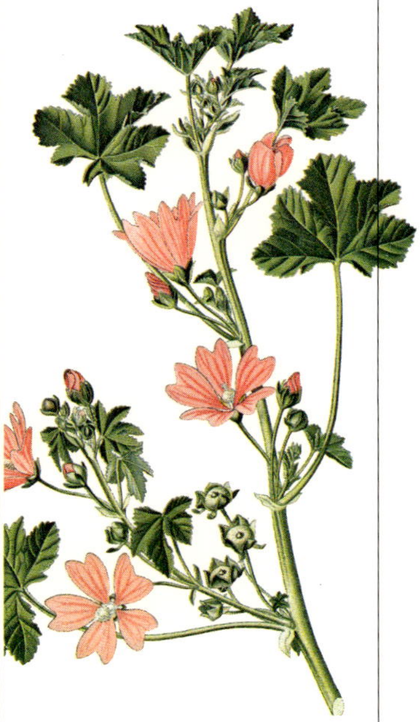

The slender tap root of the common mallow penetrates deeply into the soil, and this enables the plant to flourish in waste places, on waysides, and along walls, up to the foothills, at about 1500 m. The round, branching stem rises at an angle or grows erect to a height of 40–100 cm. The kidney-shaped leaves, lobed and hand-like and with toothed margins, are a rich green. Both stems and leaves are covered with a downy pelt, a typical feature of many mucilaginous plants. From the leaf axils grow the short-stemmed flowers with their 5 notched mauve-purple petals. The fruits are round, flattened disks which are sometimes called cheeses. A smaller species, the dwarf mallow *(Malva neglecta)*, grows to a height of about 30 cm, with smaller leaves and flowers, and is used in the same way. The leaves are still widely used for medicinal purposes, and the common mallow is cultivated.

MARRUBIUM VULGARE

HOREHOUND,
WHITE HOREHOUND

Lamiaceae, Labiatae

144 S Eur, N Af, W Asia
Warm Temperate Zones

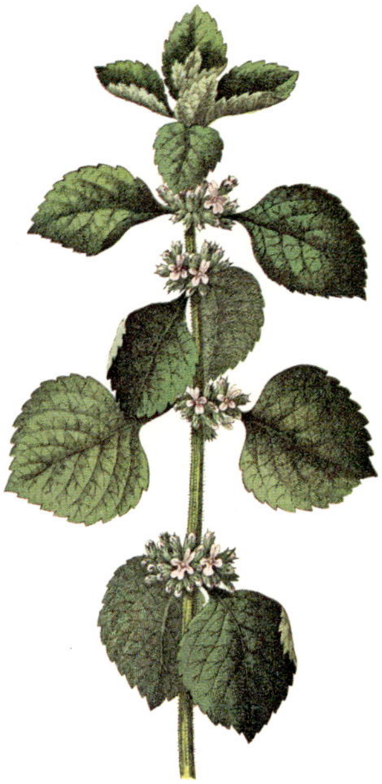

The white horehound likes dry, sunny waste places, lean pastures, and roadsides. It is also cultivated as a garden plant. The perennial herb produces hollow hairy stems up to 60 cm high. The short-stemmed, ovate pointed leaves tend to be wrinkled; they are opposite, dark green on the upper surface, and covered with a whitish pelt on the underside. Small white tubular flowers 5–7 mm in length form dense whorls in the leaf axils. The white horehound flowers from June to August. It looks rather similar to the white deadnettle, but has denser whorls of smaller flowers and the leaves have a distinctly bitter taste. For medicinal purposes, the whole of the flowering herb is used. This plant has been to some extent forgotten, but it is easily cultivated. It is known to stimulate the secretion of bile and to clear the air-passages in bronchial catarrh.

MARSDENIA
CUNDURANGO

EAGLE VINE,
CONDOR VINE

Asclepiadaceae

145 W-S Am
E Asia

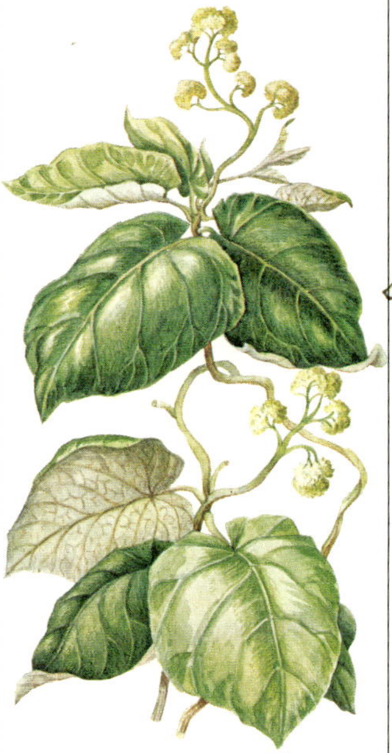

This vine pushes its pliant stem up many meters high among the deciduous forest trees, to unfold its flowers in the sun. Its stem is up to 10 cm in diameter. The heart-shaped oval leaves, 8–10 cm long and 5–8 cm wide, are borne on lateral branches. They are covered with a dense woolly down. The flowers, bell or funnel-shaped, grow in clusters on the uppermost branches. The fruits are boat-shaped follicles, their seeds bearing a tuft of hair. The leaves of the eagle vine figure large in the folk legends of the Peruvians, yet it is the bark from the branches which contains principles of medicinal value. The bark is removed from the branches, dried and cut into quilled pieces 5–10 cm long, 1–3 cm wide, and 2–5 mm thick, a pale grayish-brown, yellowish where fractured. It has a bitter, aromatic taste, similar to cinnamon, and contains a number of bitters, organic acids, and starch.

MATRICARIA
CHAMOMILLA

GERMAN CHAMOMILE,
WILD CHAMOMILE

Asteraceae, Compositae

146 C+S Eur, N Af, W Asia
Temperate Zones

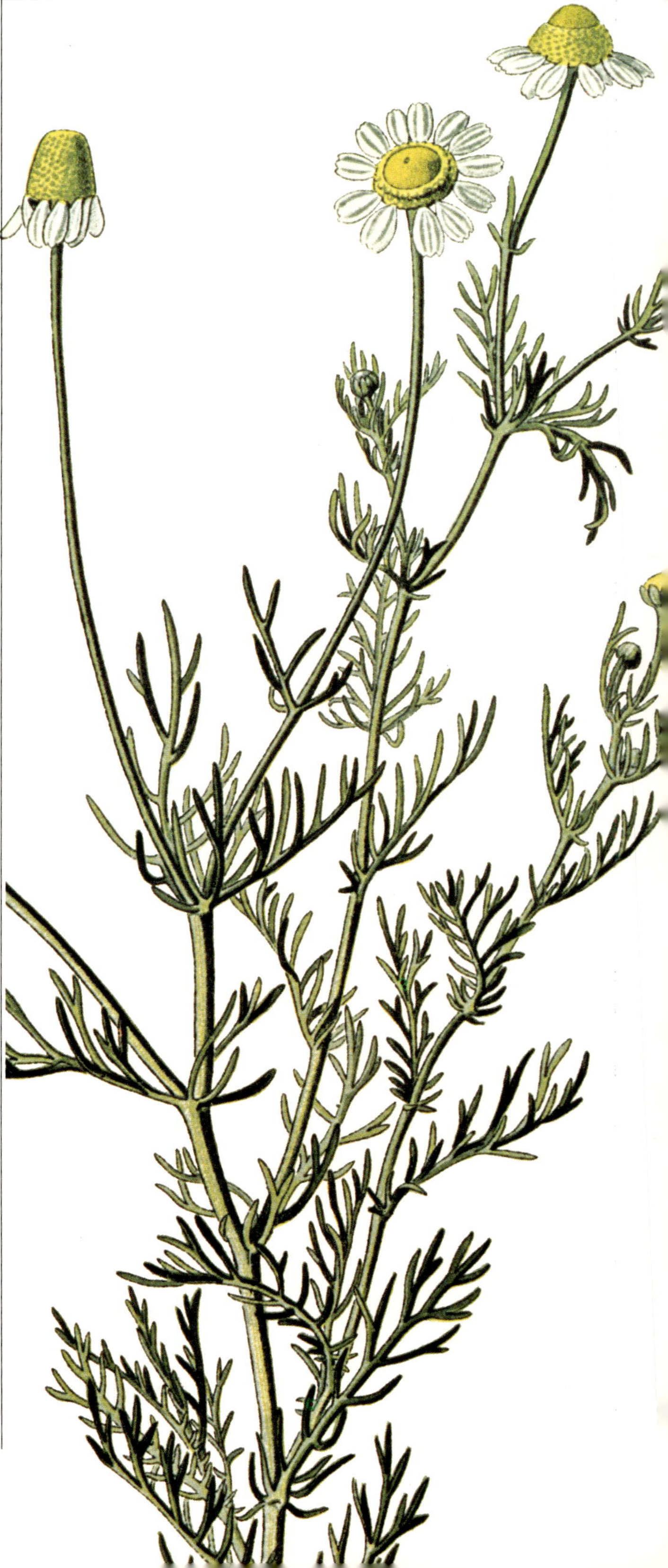

This is a versatile medicinal herb, with a wide range of uses. The name *Matricaria* (from *matrix*=womb) indicates the use made of it by the ancients, and chamomile tea still serves to relieve complaints related to childbearing and other female conditions. In southern Europe it grows wild in waste places and rubbish dumps and by the wayside and is much cultivated in gardens. It is grown on a large scale in the Balkans and South America, to meet the worldwide demand for chamomile. The plant is an annual and produces an erect, round stem 40–60 cm in height that is usually branched. The leaves are few, and much divided into thread-like pointed wisps. The flower heads with their hollow conical yellow centers grow on thin stalks. They consist of tubular disk florets surrounded by a circlet of white strap-like ray florets bent downward and out. The fully open flowers are collected for use, less commonly the whole herb. Their efficacy depends on the concentration of the volatile oil they contain, and this may vary greatly. More recent investigations have shown that the medicinal action is due not only to the main principle, azulene, but also to other constituents.

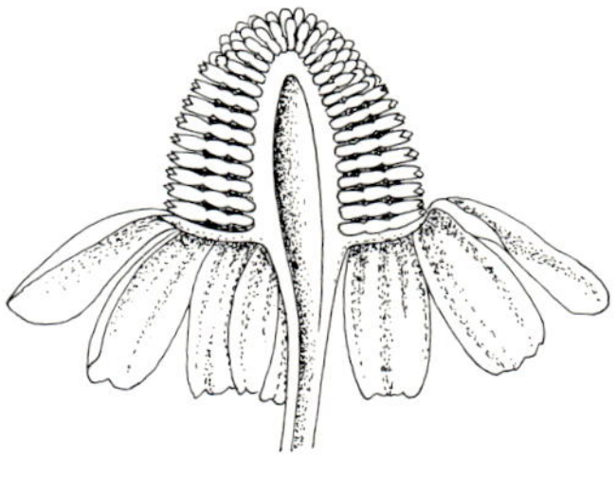

MELILOTUS OFFICINALIS

YELLOW SWEETCLOVER, RIBBED MELILOT

Fabaceae, Papilionaceae

147 Eur, Asia
Temperate Zones

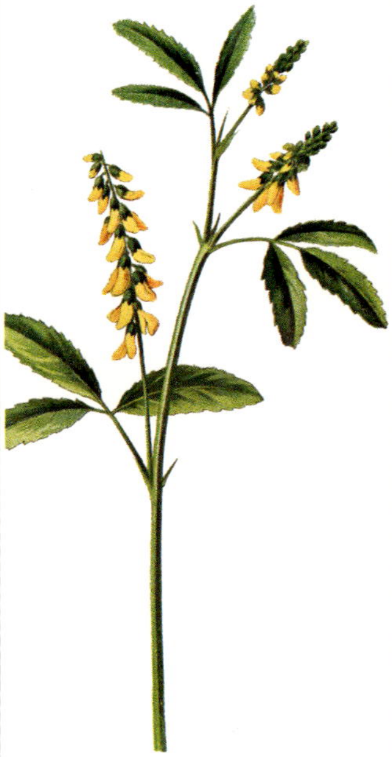

The melilot (Greek *meli*= honey) is very popular with the bees for its honey-sweet nectar. It grows from a strong tap root, the rootlets of which are covered with small nodules produced by nitrogen-fixing bacteria, as is common with leguminous plants. The tall, much branched stems grow to a height of about 1 m. The stalked leaves are elongated elliptical, a rich green, and trefoil (clover species), with lightly indented or toothed margins. Long slender spikes of flowers grow from the leaf axils; the numerous, small yellow peaflowers have large standards. The small hairless yellowish-brown pods are borne away on the wind with their seeds. The whole plant has a sweet odor of coumarin (vanilla), which becomes stronger as it dries. For medicinal use, the flowering herb (June–September) is gathered. The tall melilot *(Melilotus altissima)*, a taller and more luxuriant species, is also cultivated.

MELISSA OFFICINALIS

BALM, COMMON BALM

Lamiaceae, Labiatae

148 SE Eur, SW Asia
Temperate Zones

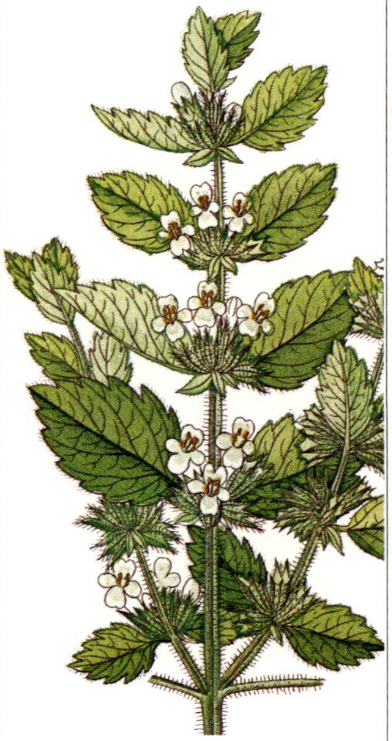

The balm grows from a persistent multiheaded rootstock which produces erect square stems, 60–100 cm in height. These branch little at first, but much more when the plant flowers. The rich foliage consists of oval to heart-shaped, stalked glossy light green leaves that grow in opposite pairs. They are toothed and bear tiny oil glands. Small bunches of whitish flowers about 1.5 cm long grow from the upper leaf axils. A delight to the bees, these open in July–August. The whole herb and above all the leaves produce a pleasant scent of lemon when rubbed between the fingers. For garden culture, balm needs a sandy clay soil rich in humus and not too dry. Before the plant flowers, the young leaves and the tips of the shoots contain most of the volatile oil. They may be used fresh in cooking, or dried in the shade and stored. Either way, this is a herb to grow in the garden.

MENTHA PIPERITA

PEPPERMINT

Lamiaceae, Labiatae

149 S Eur
Temperate Zones

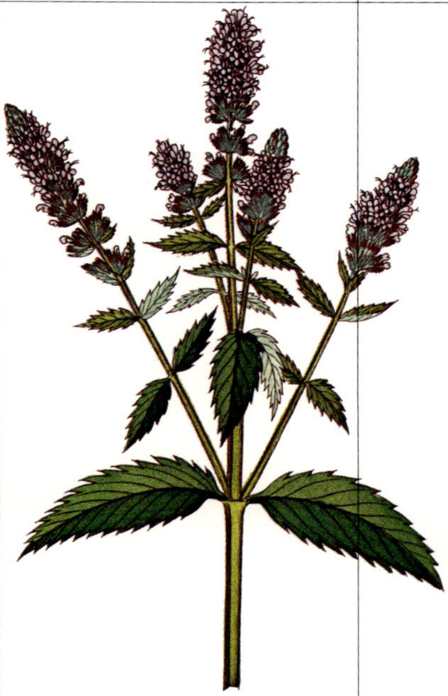

The peppermint, a cross of a number of wild mints, has been known since the seventeenth century. It differs from the wild species in that its volatile oil has a high concentration of menthol, which gives it its cooling, refreshing properties. The peppermint prefers a moist soil rich in humus, and the wild species also grow generally in damp places and marshes. The shallow underground stem, with runners above and below ground, produces square stems 50–80 cm in height and much branched at the top, which often show a reddish tinge. The plant propagates itself only by runners. The stalked leaves grow in opposite pairs. Depending on the genus, they are elliptical to lance-shaped, 4–8 cm long, with toothed margins, light or dark green, and often have a tinge of red. The leaves on the flowering shoots are very much smaller. The small violet flowers are packed close together in spikes.

MENYANTHES TRIFOLIATA

BUCKBEAN, MARSH TREFOIL, BOGBEAN

Gentianaceae

150 Eur, Asia, N Am

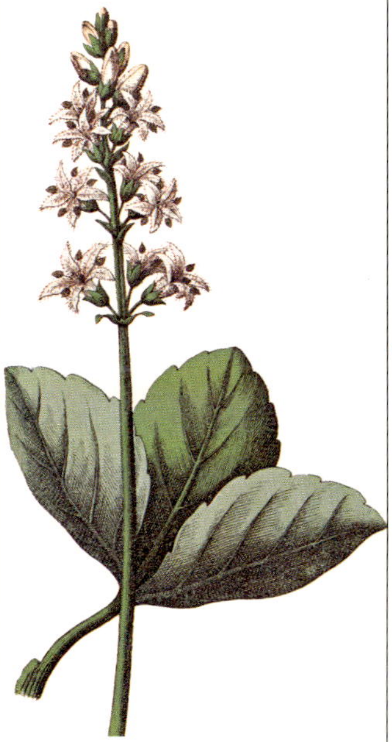

The bogbean is a member of the gentian family, though the trefoil leaf looks similar to that of clover. Botanists now classify it under a separate family, the *Menyanthaceae*. The thick, creeping underground stems are found in marshy ground, usually under water, on the edges of ponds and streams, from the lowlands up to mountain areas at altitudes of 1800 m. In the spring, shoots appear, 30–40 cm long, together with long tubular stalks bearing 3 egg-shaped leaflets held well above the water. The flowering shoot terminates in a handsome reddish-white spike of numerous 5-lobed flowers fringed with white hairs. Bumblebees fly busily to and fro. The leaves contain powerful gentian bitters, and the plant was therefore used to reduce fevers. Unfortunately it has become necessary to protect the bogbean in many areas, for it will not grow in contaminated water.

MONARDA DIDYMA

OSWEGO TEA, BERGAMOT, BEE BALM

Lamiaceae, Labiatae

151 E-N Am *Temperate Zones*

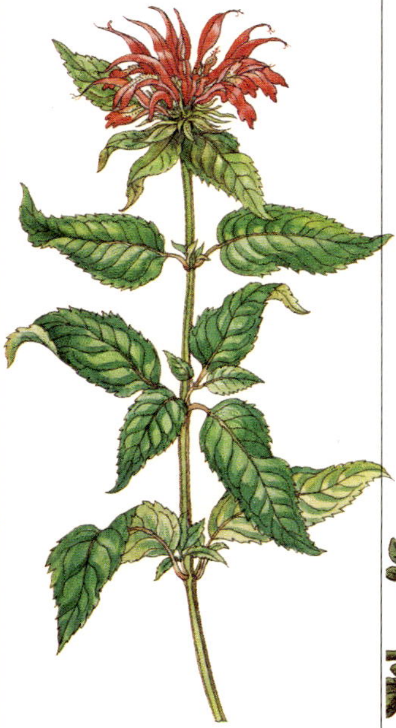

This perennial shrub is popular in country gardens.
In the last century, a plant formed part of every bride's dowry, for the tea was well known to be of great benefit to young mothers. The rootstock produces many runners in the dry, light soil the plant prefers. In spring, several square stems are produced, 60–80 cm high and often with a reddish tinge, branching only near the top. The opposite leaves grow on reddish stems; they are up to 10 cm in length, egg-shaped and pointed, with toothed margins. Narrower than the leaves of balm *(Melissa)*, they have prominent veins, are less wrinkled, and also much less aromatic. The flowers growing in terminal whorls are long, narrow, and a deep scarlet. The active principles are found in the flowers. These are gathered all through the summer, when their bright color makes them easy to find, and are dried carefully in the shade.

NASTURTIUM OFFICINALE

WATERCRESS

Brassicaceae, Cruciferae

152 Temperate Zones

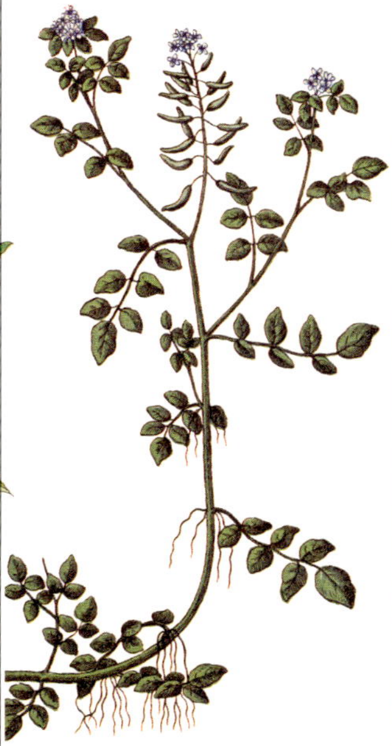

As its name suggests, watercress likes to grow in clean, slow running waters. One must wear high boots to pick it, but the reward is a whole range of valuable medicinal properties. These depend on the plant's being fresh, however, and are soon lost as it dies. This is very much a medicinal herb for springtime. The branching stems, creeping at first and later erect, produce numerous secondary roots, which in turn give rise to further angular tubular stems of a rich green. The stalked leaves are subdivided into 1–3, and higher up 5–9, fleshy ovate leaflets with small horizontal ears at the base of the stalk. The stems terminate in a pretty, erect spike of white cruciferous flowers. These develop into sickle-shaped pods, a sign that the plant is related to the mustards and to scurvy grass. The rather hot, aromatic flavor of watercress reveals the presence of many and varied active principles.

NERIUM OLEANDER

OLEANDER, ROSE BAY

Apocynaceae

153 S Eur *Warm Temperate Zones*

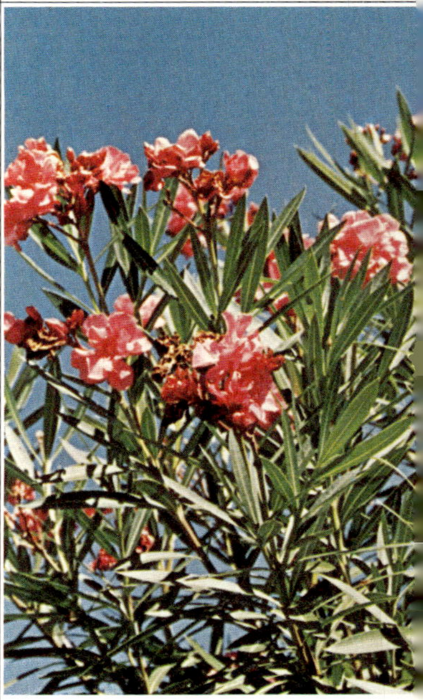

Highly esteemed as a medicinal plant in Arab medicine, the oleander was introduced to Europe as an ornamental plant in the nineteenth century. In northern latitudes, oleanders growing in the gardens of palaces and country houses still bear witness of former glory; in winter they are moved to the greenhouse, with the orange trees, for frost protection.
In southern parts the oleander is an evergreen shrub, less frequently a tree 3–8 m

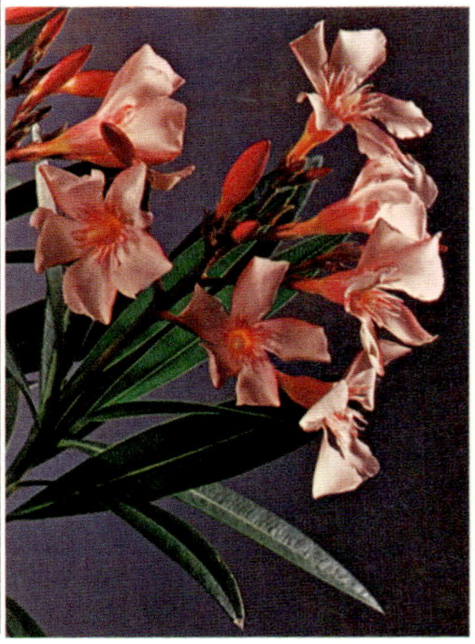

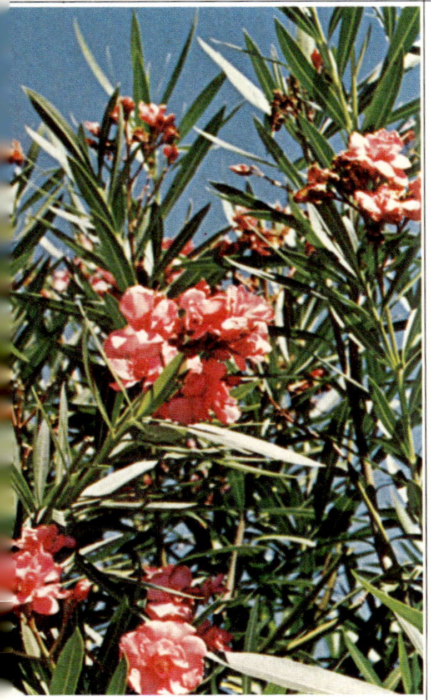

in height. A spiky shrub, it bears dark green, leathery leaves on its round woody branches. The leaves are 10–15 cm in length, narrow and lance-shaped with margins entire, and this evergreen foliage gradually renews itself. The flowers appearing at the ends of the branches are very handsome, a blazing red or white, tubular and opening into a wheel at the top. Their scent is almost narcotic. The name "rose bay" indicates that the oleander combines the severity of the baytree with the joy of life seen in the rose. The active principles in the leaves include cardiac glycosides similar to those of the foxglove *(Digitalis)*. For this purpose they are widely used in Europe instead of digitalis. To a certain extent this is based on the availability of the plant. In countries such as the United States and the United Kingdom, the preference is definitely for the cardiac glycosides of the foxglove *(Digitalis purpurea)*.

OLEA EUROPAEA

OLIVE

Oleaceae

154 S Eur, N Af, SW Asia
S Af, W-N Am, Aus

From time immemorial, people all over the world have looked for medicinal virtues in the plants they generally use for food or textile fibers. In the case of the olive tree, there is some evidence that its leaves contain a substance which, if given in suitably prepared form, brings down the blood pressure. But now as ever, the most important product of the tree is the olives, one of the few fruits to contain oil not only in the seed, but particularly also in the fleshy part. Olive trees grow extremely slowly and may become hundreds of years old. The trunk is similar to that of a willow, but may reach a height of 10 m. The branches are thin and straight, with narrow, lance-shaped leaves which are gray-green on the upper surface and silvery underneath. In April–May, small delicate yellowish-white flowers form short clusters in the leaf axils. The plum-shaped fruit, the olive, ripens very slowly and is harvested through the winter. Producing an abundance of oil seems to take up all the vitality of this tree. Fruits are not produced until the trees are 10 years old, and it is many more years before an olive tree reaches its full power.

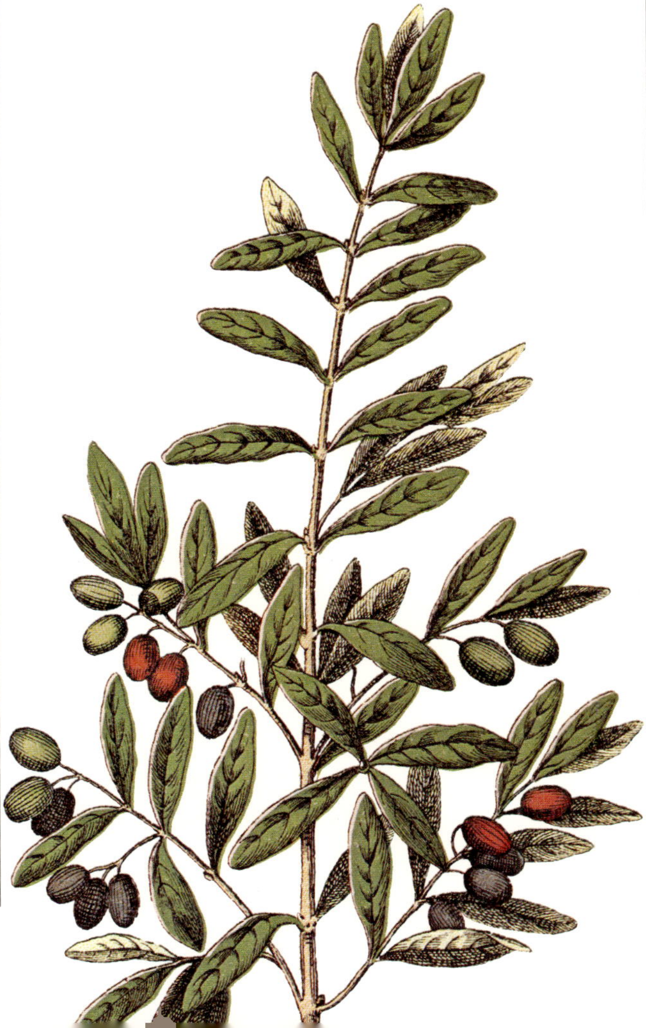

ONONIS SPINOSA

PRICKLY RESTHARROW

Fabaceae, Papilionaceae

155 Eur
N Am

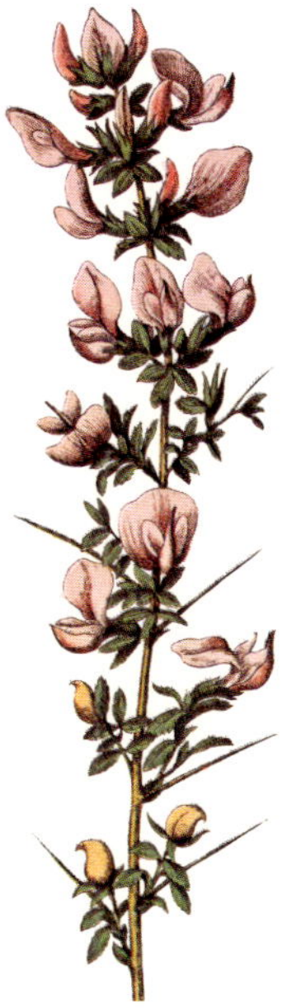

This shrub, 30–60 cm high, grows in dry grass, at the edge of woods and on roadsides, and among chalk rocks in the mountains up to 1500 m. The woody, deep-reaching rootstock produces hairy, branched, and partly woody stems, with very sharp spines on the side shoots. Lower down, the leaves are divided into 3; higher they are small, elongated oval, with toothed margins. They are pale green in color, and altogether the foliage is rather sparse. But from May until autumn the plant flowers richly, with pinkish-purple, rarely bluish, pea-type flowers on pointed green calyces in the leaf axils forming loose spikes. The active principles are found in the leaves and in the root. With its brown bark and yellow wood, the dried root is easily recognizable. Recent research has shown the plant to contain volatile oil and other principles, including the pigment found in the root.

ORIGANUM VULGARE

MARJORAM, OREGANO

Lamiaceae, Labiatae

156 Eur, C+N Asia
N Am

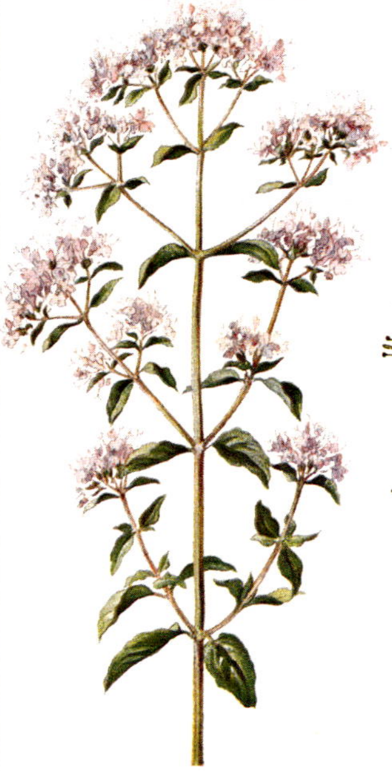

Wild marjoram grows on sunny, stony slopes, on chalky and siliceous soil, in lean grassland up to medium-high mountain regions. The much branched root produces woody runners. The square stems 40–60 cm high often have a reddish tinge and branch only at the top. The stalked ovate pointed leaves grow in opposite pairs, which follow one another at right angles. Leaves and stems are hairy and dotted with tiny glands. At the top of the stem, numerous tiny pink or purple labiate flowers grow in loose bushy clusters. The whole aromatic herb is cut and used in herbal baths. In the kitchen it serves as a seasoning for meat, like sweet marjoram. The plant shows a certain resemblance to the hemp agrimony *(Eupatorium cannabinum)*, especially in the color of the flowers, but this belongs to a different family.

ORTHOSIPHON STAMINEUS

JAVA TEA,
INDIAN KIDNEY TEA

Lamiaceae/Labiatae

157 SE Asia
Torrid Zones

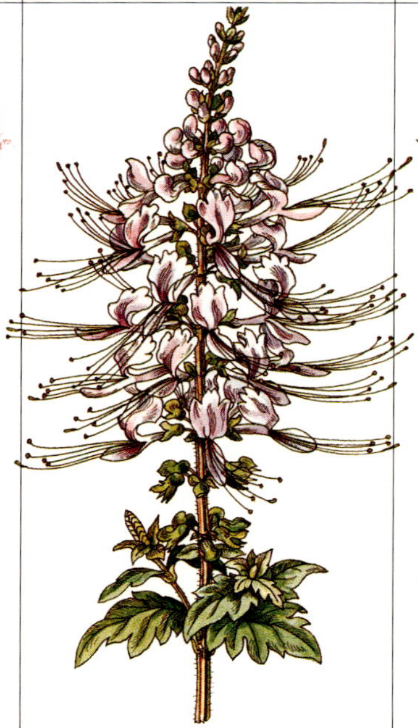

This herbaceous plant, similar to peppermint, is cultivated in the Indonesian Archipelago, especially Java, and in Australia. Valued as a medicinal plant by the natives, it was taken up by the European immigrants and brought to Holland and to Germany. The stems, 70–90 cm high, are smooth or slightly downy. They bear opposite pairs of stalked leaves, each at right angles to the one before. The leaves are wedge-shaped lower down, about 5–6 cm in length, elongated and pointed, and covered with hairs on both sides. The veining of the leaves is interesting, arising at an acute angle from the central vein and then curving in an arch toward the tip of the leaf. The flowers grow in terminal pseudo-spikes. Long stamens emerge from the pale blue tubular floral tube. These gave the plant its original name (*kumis kutjing* = cat's whiskers). The leaves are dried and cut up small for tea mixtures.

PANAX QUINQUEFOLIUS,
PANAX GINSENG

AMERICAN GINSENG,
ASIATIC GINSENG

Araliaceae

158 E Asia, E-N Am

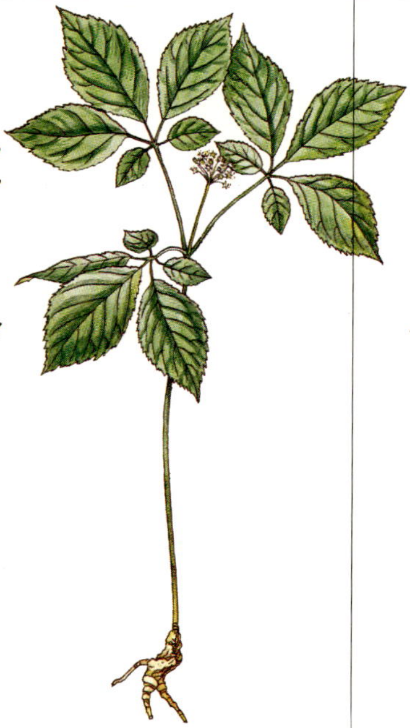

For thousands of years a panacea to the peoples of Asia, ginseng is obtained from what is really quite an insignificant woodland plant, a native of the dense mountain forests of Asia, from Nepal to Manchuria. Owing to the great demand for it, the plant is also cultivated in many countries (Korea, China, Japan, USSR, USA). *Panax quinquefolius* grows wild in Canada and the eastern United States. The multiheaded tap root forks and branches to give it an appearance similar to the human form. The name ginseng is said to come from the Chinese name Jin-chen, which means "man-like" and is derived from the fact that the roots vaguely resemble the arms, body, and legs of a human doll. The smooth round stem, 40–60 cm high, bears 2 stalked terminal leaves. These are dark green and divided into 5 leaflets, like fingers. The flowering stem terminates in a greenish-white umbel of bisexual flowers.

PAPAVER SOMNIFERUM

OPIUM POPPY

Papaveraceae

159 *Warm Temperate Zones*

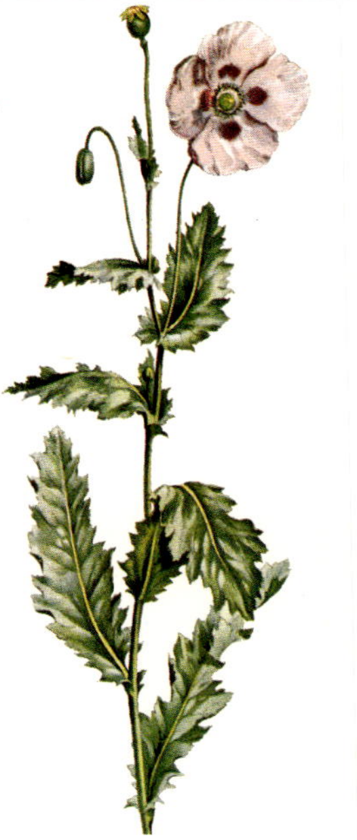

No other plant drug has played such a role in world events. Narcotics divisions all over the world are concerned to keep cultivation under government supervision. The opium poppy varies considerably in appearance. The round, blue-green stem reaches about 1 m in height. The lower leaves sit directly on the stem; they are wavy, with toothed margins. The large, strikingly handsome flowers grow on thin, hairy stalks, with 4 lilac-colored (sometimes white) petals, thin as tissue paper, surrounding a green ovary. The petals soon drop off. The ovary ripens to form a spherical capsule containing oily seeds. The stems and unripe capsules are filled with latex, which is collected and dried to give opium. In many countries, a particular black-seeded species of *Papaver* is cultivated for the seed oil. The capsules left after expressing the oil contain small amounts of opium constituents.

PASSIFLORA INCARNATA

WILD PASSIONFLOWER, MAYPOP

Passifloraceae

160 SE-N Am, C Am
S Eur, W-S Am

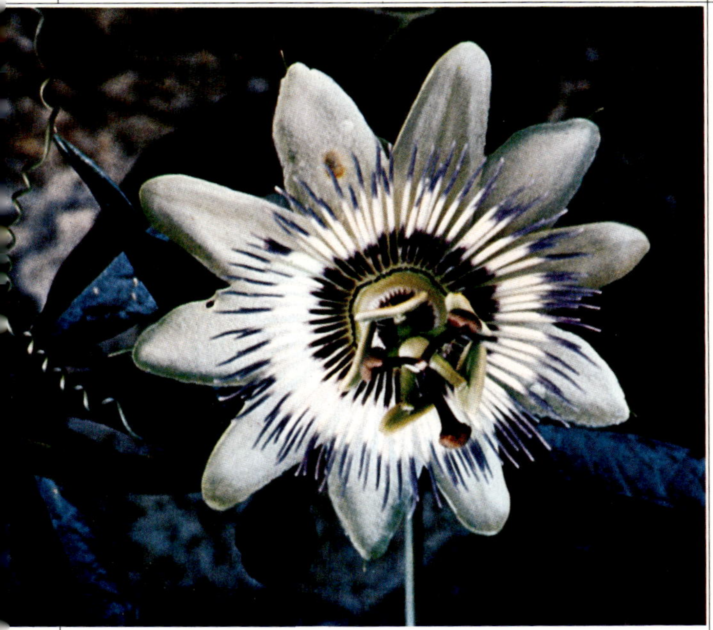

This exotic climber, with woody stems some meters in length, grows in the damp forests of South America. In northern regions it is now cultivated as an ornamental plant. The plant owes its name to the flower which resembles the instruments of Christ's crucifixion. A reddish-purple corona of filaments growing from the receptacle suggests the crown of thorns. The climbing branches bear long-stemmed, broadly oval 3-lobed leaves with toothed margins. Leafless flowering stalks bear the highly decorative white and purple flowers. By autumn the ovary has developed into a sweet-flavored egg-shaped yellow fruit. For about 100 years now medicinal use has been made of the leaves and flowers. These have been found to contain valuable principles (alkaloids) with sedative and spasmolytic properties. Passiflora tea and extracts are quite widely used to calm the nerves. The fragrant, somewhat mucilaginous fruit flesh is used in the preparation of soft drinks. This fruit, a berry, contains flat seeds with yellowish or brownish coverings. This plant is now cultivated in several parts of the Old World, especially Belgium and Italy.

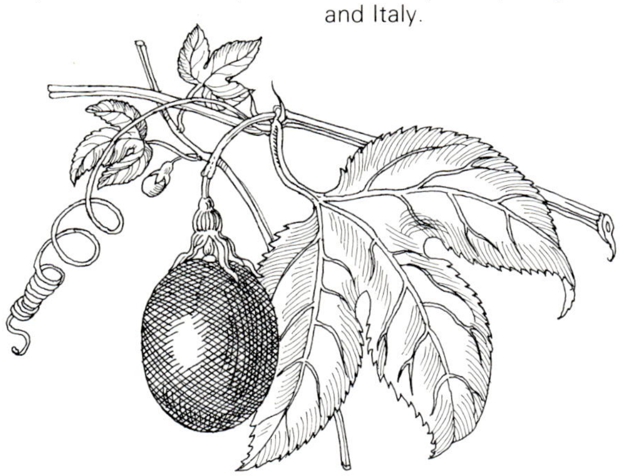

PETASITES HYBRIDUS

BUTTERBUR, SWEET COLTSFOOT

Asteraceae, Compositae

161 Eur, N+W Asia
N Am

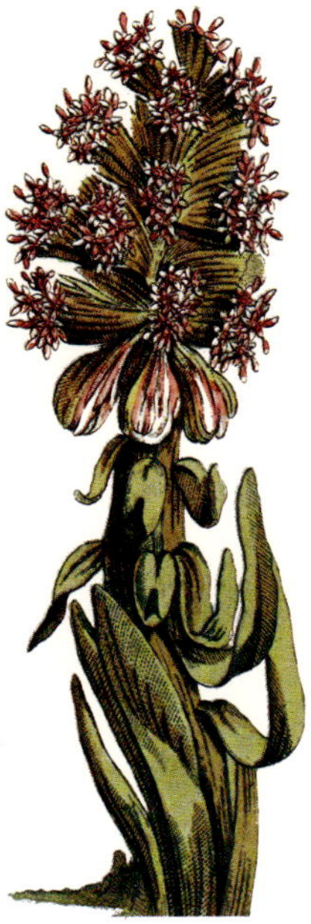

The butterbur grows in damp meadows, in the shade at the edge of woods, and on the banks of streams. The tuberous root produces runners up to 1.5 m in length. Early in spring the flowering shoots appear, scaly shafts bearing a dense, erect spike of numerous white *(Petasites albus)* or dirty-pink *(Petasites hybridus)* composite flowers. When the flowers have faded, the spikes lengthen and grow bunches of seed hairs on which the seeds are carried through the air. Meanwhile the leaf buds have unfolded, and in summer the plant has heart-shaped wavy leaves, up to 80 cm wide and curving in toward the stem. These are covered with a gray woolly pelt on the underside. The butterbur is one of the pioneering plants in mountain regions. It takes root and helps to produce humus. During the last 30 years pharmacological studies have shown it to contain antispasmodic and other active principles.

PETROSELINUM CRISPUM

PARSLEY

Apiaceae, Umbelliferae

162 S Eur, N Af, SW Asia
Temperate Zones

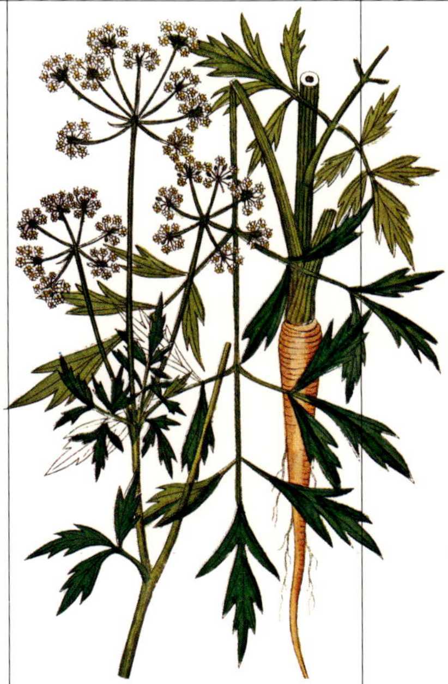

Parsley has been known for centuries, as a green kitchen herb as well as for its medicinal properties. Only the cultivated species are of interest. The fruits contain a volatile oil which promotes the blood circulation in the pelvic organs. Parsley grows from a simple beet-like root (it is related to the carrot) and likes best a deeply cultivated, rich soil. The curly-leaved type is generally preferred. The dark green, much divided leaves with their curly edges are picked as required once the plants have grown about hand-high. If the plant is left undisturbed in the second year, an erect round stem, branched at the top, will grow from the ground rosette of leaves. It reaches about 1 m in height and the leaves it bears are less divided. The long-stemmed many-rayed umbels at the top have tiny yellowish-green flowers. The egg-shaped gray-brown fruits are barely 2–3 mm in length, and break up into sickle-shaped seeds.

PEUCEDANUM OSTRUTHIUM

MASTERWORT, HOGFENNEL

Apiaceae, Umbelliferae

163 Alps

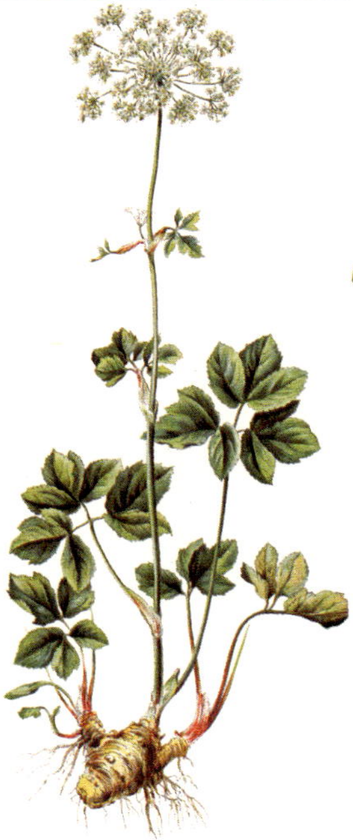

The handsome umbels of white flowers produced by the masterwort are seen in summer in damp mountain valleys and alpine meadows, on the banks of streams in chalky and siliceous soil.
In low-lying areas it is sometimes cultivated, and occasionally an escape is found. The beet-shaped fibrous root is scarred and has numerous rootlets and runners. It contains a milky juice. The fluted tubular stem has a reddish-brown tinge lower down.
It grows up to 1 m high and branches slightly at the top. The leaves are few, usually divided into threes twice, and have irregularly toothed margins. Their stalks form inflated membranous sheaths. The terminal umbels of white flowers are flat-topped. The whole plant has an aromatic, celery-like scent. Most of the volatile oil, the bitters, tannin, and resin are found in the root. The masterwort is very similar to angelica, but may be distinguished from it by the much smaller leaves.

PEUMUS BOLDUS

BOLDO

Monimiaceae

164 Chile
S Eur, N Af, W-N Am

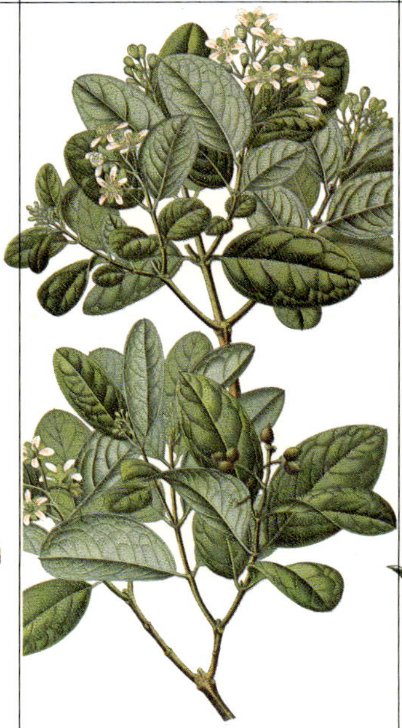

On dry, sunny slopes, this evergreen tree or shrub, up to 6 m high, grows in dense shrubberies. The numerous branches bear elongated egg-shaped leaves, 3–6 cm long, 2–4 cm wide, and with margins entire. They are short-stemmed, stiff and leathery, pale green on the upper side; and lighter in color, with prominent veins, underneath. Under a magnifying glass, numerous light-colored excrescences are visible which in the young leaves are covered with hairs. The white or yellow, bell-shaped unisexual flowers grow in loose clusters in the leaf axils or terminally. They have an aromatic scent. In autumn, the aromatic yellow stone fruits ripen. The whole plant has a peculiar scent, somewhat like peppermint. The leaves are cut up small for commercial use, and their various active principles make them of medicinal value. In the countries of origin, the bark is used for tanning and for the dyeing of fibers.

PHASEOLUS VULGARIS

BEAN, KIDNEY BEAN, COMMON HARICOT

Fabaceae, Papilionaceae

165 C Am, S Am
Temperate + Warm Temperate Zones

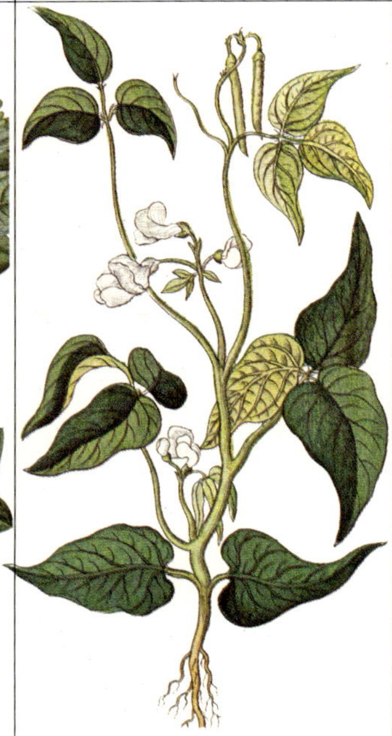

They are many varieties of this vegetable, which hardly needs to be described. An interesting and less well-known fact is that uncooked green beans contain a toxic protein (phasine) which is not destroyed on drying. Beans should be properly cooked, or they can cause poisoning. Depending on the variety, the fleshy pods with the seeds are prepared as a vegetable, or the seeds are shelled and cooked without the pods. Green beans are the unripe pods. These turn yellowish-white as they ripen, and loose their chlorophyll. The empty pods have been used for medicinal purposes for some time. In recent years they have been analyzed for their active principles, and were found to contain substances that reduce blood pressure, and others which encourage metabolism and kidney function.

PHYSOSTIGMA VENENOSUM

CALABAR BEAN, ORDEAL BEAN

Leguminosae

166 W Af

Calabar beans are the ripe seeds of *Physostigma venenosum*, which is indigenous to the west coast of Africa, especially near the mouths of the Old Calabar and Niger rivers. Hence their popular name. They owe their alternative name "ordeal bean" to the fact that they were used by the natives in trials. The beans were given to the accused to eat. If he died, this confirmed his guilt and also served as his execution. If he was able to withstand the poison by vomiting, his innocence was proven. The plant is a creeper reaching a height of up to 16 m. The woody branches are herba-

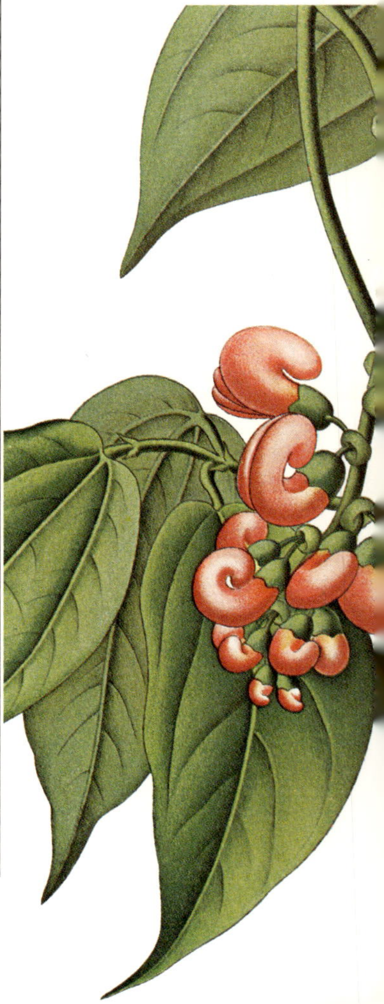

ceous in the upper regions, bearing large trifoliate leaves with small lance-shaped leafy bracts. From the upper leaf axils hang loose clusters of unusually shaped purple butterfly-type flowers. The fruits are flat woody pods narrowing at both ends and containing 1–3 kidney-shaped dark brown seeds with a silky sheen. Calabar beans are about 3 cm long, 1.5 cm wide, with a finely wrinkled surface. They contain starch, protein and a fatty oil. Their principal alkaloid is physostigmine, an intensely toxic substance whose principal use today is in eyedrops to constrict the pupils.

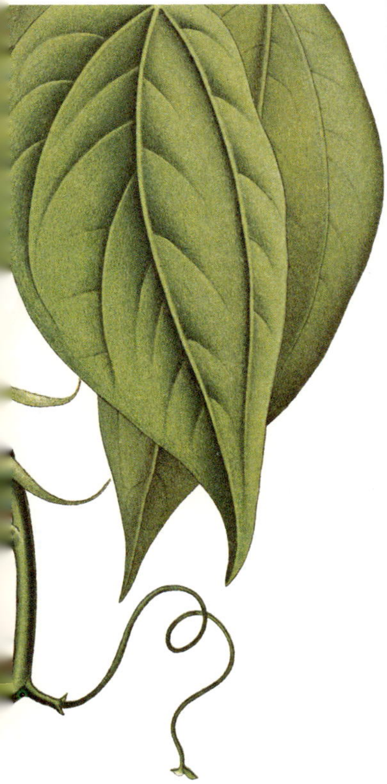

PHYTOLACCA AMERICANA

POKE, POKEWEED

Phytolaccaceae

167 SE-N Am
Warm Temperate Zones

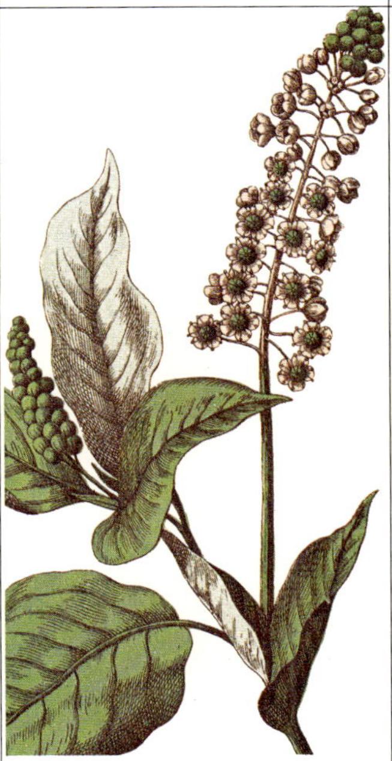

The poke, an American perennial shrub up to 3 m high, grows in damp woodlands, hedges, and waste places. It has been introduced to some parts of Europe. The root with its irregular branches is unusually large. The shoots produced from it in spring are cut off just above soil level and cooked like asparagus. The stems are erect, round, and hairless. They branch near the top and often have a reddish tinge. The short-stemmed light green leaves are 12–20 cm long, a pointed egg-shape or oval, their margins entire and wavy. The leafless flowering stem bears an extended spike of small greenish-white flowers. The deep purple or black berries ripen in autumn. About 1 cm in diameter, they contain a purple juice that makes a powerful dye. Unripe berries are slightly poisonous. The root contains saponins with powerful antirheumatic and purgative properties.

PILOCARPUS PENNATIFOLIUS

JABORANDI

Rutaceae

168 C-S Am

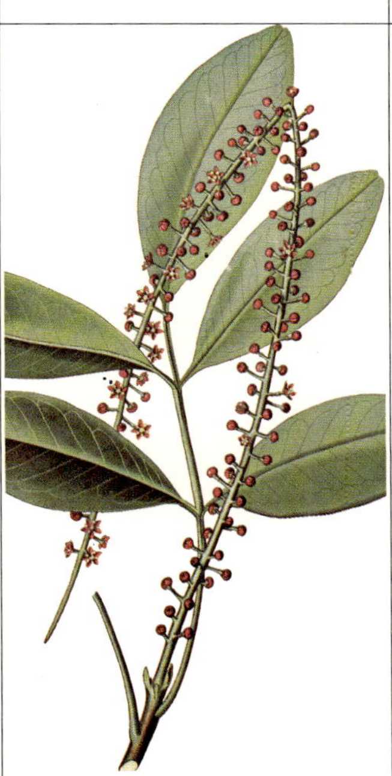

The jaborandi leaves are used chiefly to obtain the alkaloid pilocarpine. The much-branched shrub is densely foliated. The leaves have a short, winged stalk and are divided into pairs of leaflets, sometimes with an odd one at the top. These are 2–5 cm long, 1–2.5 cm wide, a pointed egg-shape, the margin notched to form 2 lobes at the tip. The upper surface is a brownish-green, the underside pale green with prominent veins. The leaflets are dotted with secretory glands containing volatile oil. The flowers are small, sitting on a leathery crown, and arranged in spikes growing from the axils. The leaves have an aromatic scent and bitter taste. The leaves of various jaborandi species are official; they must contain a specified amount of alkaloid. The dried leaflets are thin, leathery or parchment-like, brown to pale green. Against the light they are seen to be dotted with numerous glands.

PIMPINELLA ANISUM

ANISE

Apiaceae, Umbelliferae

169 SW Asia
Warm Temperate Zones

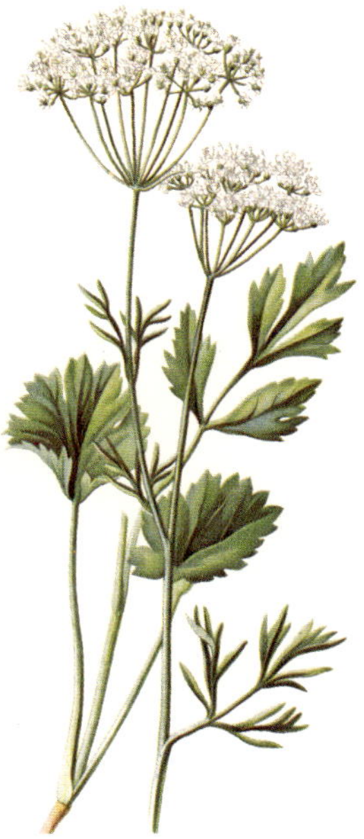

This flavoring herb is cultivated in many countries and is only occasionally found growing wild, as a garden escape. It belongs to the large family of Umbelliferae (carrot family) which are often difficult to tell apart. Fortunately recognition is made easier by the scent and appearance of the parts used medicinally. The annual herb grows to a height of 40–60 cm from a thin spindle-shaped root. The round, ridged stem branches higher up and terminates in flat-topped double umbels of white flowers. The shape of the leaf varies, with long-stemmed, deeply incised heart-shaped leaves lower down, and much divided feathery wisps halfway up the stem. The fruits are densely covered with short hairs and contain two gray-brown seeds with light-colored ribs.

PIMPINELLA SAXIFRAGA

BLACK CARAWAY,
BURNET SAXIFRAGE

Apiaceae, Umbelliferae

170 Eur, C+W Asia
N Am

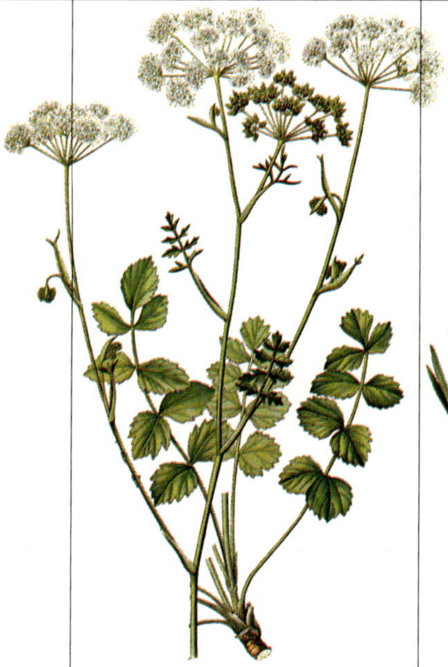

Black caraway grows in dry, lean meadows, in open woodlands, and among bushes, from the lowlands up to altitudes of 2000 m. From the thick, often branching tap root which is about 2 cm across, grow ridged stems, usually filled, to a height of 30–50 cm or, in the case of the bigger species, 50–100 cm. The foliage leaves lower down are divided into an odd number of elongated oval leaflets with pointed tips and toothed margins. The stem usually bears only a few leaves, on membranous leaf-sheaths. The terminal umbels bear white flowers (sometimes pink in mountain regions), which in autumn develop into ribbed fruits. The plant is easily recognizable from the tap root, usually growing in friable soil, which may reach 20 cm in length and has a pungent smell of billygoat. Black caraway has been used for medicinal purposes since ancient days.

PINUS SYLVESTRIS

SCOTCH PINE

Pinaceae

171 Eur, N+W Asia
Temperate Zones

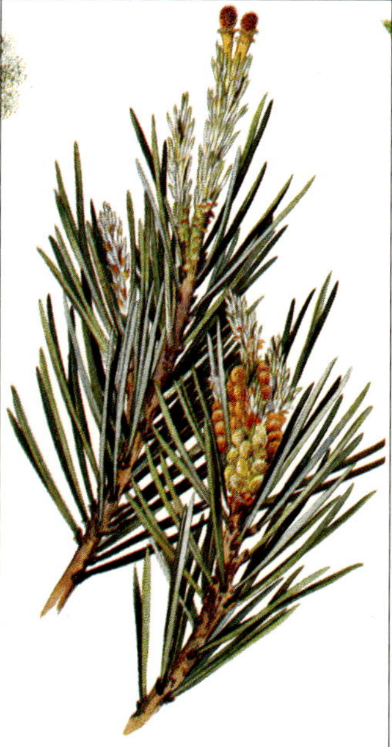

The coniferous (cone-bearing) trees include about 100 species from different plant families. In the lowlands, the trunks of pines may reach a height of 40 m. In the mountains, the knee pine still manages to grow above the tree line, as a low shrub (dwarf mountain pine). The characteristic features of pines are as follows: lofty trunks, with the branching conical crown set high; smooth bark that is gray-brown and later reddish, flaking; depending on the species, older trees have fissured bark, gray-brown outside and reddish inside; needles twisted, dark green or blue-green, remaining for 3–6 years; cones conical, stalked, erect or hanging. Pines may grow 600 years old. Medicinally, young stem shoots gathered in spring *(Turio pini)* are used, also the resin seeping from the trunks of larches *(Terebinthina laricina)*, pine oil distilled from fresh branches, and oil of turpentine obtained from the crude resin.

PIPER METHYSTICUM

KAVA, KAVA-KAVA

Piperaceae

172 Polynesia
New Guinea, Hawaii

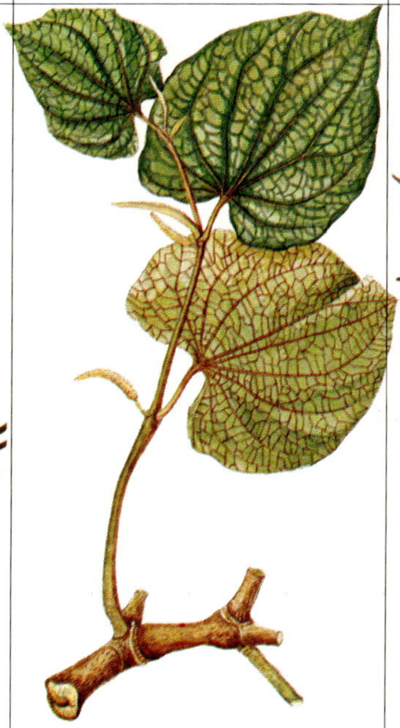

In the countries of its origin, kava plays an important role in the religious and social life of the natives. Kava or Ava liquors containing a limited quantity of the rhizome (underground stem) are taken as a stimulant or to improve the appetite. Stronger doses are intoxicating, and so dangerous that legal restrictions had to be imposed on the use of the drug. The kava shrub grows to a height of 1.5–4 m, with a large, woody, often knotty rhizome sometimes weighing several kilograms producing smooth, reed-like, knotty branches. The short-stemmed leaves are about 20 cm wide, and broadly heart-shaped, with prominent veins. The stem nodes have occasional spines. The flowers are small and unisexual, the male growing in dense spikes on the upper stem nodes. Reproduction is entirely vegetative, by runners. The drug-containing part consists of the root, very juicy when fresh.

PLANTAGO PSYLLIUM

PSYLLIUM, FLEA SEED

Plantaginaceae

173 S Eur, N Af, SW Asia

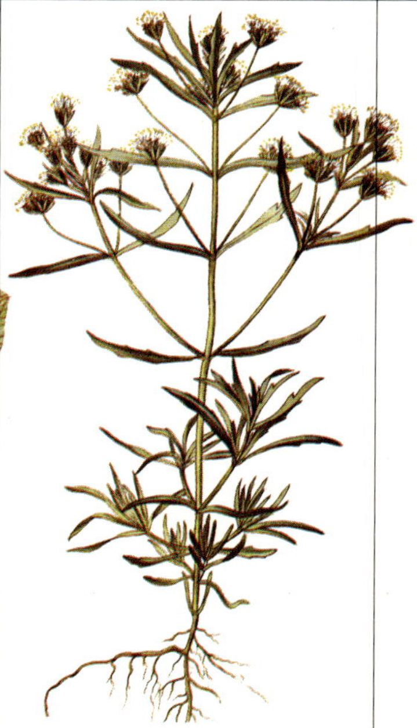

Some species of *Plantago* contain mucilage of great swelling power, particularly in the seeds. Hence their medicinal value as a mechanical or bulk laxative. Medicinal use is made primarily of seeds obtained from plantain species native to southern France *(P. psyllium)*, North Africa *(P. Indica)*, and India (*P. ovate* Forsk). Psyllium comes from an annual herb growing 20–40 cm high. The pale green, herbaceous, hairy stem is erect or sloping and branches only little. The narrow linear leaves grow in whorls up the stem, with those at the base slightly downy. The tiny whitish to brownish flowers are in long-stemmed spherical heads growing from the upper leaf axils. The ovary is surrounded by 4 pointed, rough, green sepals. The fruit, a membranous lidded capsule, contains small brown elongated elliptical seeds which are 1.5–2 cm in length.

PLANTAGO LANCEOLATA

ENGLISH PLANTAIN, RIB GRASS

Plantaginaceae

174 Eur, Asia
Temperate Zones

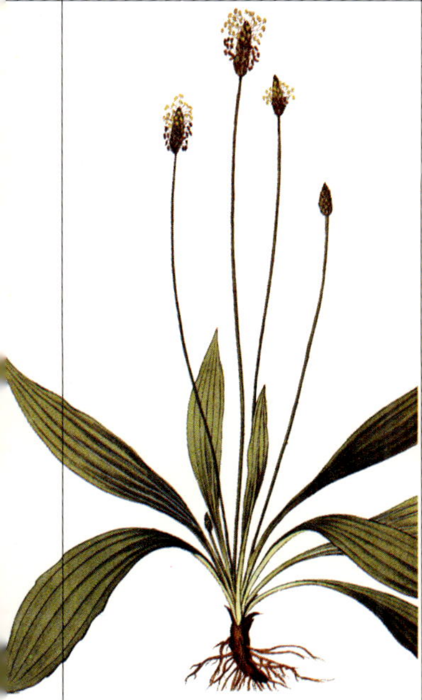

There are more than 200 species of plantain found all over the world. The family name derives from the Latin for "sole of the foot," because the shape of the leaves, which in some species lie close to the ground, resembles a footprint. The perennial herb grows anywhere in dry, sandy soil, on roadsides, in lean meadows, and along the shore. In eastern Europe the ribwort plantain is cultivated as a medicinal plant. From the underground stem grows a flat or partly upright rosette of robust stalked leaves with parallel longitudinal ribs, their blades being narrow and pointed *(Plantago lanceolata)*. The basal leaf stems are covered with woolly hairs. Elongated or spherical brownish flower spikes rise on erect, furrowed, leafless stalks. Other species have rose pink flowers. Recent investigations have shown that some of the active principles have antibiotic properties.

PODOPHYLLUM PELTATUM

MAYAPPLE, AMERICAN MANDRAKE, WILD LEMON

Berberidaceae

175 E-N Am
NE Asia

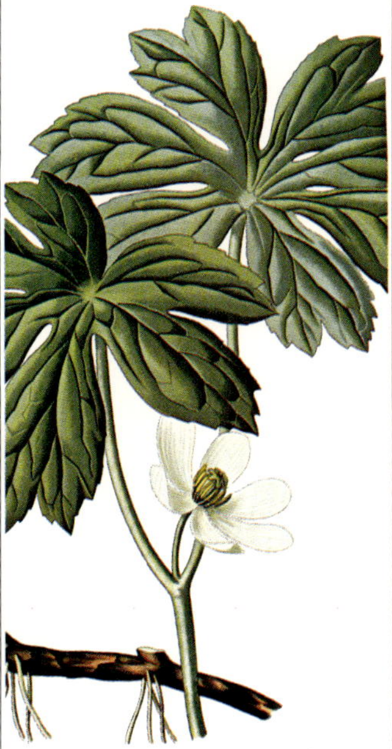

Mayapple is found in the damp woodlands and tree-shaded pastures of the Atlantic region of North America. A much-branched underground stem, its rootstock barely 1 cm in diameter and with numerous long-jointed brown runners, produces 2 kinds of stem. One of these is 30–50 cm high and sterile, and bears a single leaf, 15–30 cm in diameter, composed of 7–9 wedge-shaped divisions and borne like a shield (peltatum); that is, the stalk attaches at a point beneath. The upper surface is dark green and slightly hairy. The fertile, fruit-bearing stem terminates in 2 leaves that are similar in shape, with 5–7 lobes. Between these grows a single, short-stemmed, pendant white flower, its corona made up of 6–9 inverted egg-shaped petals. It has an aromatic scent. The fruit is a yellow berry 4–5 cm long containing 12 egg-shaped seeds. Its taste is sweet and slightly tart.

POLYGALA SENEGA

SENECA SNAKEROOT

Polygalaceae

176 N Am

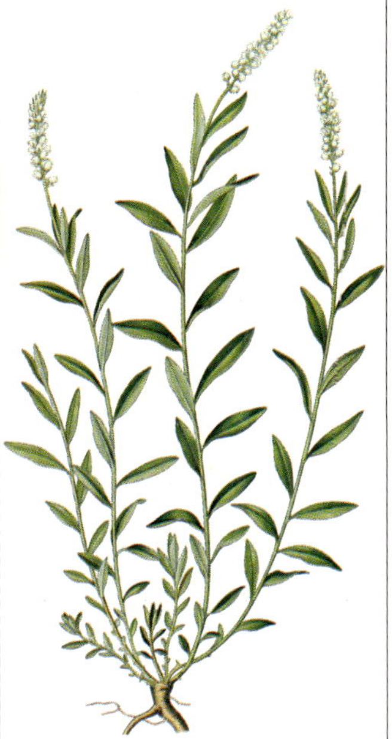

Seneca snakeroot is a native of the dry, stony open woodlands of North America. The specific name *senega* is probably derived from Seneca, the name of the North American Indian tribe who used the root as a treatment for snake bite (because the root resembles a snake). Hence the popular name "snakeroot." A perennial, creeping rootstock produces simple erect herbaceous stems which reach 40 cm in height. These stems grow from the axils of scale-like base leaves. The leaves are alternate, 5–8 cm in length, 3 cm wide, egg-shaped to lanceolate and pointed, with toothed margins. The upper surface is a rich green, the underside lighter in color. Near the ground the leaves are smaller and often reduced to scale leaves. The stems terminate in extended spikes of whitish-pink flowers The knotted root, often up to 5 cm in diameter, is usually divided into several spindles and twisted.

POLYGONUM HYDROPIPER

SMARTWEED, WATERPEPPER

Polygonaceae

177 Eur, NW Af, Asia, N Am

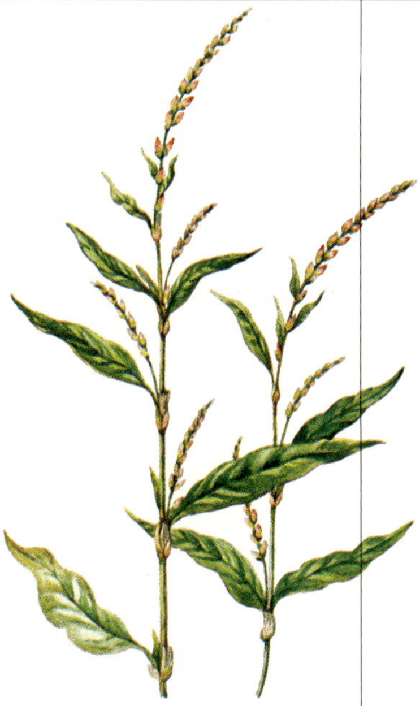

The plants of this family owe their botanical name *Polygonum* to the many nodes in their stems (*poly*=many, *gony*=knee, knot). The peppery taste and the fact that this herb likes to grow in damp places and by streams are responsible for the alternate name "waterpepper." It is an annual, producing an erect, branching stem up to 80 cm high, with the aforementioned in the stems. There are only a few leaves, elongated and broadly lance-shaped, their underside dotted with glands or black spots. The tiny flowers in their reddish or greenish calyces are 3–4 mm in length and dotted with numerous yellow glands. They grow on thin stems in a slim, nodding spike. Flowering time is July–August. The fresh herb has a sharpish, peppery taste. The roots of the bistort or snakeweed *(Polygonum bistorta)* have the reputation of stopping hemorrhages when used internally.

POLYPODIUM VULGARE

EUROPEAN POLYPODY,
SWEET FERN

Polypodiaceae

178 Eur, N Asia

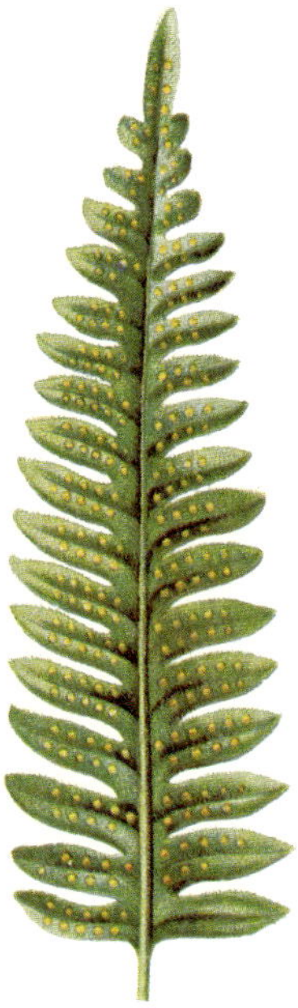

The polypody species form the largest group among the ferns. The common polypody likes to grow in places rich in humus where there is little lime, among mosses, on rocks and tree stumps, but always in shady woods and slopes. Immediately beneath the surface lie the pencil-slim, slightly flattened underground stems, brownish-red in color and still bearing the marks of the old leafy shoots. In spring, the scaly, curled-up shoots unfold into fronds 30–40 cm in length, which are divided into simple leaflets with rounded tips ranged along a center rib that stands out underneath. On the underside of the leaflets are 2 rows of sori, groups of spore-carrying bodies, orange-colored at first and later brown. The shape of the frond is that of a gently curving, pointed lance. The fresh roots have a sweetish taste. Apart from sugar, the active principles are bitter resins, a volatile oil, a sweet saponin, and mucilage.

POPULUS NIGRA

BALSAM POPLAR

Salicaceae

179 Eur, N Af, M+W Asia
Temperate Zones

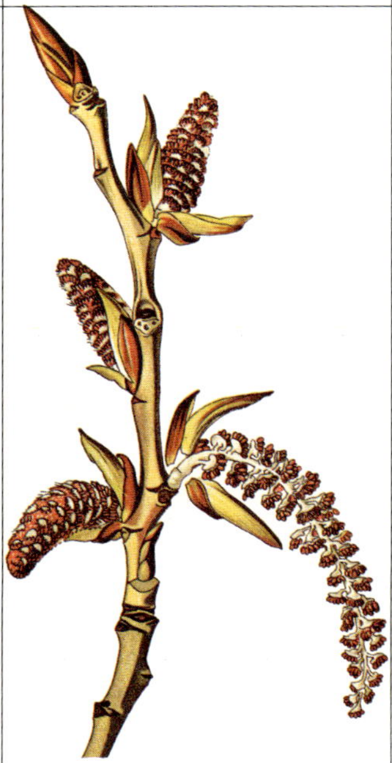

These trees are related to the willows and require a friable soil, with plenty of moisture at some depth, to achieve the rapid growth that is characteristic of them. Populars are often planted to line avenues. In the young trees, the bark is gray and smooth; in older trees it grows rugged and grayish-black. The trees grow to a height of 20–30 m and may be a few hundred years old. The leaves on their long flattened stalks are usually more or less round or triangular. Male and female flowers grow on different trees, the male in fat, cylindrical hanging catkins with crimson stamens, the female in shorter, greenish spikes which may be hanging or erect. The fresh bark of young branches and the young leaves are used to obtain homeopathic tinctures and extracts containing salicin. On the Continent, particular use is made of popular buds *(Gemmae Populi)* which contain a volatile oil and tannins.

POTENTILLA ANSERINA

SILVERWEED,
SILVERY CINQUEFOIL

Rosaceae

180 Temperate Zones

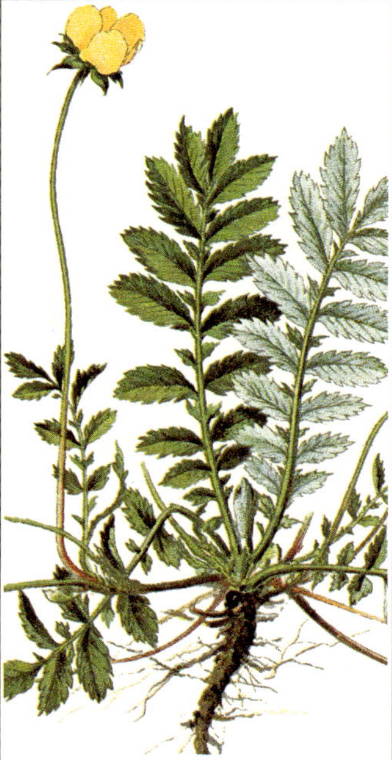

The cinquefoils are small, often creeping herbs, with many different species growing anywhere from the lowlands up to high altitudes. The Latin name derives from *potentia,* power, and the diminutive *illa,* to signify great power in a small plant. The silverweed grows in abundance in waste places, on roadsides, and around poultry yards, where it covers the broken ground with its shapely divided leaves. The perennial, branched, and often woody rootstock produces extensive runners that root easily, producing whole carpets of rich green foliage. The leaves grow to 20–25 cm in length; they are divided into pairs of leaflets with an odd one at the top, stalked, and have toothed margins. The undersides of the leaves are covered with silvery white hairs, a protection, as it were, against the dampness of the ground. The golden-yellow flowers with their 5 oval petals grow singly on long leafless stalks.

POTENTILLA ERECTA

TORMENTIL, BLOODROOT

Rosaceae

181 Eur, NW Af, N Asia,
NE-N Am

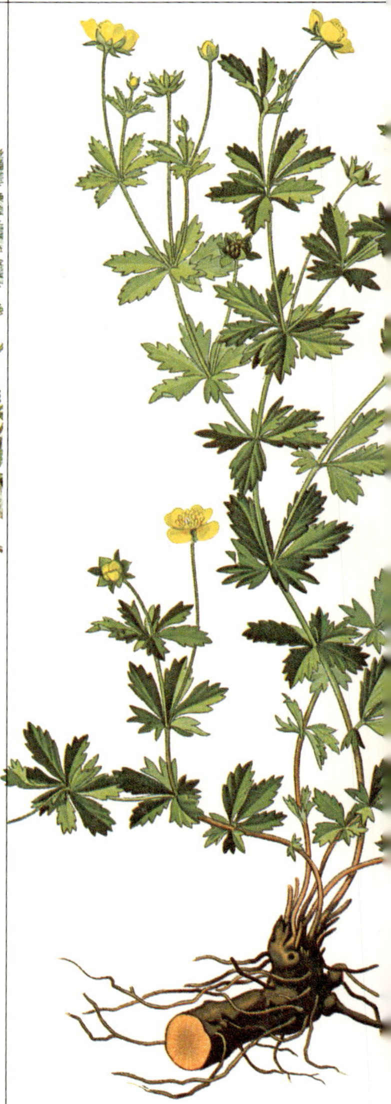

The tormentil, one of the most unassuming members of the great rose family, grows to a height of 10–20 cm in dry or damp lean meadows and in marshy ground on the edge of woods, from the lowlands up to 2500 m. The gnarled rootstock produces thin branching stems, creeping at first and then erect. The stalked ground leaves are trefoil; the stalkless stem leaves also have 3 leaflets

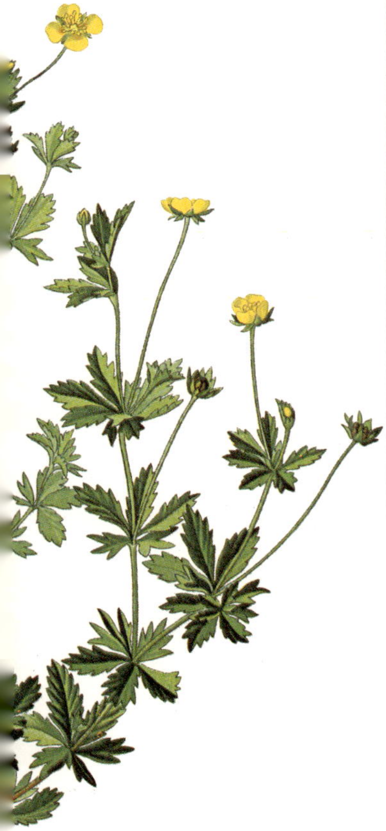

which are narrower and toothed; the side leaflets are only a little smaller. The stems terminate in green calyces of 4 sepals holding 4 bright yellow petals, a rarity in the rose family which normally has 5 petals, so that the tormentil may be recognized by their number. Another feature of this plant is the reddish-brown color of the root, which contains tormentil red, a special tannin with astringent, styptic properties. The rootstocks, 1–3 cm in diameter, are tedious to collect. Rhatany root is equally effective, as is the bistort root *(Radix bistortae)*. Tinctures prepared from them are more effective than teas.

PRIMULA VERIS
PRIMULA ELATIOR

COWSLIP OXLIP

Primulaceae

182 C Eur
Temperate Zones

Cowslips and oxlips, heralds of spring as well as medicinal herbs, are often found in meadows, open scrub, and on roadsides, up to a height of 2000 m. The golden-yellow species *(Primula veris)* prefers a dry site; the larger sulfur-yellow species *(Primula elatior)* grows in damper meadows and open woodland. From a short rootstock grows a ground rosette of leaves with variable, usually egg-shaped leaves narrowing into a winged stem. The leaves are wrinkled, with marked veins, and covered with downy hair on the underside. The flowers form one-sided clusters, erect or hanging, on thin flowering stems up to 20 cm high. A whitish-green angular calyx holds the sweet-scented golden-yellow corolla tube which opens out into 5 lobes. The sulfur-yellow flowers of the oxlip *(Primula elatior)* have less scent. The dried flowers are used, with or without the green calyx. Those who gather their own, prefer the golden-yellow scented flower. The dried rootstock contains saponins and also active principles similar to salicylic acid.

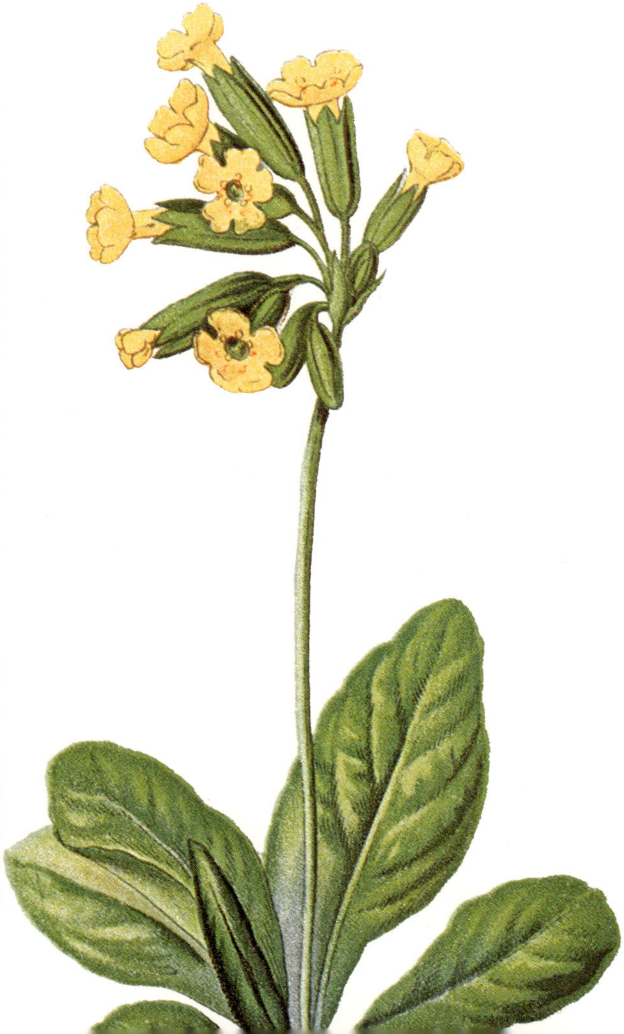

PRUNUS DULCIS
VAR. AMARA

BITTER ALMOND

Rosaceae

183 C Asia
S Eur, N Af, C Am

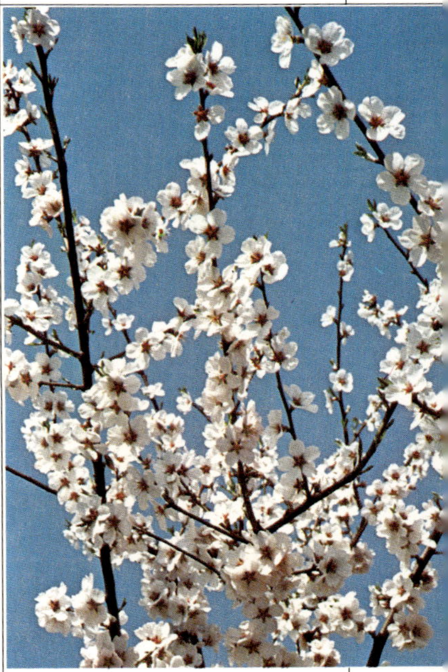

Almond trees are widely cultivated in the Mediterranean regions, as far as Morocco (and in the southern United States). This tree gives further proof of the wide variety of form produced within the rose family.
It grows best in dry, stony soil containing lime. The trunk usually leans at an angle, is 4–6 m high and often bent; it has a smooth bark and a flat spreading crown. Toward the end of winter, and before the leaves appear, white or pink flowers with 5 petals and numerous stamens cover the shoots of the previous year. Later the stalked, elongated, pointed leaves develop, 4–8 cm in length, and with finely toothed margins. The longish oval, plum-shaped fruits are pale green and covered with a silvery down. Each holds a single almond (i. e., 1, rarely 2, seeds) in the hard, deeply pitted shell.

PRUNUS SEROTINA

BLACK CHERRY, WILD CHERRY

Rosaceae

184 E-N Am
Temperate Zones

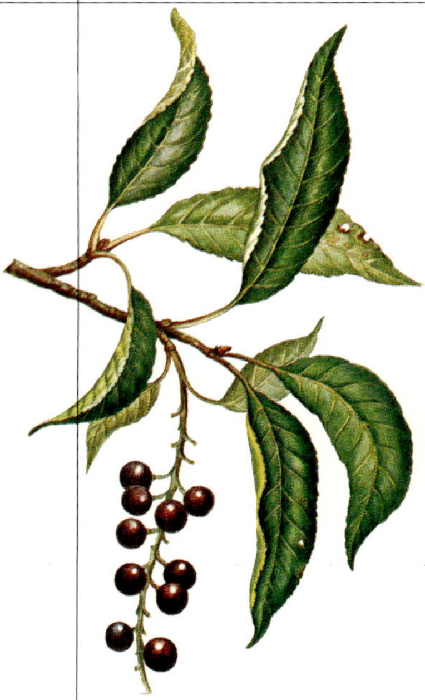

In its country of origin, the black cherry grows on rocky hillsides, in open woodlands, and on the edges of woods. In the wild state it will often grow only as a shrub, otherwise as a tree up to 30 m high. The bark of the trunk and major branches is gray to gray-brown, that of the smaller branches brown to gray-brown. The leaves are short-stemmed, elongated, lance-shaped, dark green and leathery, with serrated margins. The underside is pale green. The midrib bears yellowish hairs. The small white flowers grow in short clusters, erect at first and later hanging. The fruits ripening in autumn are small purple-black cherries, aromatic and slightly bitter, which are used in the manufacture of soft drinks. The leaves contain hydrogen cyanide and are poisonous to cattle. The bark of the young trunks and branches is used in medicine.

PRUNUS SPINOSA

BLACKTHORN, SLOE

Rosaceae

185 Eur, N Af, W Asia
N Am

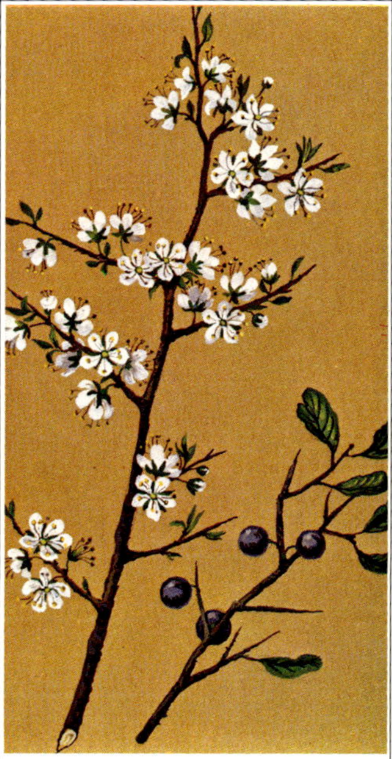

The blackthorn flowers in spring, often as early as March or April, before the leaves appear. Then the short gnarled branches armed with sharp spines are adorned with numerous small white 5-petaled flowers. The compact, spiky shrub reaches a height of 2–3 m. It prefers a dry, stony, calcareous soil and a sunny site in hedges and on the edges of woods. The bark is a dull, sooty brownish-black. The branches have short lateral shoots bearing either short dense spikes of flowers or long straight spines. The small soft stalked leaves are alternate. Wedge-shaped at the base, they terminate in a blunt point and are sharply toothed. The upper surface is dark green, the underside lighter in color. The leaves are frequently accompanied by smaller bract leaves. The fruits (sloes) develop very slowly into cherry-sized plums which contain a large wrinkled stone.

PULMONARIA OFFICINALIS

BLUE LUNGWORT

Boraginaceae

186 Eur, W Asia

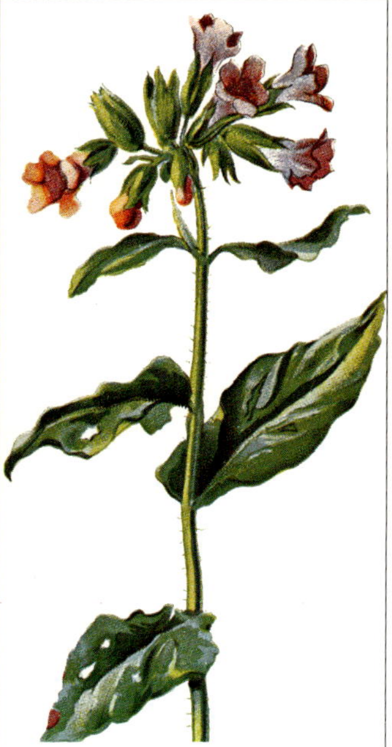

The lungwort prefers shady deciduous forests, banks of streams, and bushes on chalky soil, up to an altitude of 1700 m. The thin branching underground stem produces erect flowering stems 20–30 cm in height. These bear a few unstalked, elongated oval hairy leaves with pointed tips. Leaves and stem are roughly hairy, as in most members of the borage family, and the leaves often have whitish spots. The stems are usually branched and bear small clusters of short-stemmed flowers with a green calyx and the corolla opening out into 5 petal lobes. The color of the flowers changes from pink to purple and a pure blue; 2 or 3 colors are usually present at the same time. When flowering is over, the stalked, ovate heart-shaped, roughly hairy basal leaves, like the stem leaves often spotted white, remain until autumn. The Latin and English names indicate that the plant is considered beneficial in lung complaints.

PULSATILLA VULGARIS

PASQUE FLOWER

Ranunculaceae

187 Eur

Pulsatilla likes warm, dry sites, even at altitudes to 1200 m. The sturdy rootstock sends a long tap root into the dry ground. Early in spring the flowering stems appear, 10–30 cm high, with 3 leaves, frayed into narrows wisps and covered with silvery down, forming a ruff around the upper stem. The deep-purple bell-shaped flower usually has 6 petals, and numerous golden-yellow stamens. The fruits are a tassel of silvery plumes. The basal leaves develop only after the flower; they are divided 2 or 3 times and feathery. The whole plant is densely hairy. The fresh herb is poisonous and can cause marked skin irritation.

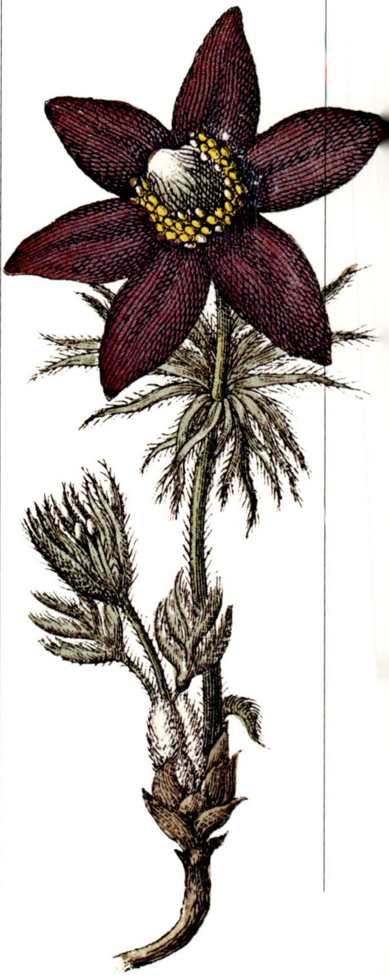

QUERCUS ROBUR

OAK, ENGLISH OAK

Fagaceae

188 Eur
Temperate Zones

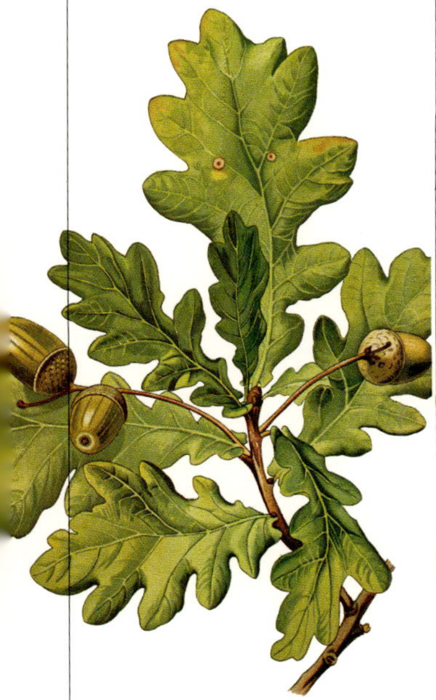

Different species of oak grow in north and south. This mighty tree grows to a height of 35 or 40 m, with trunks 2 m in diameter, and remains viable for centuries. It provides very durable timber. In soils rich in minerals, in temperate areas of lowlands and hill country, the trunks grow rapidly at first and then very slowly, with a spreading, much branched crown. The bark has a silvery gray sheen (mirror bark), and from the twentieth year onward is deeply fissured and gray-brown. The leaves grow in alternate bunches or are distributed along the twig. They are a glossy dark green on the upper surface and are easily recognizable by their lobed outline. The male flowers are in greenish hanging catkins, the females in red clusters sitting on the twig. Oaks do not flower every year. The fruits are the well-known acorns sitting in scaly cups. Tannins are obtained for medicinal purposes from the bark of twigs and side shoots.

RAUVOLFIA SERPENTINA

INDIAN SNAKEROOT, RAUVOLFIA

Apocynaceae

189 SE Asia
Torrid Zones

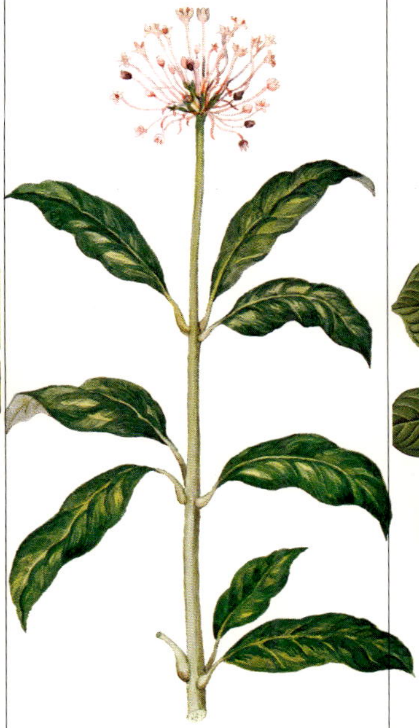

In Indian folk medicine this plant has been used for centuries as a remedy for snake bite. Indian doctors have long used it for nervous conditions, mental illness, and more recently to treat high blood pressure. The first mention of it in European herbals dates form the eighteenth century, but it was not until the twentieth century (1949) that it was introduced to western medicine. This is a low perennial shrub, 50–100 cm in height, growing from a broad rootstock. The root and branches contain a milky juice. The leaves are opposite or grow in 3–5 nodular whorls on the stem. They are elongated, elliptical and 10–15 cm in length, terminating in a point at either end. The small white tubular flowers grow in a multiple terminal pseudo-umbel. The valuable active principles are obtained mainly from the root and occasionally also from the leaves.

RHAMNUS FRANGULA

ALDER BUCKTHORN

Rhamnaceae

190 Eur, C+N Asia
N Am

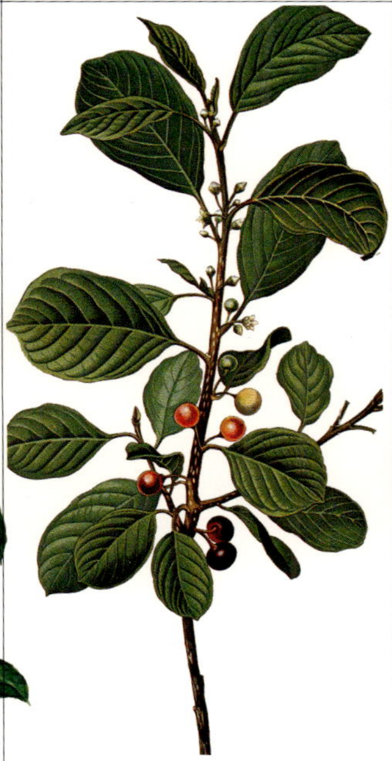

This handsome shrub, 1–6 m in height, lines the banks of lakes and rivers and damp woods in river valleys from the lowlands up to medium high altitudes. The upright branches are long and slender, their bark is smooth on the outside, dark brown to brownish-gray, with striking light-colored markings (lenticels). The inside of the bark has a yellow layer of bast that turns brown as it dries. The firm oval leaves, shiny green on the upper surface and delicately veined, appear in April. From the leaf axils at the upper ends of the branches grow short-stemmed, inconspicuous greenish-white flowers. The globular berries are green in summer, turning red and finally a glossy blue-black. The bark provides valuable principles for the treatment of sluggishness of the bowels. Other buckthorn species *(Rhamnus purshiana DC.)* are used for the same purpose in America.

RHAMNUS PURSHIANA

CASCARA SAGRADA

Rhamnaceae

191 C Am

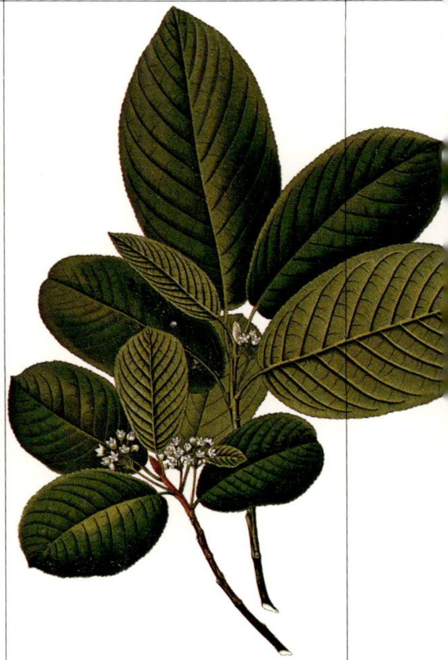

Only few *Rhamnaceae* species grow in the north, among them the cascara sagrada. Another species (*Rhamnus frangula* L. or *Frangula alnus* Mill., also known as the alder buckthorn) is found in Europe and western Asia. The term "cascara sagrada" derives from the Spanish for "sacred bark." The tree grows to a height of 6–12 m, usually forming the undergrowth in the great forests. The bark of the trunk and numerous branches is gray, with white markings (lenticels); the upper branches are covered with a downy pelt. The elongated, rich green leaves are an inverted egg-shape, 6–10 cm long, with promiment veins and toothed margins. Short-stemmed clusters of inconspicuous small whitish flowers grow from the upper leaf axils. The ovaries develop into green fruits, cherry-sized and a glossy black when ripe. These are poisonous.

RHEUM PALMATUM
RHEUM OFFICINALE

RHUBARB, MEDICINAL RHUBARB

Polygonaceae

192 E Asia
Temperate Zones

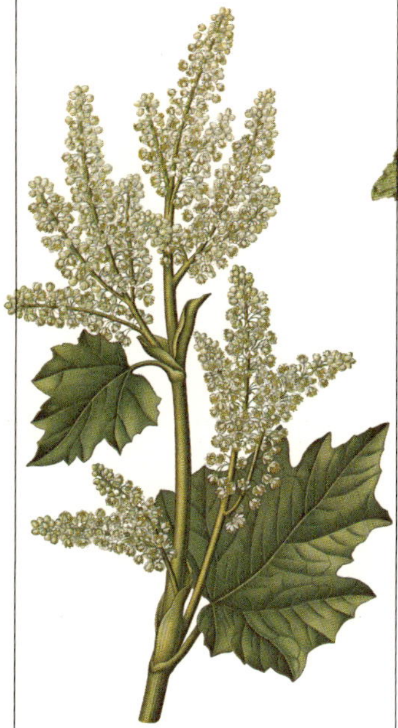

Rhubarb (Rheum rhabarbarum L.) is popular as a garden plant in almost all northern countries and is used for desserts and in jam. Phytotherapy makes use of the gently purgative principles in the roots. During the first years, the large rootstock produces only a rosette of ground leaves, while the root produces numerous branch roots. After 3–4 years, the stalked leaves grow to a length of up to 1 m. They differ from garden rhubarb *(Rheum palmatum* = hand-shaped). At this time the flowering stem also appears and grows up to 2 m high. It bears large, branched spikes of numerous small greenish or reddish flowers. Poke-shaped leaves sit at the nodes. For the plant drug, roots and branch roots are cut into small pieces. These look granular, yellowy, and reddish where cut across. The bitter aromatic principles are used in pharmaceutical preparations.

RIBES NIGRUM

BLACK CURRANT

Saxifragaceae

193 Eur, Asia
Temperate Zones

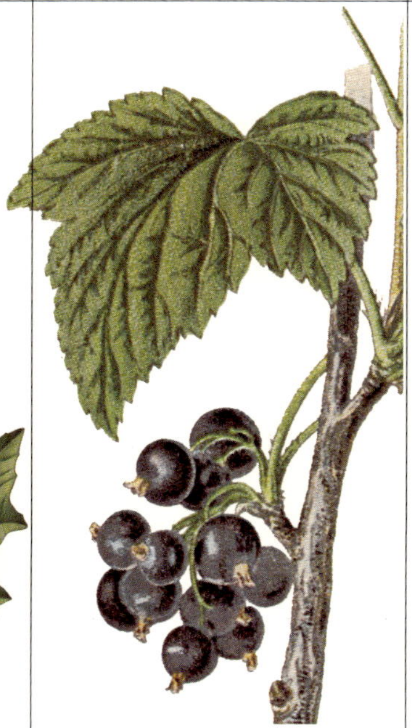

Currants, either black or red *(Ribes rubrum),* are a popular soft fruit grown in many gardens; they occasionally may be found growing wild in hedgerows and damp woodlands. The black currant bush, an erect, spine-free shrub, reaches a height of 1.3–1.5 m. The alternate leaves have 3–5 lobes, are a rich green, and are dotted with yellow glands here and there on the underside. Their margins are lightly serrated. The small greenish-red flowers grow in drooping, softly downy spikes. The berries turn a deep black. They have a small remnant of the dried calyx at the tip. The whole plant has a distinctively peculiar smell. A volatile oil, tannins, and organic acids are obtained from the leaves. The berries have a high concentration of vitamin C. They are also used to produce full-bodied liqueurs.

RICINUS COMMUNIS

CASTOR BEAN, CASTOR OIL PLANT

Euphorbiaceae

194 Af, S Asia
Torrid + Warm Temperate Zones

In its native habitat, the castor oil plant grows as a tree which reaches a height of 10 m; cultivated, it is grown in bushes 2–3 m high. In northern latitudes, it is popular as a rapidly growing shrub which reaches a height of 2 m. With its large, handsome leaves, it is very ornamental. The leaves of the castor oil tree may be 1 m in diameter and are divided into 7–11 segments. They sit like shields on their long, sturdy, hollow footstalks. The shoots terminate in a spike bearing the stalked female flowers above and small bunches of male flowers below. These very attractive flowers tend to disappear among the rich foliage. The fruit is a capsule covered with soft prickles. Within it are the speckled oval seeds. The seeds contain a high proportion of fats and protein and a highly toxic albumin (ricin) which, however, remains behind in the cake when the oil is extracted. Castor oil has purgative properties. It differs from other vegetable oils in that it is soluble in alcohol, and therefore it is used widely in cosmetics and industry. Being rather unpalatable, it is now infrequently used as a laxative.

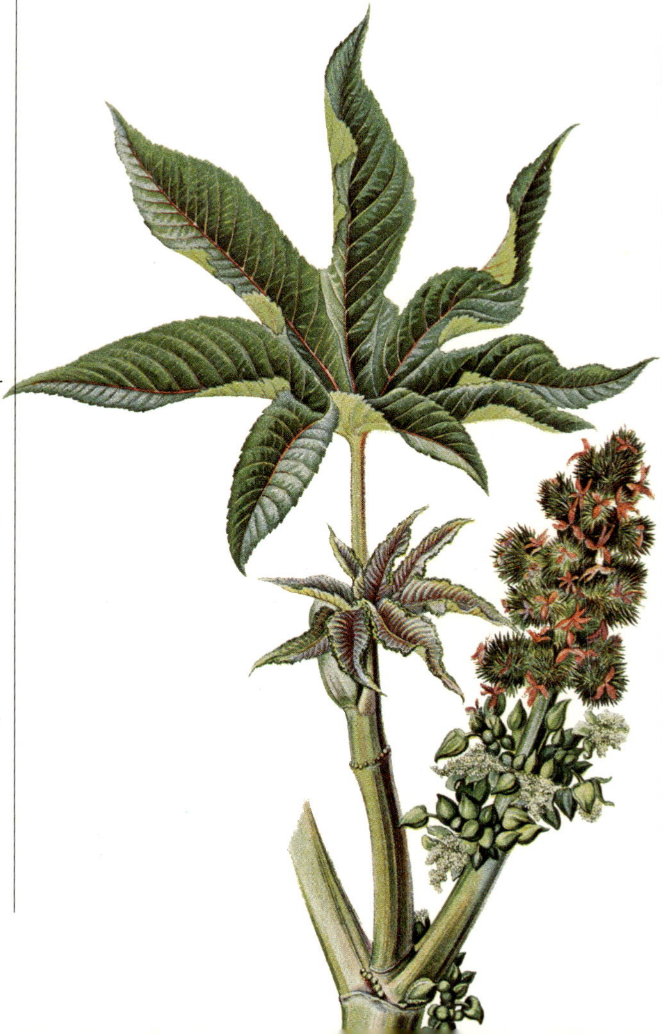

ROSA CANINA

DOG ROSE

Rosaceae

195 Eur, NW Af, C+W Asia
N Am

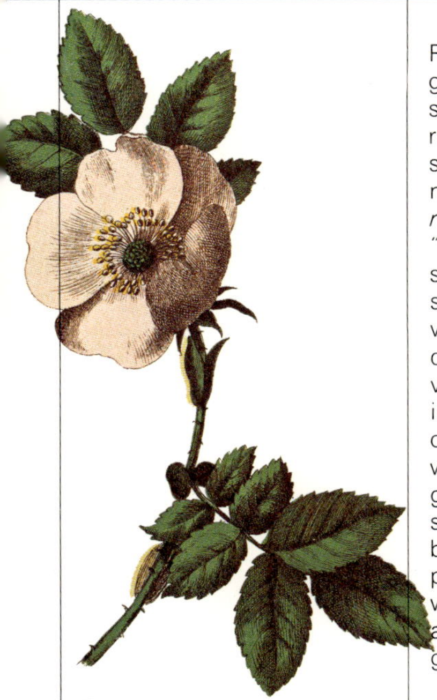

The dog rose likes firm, stony soil in hedgerows and on the edge of woods and embankments. Directly from the root grow robust small trunks which continually produce new shoots. They stand stiffly erect and divide into numerous arching, downward curving branches which form bushes 2–4 m in height. The leaves are divided into 2–3 pairs of leaflets with an odd leaflet at the tip which is egg-shaped, a fresh green, hairless on the upper surface, and with toothed margins. The leafstalks bear prickles and small leaflets at the base. The branches also are well endowed with thorns. The stalked flowers have 5 petals, usually rose pink, and are sweetly scented. The scarlet hips do not ripen until autumn, at which time they become fleshy, berry-like fruits with smooth skins containing hairy nutlets. The skin has a high content of vitamin C. The petals of other rose species are used in pharmaceuticals.

ROSMARINUS OFFICINALIS

ROSEMARY

Lamiaceae / Labiatae

196 S Eur, N Af, SW Asia
Warm Temperate Zones

Rosemary may be found growing wild on the rocky shores of the Mediterranean—a woody evergreen shrub up to 2 m high. The name derives from the Latin *ros marinus*, which means "sea dew." The herb is also specially cultivated in the south, for much light and warmth are needed to produce the highly aromatic volatile oil which is the most important active principle of rosemary. Rigid branches with scaly or fissured bark grow from a woody rootstock. In spring, these branches produce square pale green shoots covered with a soft down. The small, almost needle-like leaves grow in whorls; they are 2–4 cm in length, leathery, rolled inward and covered with a pelt of small stellate hairs on the underside. Five to 10 small, pale blue, 2-lipped flowers grow in apparent whorls on short lateral spikes. Both fresh and dried leaves have an aromatic, camphor-like scent. Apart from the volatile oil they contain bitters and tannins. In northern gardens, rosemary needs some frost protection in winter. The young shoots are popular as a culinary herb. For pharmaceutical use, young shoots from shrubs grown in southern regions (Dalmatia) are preferred, because their aroma is stronger.

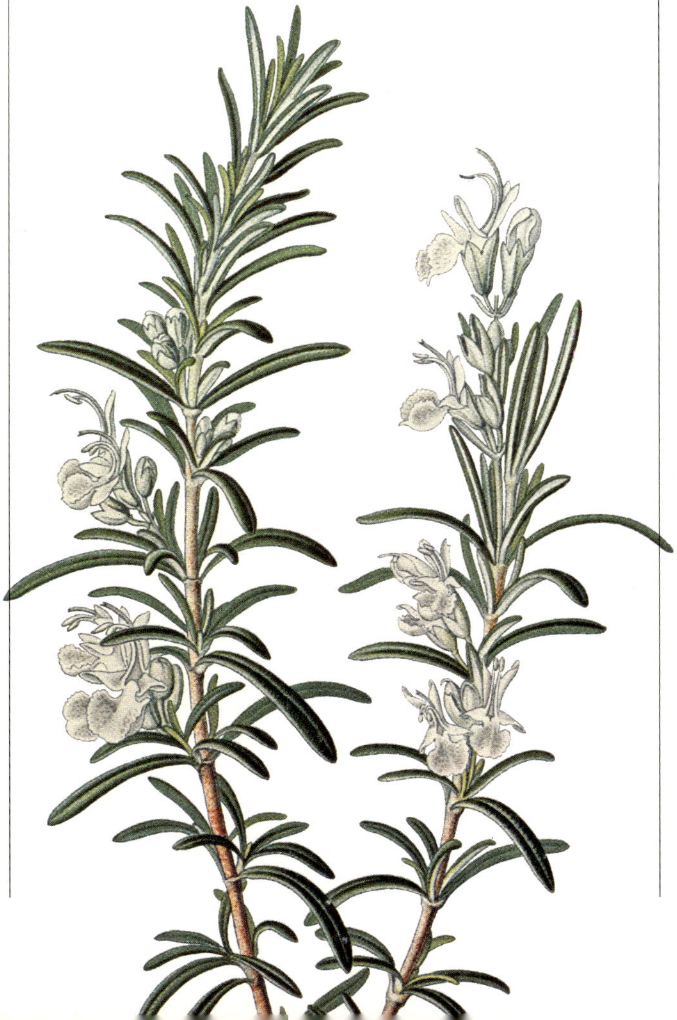

RUBIA TINCTORUM

MADDER, COMMON MADDER

Rubiaceae

197 S Eur, SW Asia
C Eur

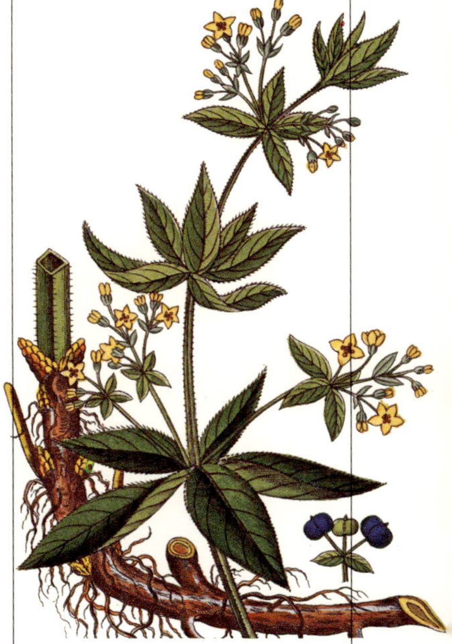

When red was the color for military uniforms, madder roots were much in demand for the dye known as turkey red. The deeply penetrating yellow underground stem may reach a length of 1 m. It is much branched and jointed, with pale red fibrous roots growing from the nodes. The stem, 60–90 cm high, is quadrangular and roughly hairy. Parts of it may be tinged with red. The edges have small hooked spines. Narrow, lance-shaped leaves of a rich green color grow in whorls of 4 or 6 up the stem. Their margins and the ends of their ribs are also prickly. The stems branch at the top and terminate in loose pseudo-umbels of small greenish-yellow flowers. The fruits are stalked purple berries the size of peas. The coloring matter is also the principle with medicinal activity; it is found in the roots, but also in the stems and leaves.

RUBUS FRUTICOSUS

EUROPEAN BLACKBERRY, BRAMBLE

Rosaceae

198 Eur, N Af, Asia, N Am
Temperate Zones

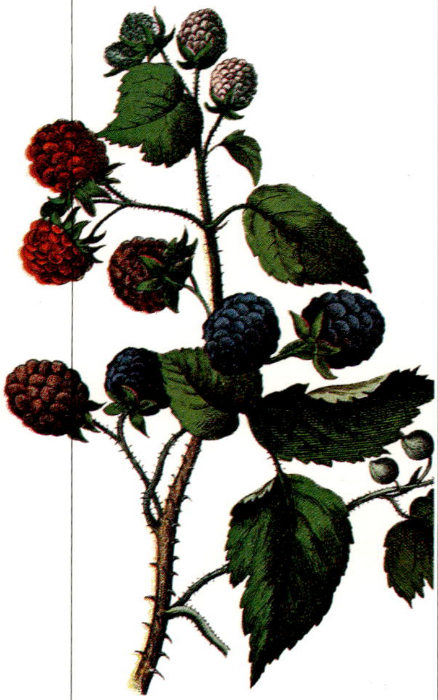

Wild and prickly, the bramble is not easily tamed. Its many varieties grow prolifically in hedgerows, woods, rubbish heaps, and neglected fields and gardens, rooting where they touch the ground. The branching rootstock produces long curving branches which are erect or sprawling and armed with backward-facing thorns. In their first year, these bear only dark green foliage leaves divided into 5–7 leaflets, usually a pointed oval, with toothed margins and covered with a whitish down on the underside. The stalks and veins of the leaves are also prickly. In the second year, side shoots appear which bear the handsome pink or white rose-type flowers with 5 petals and numerous stamens. The plant flowers throughout the summer. The berries ripen on other branches, first turning red and finally a glossy black. They have a high content of sugar, pectin, and vitamin C. The leaves contain tannins and flavones.

RUMEX CRISPUS, RUMEX ACETOSA

CURLED DOCK, COMMON SORREL

Polygonaceae

199 Eur, Asia
Temperate Zones

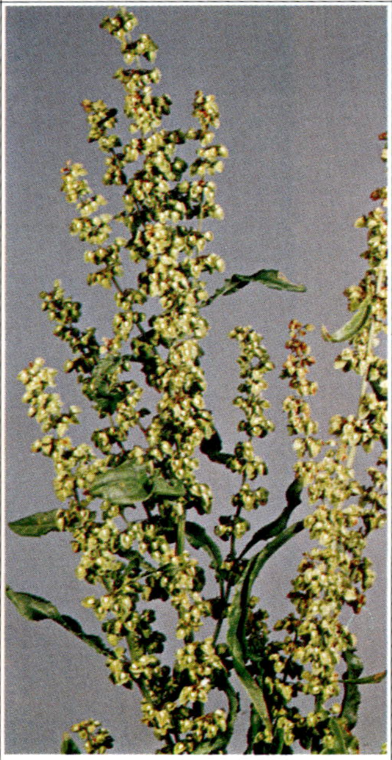

The docks and sorrels are a prolific genus commonly found in damp meadows, pastures, and ditches. They belong to the same family as rhubarb, and as in the case of rhubarb, their stems and leaves contain oxalic acid and vitamin C. The roots of some species (particularly *Rumex alpinus*) contain active principles with aperient properties, but a higher concentration of these principles is found in the Turkey rhubarb *(Rheum palmatum)*. A tincture prepared from the fresh roots is still used to some extent in homeopathy. The various species differ mainly in the shape of the leaf. The multiheaded branching rootstock produces ridged stems 30–80 cm in height. The lower leaves are long-stemmed and frequently arrow-shaped while those growing on the stem are stalkless, slim, pointed, and have wavy or curled margins. The reddish flowers grow in long spikes at the end of the stem and branches.

RUTA GRAVEOLENS

RUE

Rutaceae

200 SE Eur
Warm Temperate Zones

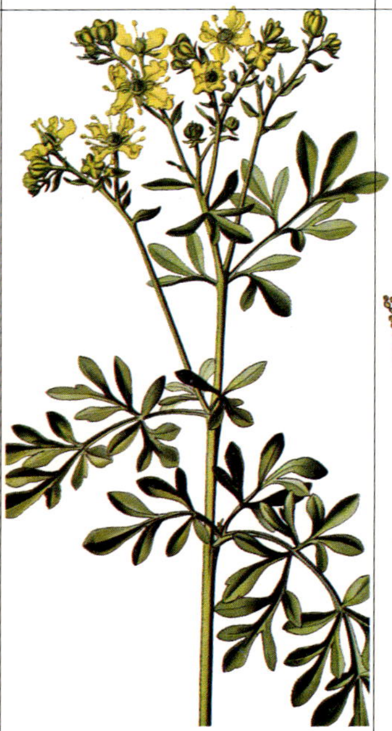

The *Rutaceae* family has more than 900 species, most being tropical plants. These include lemon and orange trees. Only the rue and the dittany have dared to venture farther north, where they grow as woody shrubs in warm situations. The sturdy perennial shrub has hard, round stems which do not branch much and bear alternate, much divided leaves with pairs of leaflets and an odd leaflet at the tip. The leaves are 10–15 cm long, tough, and dotted with glands. Both leaves and stem are a striking yellow grayish-green. The stems terminate in pseudo-umbels of yellowish-green flowers which are also dotted with glands. The whole plant has a somewhat harsh aromatic odor and tastes bitter. The leaflets are used as a seasoning. In winegrowing areas, leaves of rue are put in brandy to produce a liqueur used to aid digestion. Taken in large doses, rue may cause poisoning.

SALIX ALBA

WHITE WILLOW

Salicaceae

201 Eur, Asia
N Am

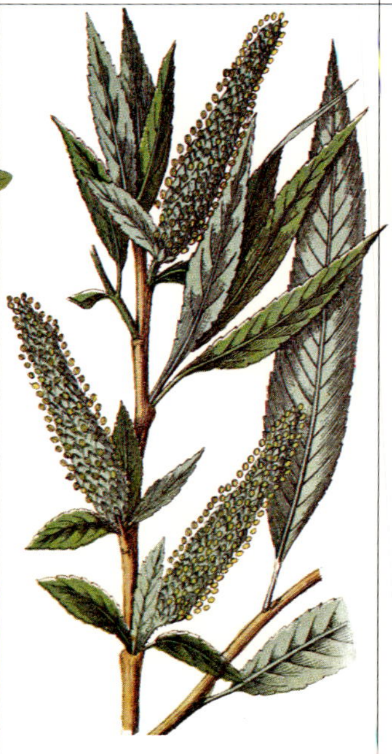

Along river banks, the willows grow as trees or shrubs; in mountain areas, as rather low, deep-rooted shrubs; and in snow-covered regions, as low spreading carpets, barely 5 cm high. The white willow is a medium-sized tree growing on river banks, in damp low areas, and frequently in parks. The trunk is slim and straight with a whitish-gray bark which, in old trees, is fissured lengthwise. The thin straight branches bear close-held buds which open outward into lance-shaped, finely toothed, light or dark green leaves. These are covered with a silvery down on the underside (white willow). Male and female flowers grow on different plants, in upright catkins, and have golden-yellow stamens. The active principle is salicin, a precursor of salicylic acid. This was isolated from willow bark as early as 1830, and a whole range of medicaments, including aspirin, have been prepared from it.

SALVIA OFFICINALIS

GARDEN SAGE

Lamiaceae, Labiatae

202 S Eur
Temperate Zones

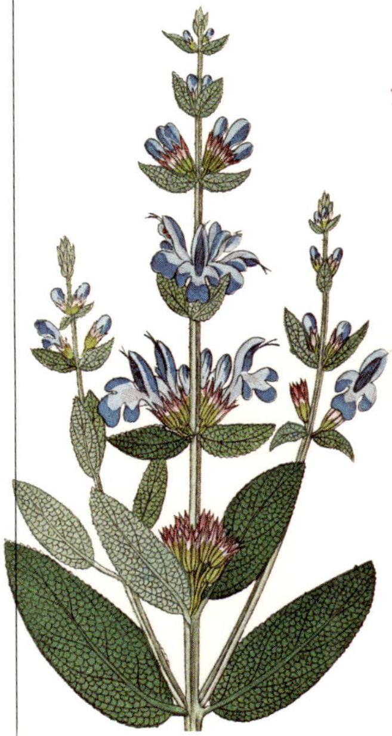

The Latin name *Salvia* derives from *salvare,* to heal. Sage has been cultivated from earliest times and the cultivated species, garden sage, is used medicinally. The plant drug offered on the market consists chiefly of plants gathered in the wild. Both the wild and the cultivated species prefer dry, chalky soils and a sunny climate. The tap root, often woody, produces square stems, herbaceous at the top, 30–80 cm long, woody near the base, and densely hairy. The stalked opposite leaves are elongated, oval, and pointed; leathery, hairy, and grayish-green in color; and have lightly toothed margins. Whorls of purplish-blue flowers at the top of the stem are visited frequently by bees and bumble bees. The leaves are used fresh for seasoning or chewed for infections of the mouth and throat. The volatile oil is concentrated in the leaves, as are the tannins and bitters.

SAMBUCUS EBULUS

DWARF ELDER

Caprifoliaceae

203 Eur, NW Af, W Asia
N Am

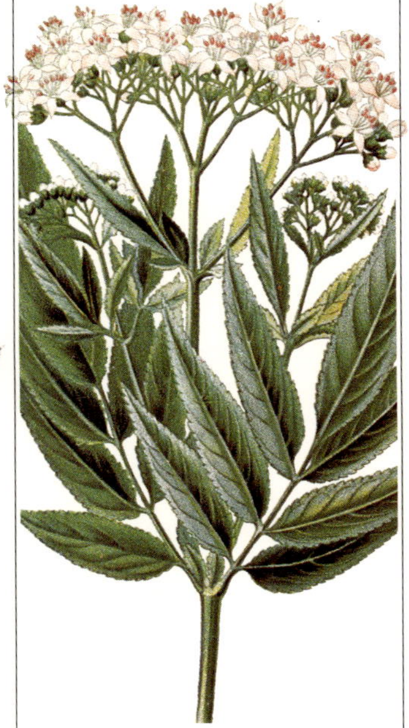

Only the rootstock and roots of the dwarf elder survive the winter. It produces a herbaceous, upright, furrowed hollow stem which grows to a height of 100–150 cm. The stem does not become woody and dies back in autumn. The large dark green leaves are divided and narrower than those of the European elder *(Scambucus nigra)* and have toothed margins. At the base of the leafstalk grow two small egg-shaped leaflets (stipules). The stem terminates in a flat, umbel-like cluster of numerous strongly scented, reddish-white flowers. The leaves have an unpleasant smell. Small, matt-black berries ripen in autumn. They are inedible, having an unpleasantly bitter taste, so that they may be distinguished easily from the berries of the common elder. The ground elder *(Radix ebuli)* grows wild in hedgerows and ditches, damp places, open woodlands, and waste places.

SAMBUCUS NIGRA

EUROPEAN ELDER

Caprifoliaceae

204 Eur
W Asia, N Am

This large shrub, also often growing as a tree, is common in southern and northern regions, generally growing uncultivated by a wall. It may also!be cultivated. The roots are very branched and will penetrate walls. The trunk often is crooked with a pale gray, deeply fissured bark. A shrub 4–7 m high is formed by the branches arching outward. The core of the trunk and branches consists of snow-white pith. The divided, opposite leaves usually have 5 pointed egg-shaped leaflets with jagged edges, dark green on the upper surface, and a lighter color underneath. The numerous creamy-white flowers, with their strong and rather strange scent, are borne in flat-topped terminal clusters. They later develop into small, round, glossy black berries on dark red stalks, filled with blood-red juice. Country people use the flowers to make aromatic summer drinks. The flowers are used medicinally to promote sweating. The fruits contain vitamins C and P and also a coloring matter with medicinal properties; syrups and robs (i.e., juice thickened by heat) are made from them and used as a home remedy for colds.

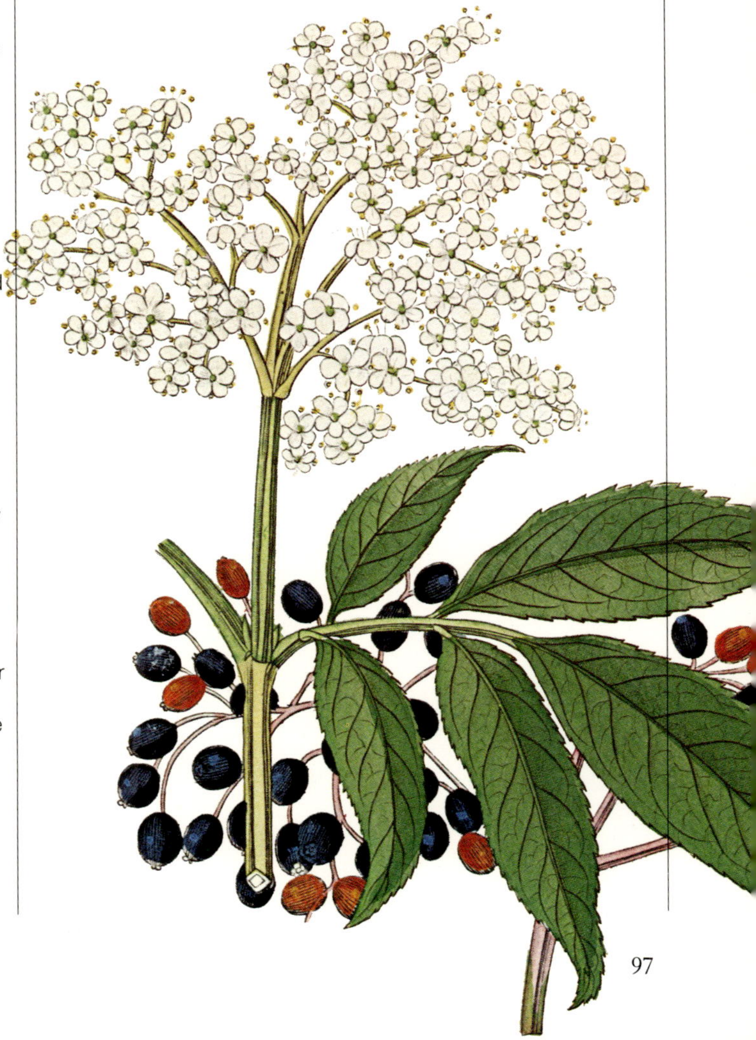

SANGUINARIA CANADENSIS

BLOODROOT

Papaveraceae

205 E-N Am

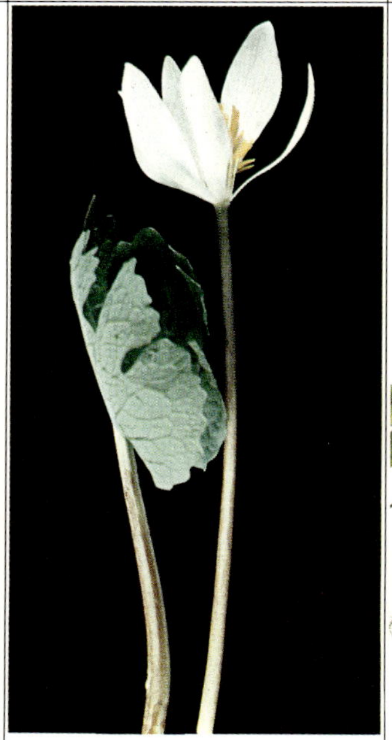

This North American member of the poppy family is named for the color of its perennial, woody rootstock. The root was used by the Red Indians to cure many of their ills including cancer of the breast and also to dye their skin. The creeping rootstock, 5–8 cm long and reddish-brown on the outside, contains a reddish milky juice. At its upper end, just above ground level, grows a poke of basal leaves, with the angular flowering stem rising from the center of it. The stem reaches a height of about 25 cm. It bears lobed leaves the shape of a hand, with the leaflets egg-shaped and serrated. The leaves are soft, yellowish-green on the upper surface, and lighter in color on the underside, which is patterned with strong, orange-colored veins. The long-stemmed flower is 2–5 cm in diameter, usually white and occasionally pink. The fruit is a capsule 3–5 cm in length.

SANICULA EUROPAEA

SNAKEROOT, SANICLE

Apiaceae, Umbelliferae

206 Eur, W Asia

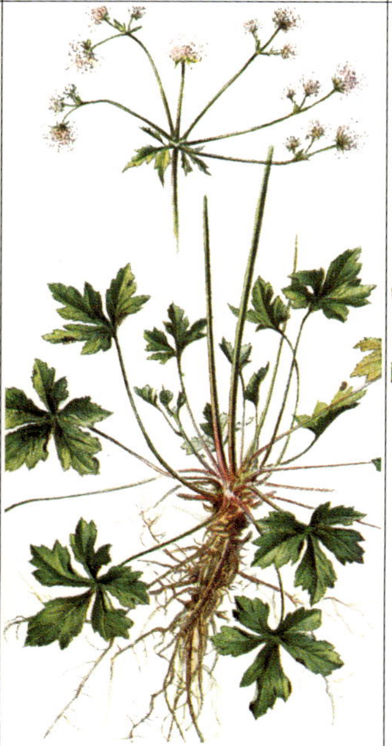

The snakeroot or sanicle (from *sanus*, "healthy") prefers shady sites in the humus-rich soil of deciduous woods to an altitude of 1400 m. The fibrous, brown rootstock produces long-stemmed ground leaves, deeply divided into 3 or 5 lobes of a deep glossy green, with regular veining. They look extraordinarily decorative against the brown woodland floor. The flowering stems generally are leafless, grow to a height 20–40 cm, and bear tiny umbels of white to pale pink. As the leaves are similar to some buttercup species, inexperienced persons should gather snakeroot at flowering time, when the umbels are quite distinctive. The whole-cut plant is medicinal, as are the roots; however, the roots should be left to produce the next year's crop. It contains a volatile oil, saponin, tannin, and allantoin and is effective in preventing inflammation, healing infected wounds, and soothing the mucous membranes.

SAPONARIA OFFICINALIS

SOAPWORT, BOUNCING BET

Caryophyllaceae

207 Eur, W Asia *C+E Asia, N Am*

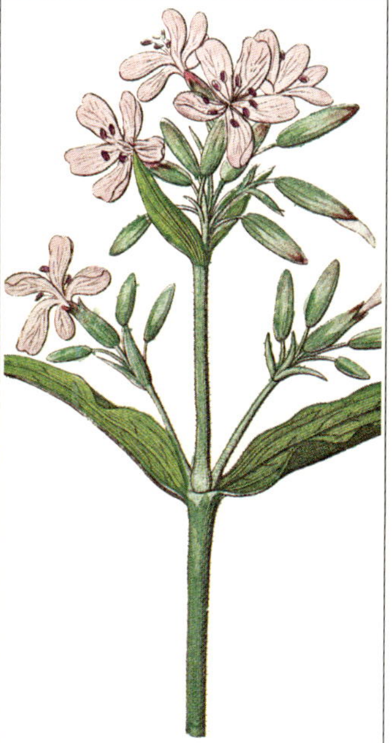

This decorative plant produces beautiful flowers and is also grown in gardens. It may be found growing wild in waste places, on embankments, in hedgerows, among shrubs, and in open woodlands, but prefers a fairly warm location. The rootstock is very branched, produces simple nonflowering shoots, and has an upright flowering stem branching at the top. Both are downy and show a tinge of red in places. The leaves grow in opposite pairs, standing at right angles to each other, on the enlarged nodes of the stem. They are elongated and lance-shaped with 3 veins running lengthwise. The flowers grow in clusters from the leaf axils and, particularly at the top of the stem, are quite typical for the pink family, with 5 petals, white or soft pink, opening into a wheel shape on top of the cylindrical, often reddish calyx. The active principle, saponin, is found mainly in the root, but also in the herb.

SASSAFRAS ALBIDUM

SASSAFRAS, COMMON SASSAFRAS

Lauraceae

208 E-N Am

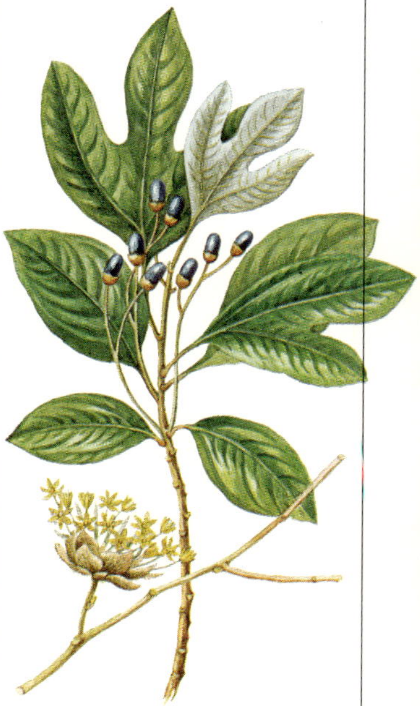

This is a unisexual tree growing in mixed deciduous forests in the Atlantic states of North America. In southern latitudes it may reach a height of 30 m. The rich foliage is pale green, or it may have a reddish hue. The shape of the leaf varies according to the species and subspecies, and one and the same tree may have oval, entire leaves as well as others divided into 2 or 3 rounded lobes. The wood and root have an aromatic smell of fennel and a sweetish taste. The drug-containing part consists of irregular, thick, gray-brown or reddish pieces or slices which easily split into smaller pieces, often with the brittle, cinnamon-brown bark still attached. The volatile oil obtained from the drug by distillation is used to flavor soft drinks in the United States.

SCOPOLIA CARNIOLICA

SCOPOLIA

Solanaceae

209 SE Eur
C Eur

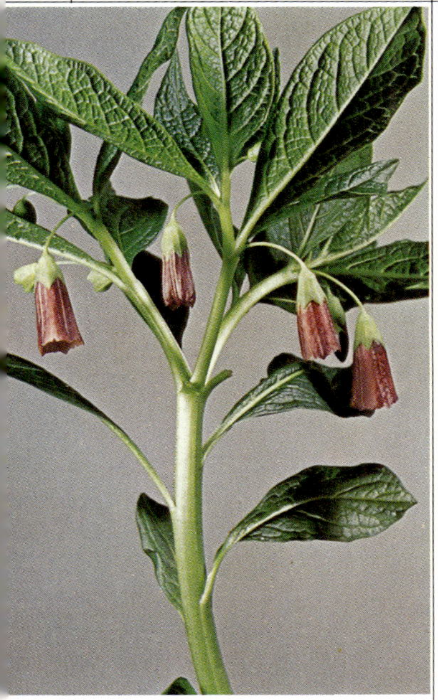

A relative of the henbane *(Hyoscyamus),* this plant has been introduced to the southern United States, chiefly because it yields scopolamine, an alkaloid of considerable medicinal value. Scopolia is a perennial with a knotty underground stem branching horizontally. The leaf-bearing stems are smooth and hairless. The grow to a height of 20–60 cm and branch only slightly. The lower leaves are alternate, elongated and pointed, 20 cm long and about 6–8 cm wide. Higher up, the shape of the leaf changes to a stalked, broadly ovate form ending in a point, with margins entire.
The short-stemmed flowers grow singly from the leaf axils, with a 5-pointed calyx cupping the bell-shaped yellow or greenish-yellow corona. The fruits are roundish capsules 1 cm in diameter.

SCROPHULARIA NODOSA

FIGWORT

Scrophulariaceae

210 Eur, Asia
N Am

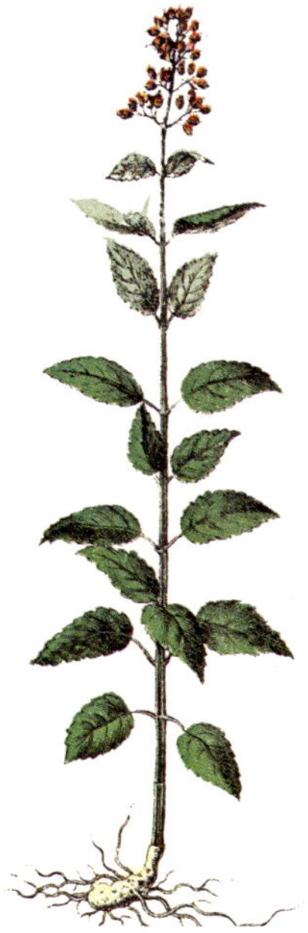

The common figwort may still be found distributed widely in damp ditches, on stream banks, in woods, and among shrubs. The knobbed horizontal rootstock produces square stems, usually unbranched, which reach a height of 50–90 cm. Further down, these bear opposite, short-stemmed, pointed, egg-shaped leaves with double-toothed margins. At the upper end of the stem, narrow lance-shaped leaves support long-stemmed clusters of flowers which combine to form an elongated terminal spike. The 4-square flower stalks bear a spherical calyx of 5 green sepals which holds the muddy-brown, 2-lipped flower shaped to fit an insect commonly visiting this plant, the wasp. An egg-shaped capsule with a pointed tip holds the seeds, which are dispersed by the wind in autumn.

SEDUM ACRE

MOSSY STONECROP,
WALL PEPPER

Crassulaceae

211 Eur, N Af, SW Asia
Temperate Zones

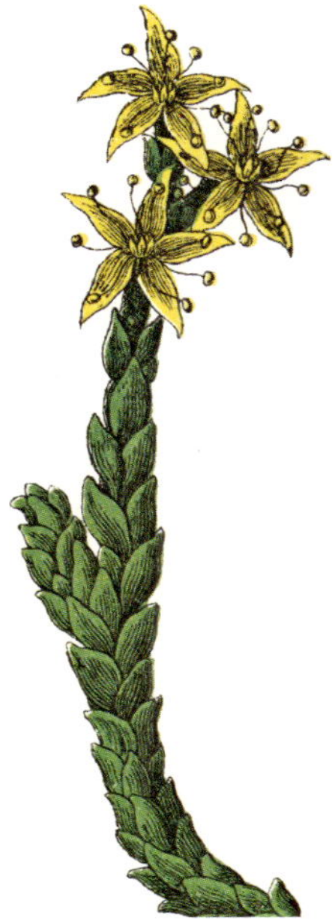

The stonecrops form tufts and cushions on rocks, walls, sandy soil, and dry roadsides. They are succulent plants. Many species may vary in the color of the flower and the shape of the leaf. An evergreen herb, the wallpepper, grows in a creeping manner from many-branched shoots and reaches a height of barely 10–15 cm. Small, fleshy, pale green cylindrical leaves cover the short branches like scales. The branching, flowering stems are short, have fewer leaves, and bear yellow (in some species white) star-like flowers of 5 small pointed petals. The tiny seeds are washed away by rain or borne away by wind. Broken-off shoots will take root quickly if they are left lying on the ground. Despite its hot, peppery taste, which would seem to suggest medicinal properties, the biting stonecrop is of little medicinal value.

SELENICEREUS GRANDIFLORUS

NIGHT-BLOOMING CEREUS,
QUEEN OF THE NIGHT

Cactaceae

212 C Am

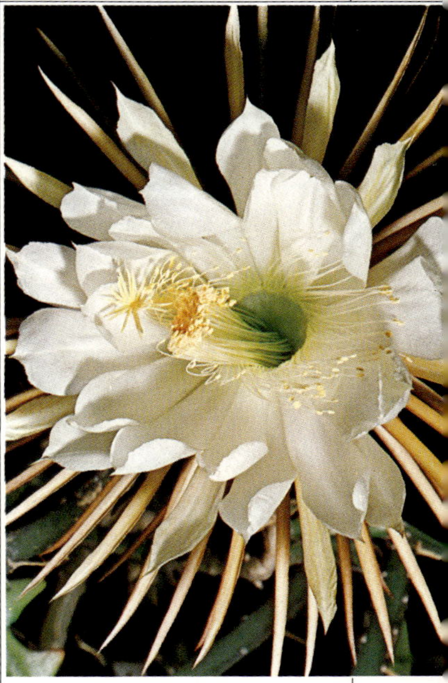

The *Cereus* and *Selenicereus genera* of cacti form upright cylindrical stems. Those of the night-blooming cereus are a succession of thin elongated sections. Instead of leaves they have angular ribs, with numerous aerial roots which keep a hold on rocks and trees, and also absorb humidity from the air. After a number of years, when the much-branched, swollen stems have reached a certain maturity, lighter-colored buds appear here and there among them. These increase rapidly in size, taking almost the form of a small, spiny barrel cactus. They are the ovaries of the flowers now developing, 12–15 cm in length and growing horizontally, facing the light. The flower is 20 cm in diameter, with cream-colored sepals bearing a tinge of red which on the inside merge into the white corolla. Only for a few hours of darkness does the "queen of the night" flower and give off its delicious perfume.

SENECIO FUCHSII

ALPINE RAGWORT

Asteraceae, Compositae

213 C Eur

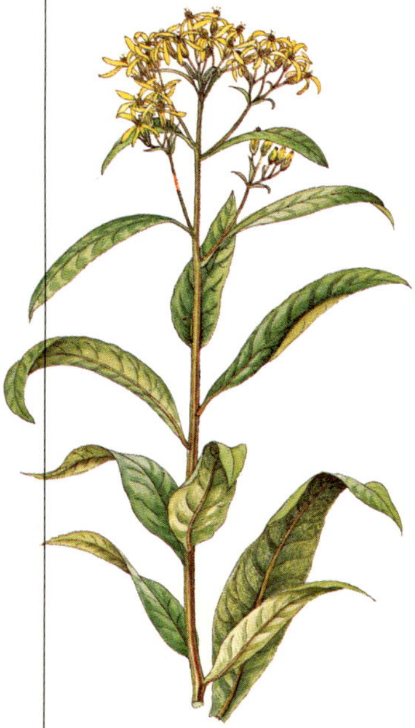

The name *Senecio* refers to the whitish shocks of seed hairs that appear during the fruiting stage (*senex*=old man). While groundsel *(S. vulgaris)* is an unwelcome weed which is widespread in fields, on rubbish dumps, and along roadsides, the alpine ragwort is a very handsome plant growing to a height of 70–120 cm. It has reddish stems bearing large, lance-shaped, alternate leaves with saw-toothed margins. From the upper leaf axils grow umbel-like stalked clusters of yellow star-shaped flowers which together form a broad terminal umbel. This plant was often confused with the goldenrod and was called heathen's woundwort. Today, only the goldenrod *(Solidago)* bears that name. The common ragwort *(S. jacobaea)* is not as tall but otherwise is similar to the alpine ragwort. The active principles are powerful alkaloids and are obtained from the whole plant, either fresh or dried.

SERENOA REPENS

SAW PALMETTO

Palmaceae

214 S-N Am

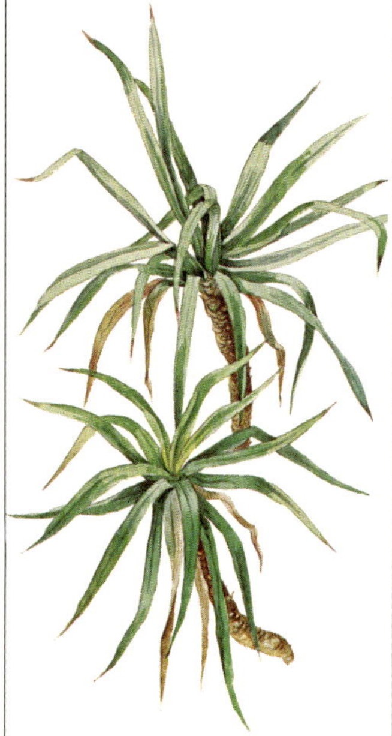

This palm, 4–6 m high, grows in the sand dunes and coastal regions of Florida and Texas, where its fruits are a valuable source of food for the local population. They are also gathered for the extraction of their medicinal principles. The rough trunk is covered all the way round with the leaf bases of withered leaves; these will often grow stunted or form twiggy branches creeping along the ground. The long, stiff leaves are about 1 m long and grow in fans; they are yellowish- or grayish-green, narrow and pointed, and frequently coated with wax. The ivory-colored flowers grow in fragrant clusters The stone fruits are 2–3 cm in length and black when ripe. Their fruit flesh is light brown and spongy and contains a brown seed. The leaf buds are also edible.

SILYBUM MARIANUM

MILK THISTLE, MARIAN THISTLE

Asteraceae, Compositae

215 S Eur, N Af, SW Asia
Warm Temperate Zones

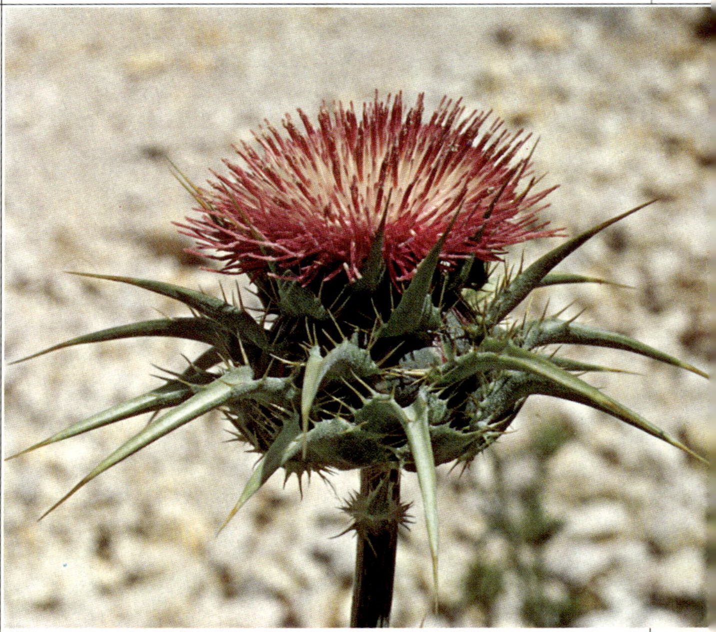

The milk thistle is one of the most decorative thistles. In dry southern locations, it still may be found growing wild, but in the north, it generally is cultivated. According to legend, the white veins marking the leaves originated in the milk of the Virgin falling on a thistle; hence the name Marian thistle. John Evelyn described it as "a great breeder of milk and a proper diet for wetnurses." The erect stem, branching at the top, reaches a height of up to 150 cm. The broad, very wavy leaves are lance-shaped, pointed, and a glossy green with conspicuous white markings. Their margins and tips are spiny. The upper leaves are partly divided and clasp the stem. The stem terminates in a spiny spherical head bearing a thick brush of purple tubular florets. The fruit (i.e., seeds) of this plant contain several very interesting active principles which, recent research has shown, benefit the liver. In Europe the principles from these seeds are used in many pharmaceutical preparations. The young shoots, known in Arabic as *Khurfesh*, are a favorite with Bedouins.

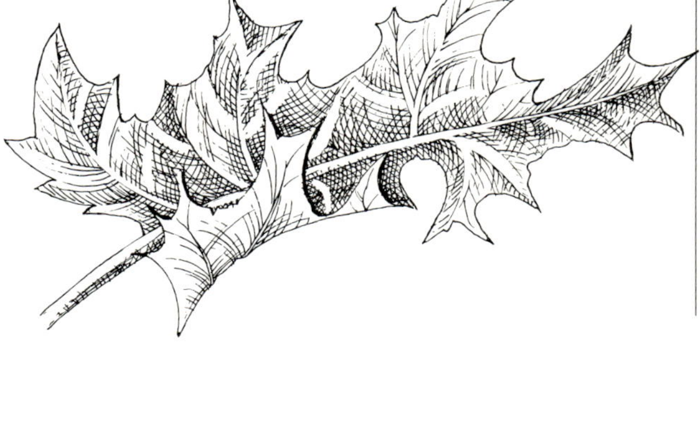

SMILAX UTILIS

SARSAPARILLA

Liliaceae

216 Salomon Islands
S Am

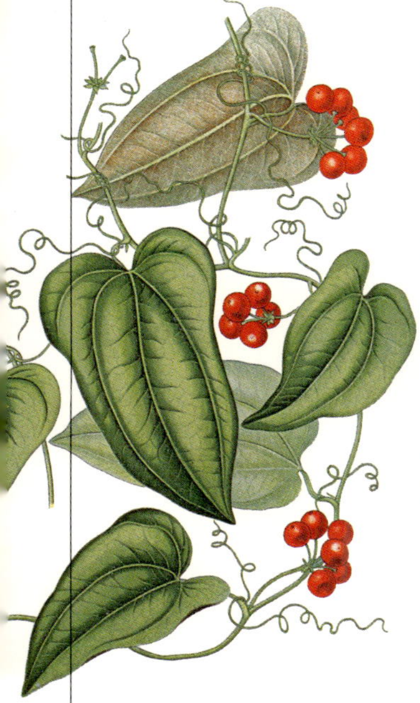

This large perennial climber may reach a length of 40–50 m. It clambers up forest trees in the humid climate of the Central American countries and neighboring parts of South America. The plant has a large underground stem with roots 1 m long. The climbing stems are sharply quadrangular, their winged edges bearing sharp prickles. The glossy dark green leaves are heart-shaped and may reach a length of 35 cm. Their 3–7 cm long stalks arise from a sheath-like leaf base with lateral tendrils. From the upper leaf axils grow stalked clusters of small, star-shaped greenish-white flowers. The ovaries develop into red berries. Medicinal use has been made of the root for centuries. The Spaniards brought the roots to Europe during the sixteenth century, hoping that it might serve as a cure for syphilis. Today it is largely used in the making of soft drinks.

SOLANUM DULCAMARA

EUROPEAN BITTERSWEET, BITTER NIGHTSHADE

Solanaceae

217 Eur, N Asia
N Am

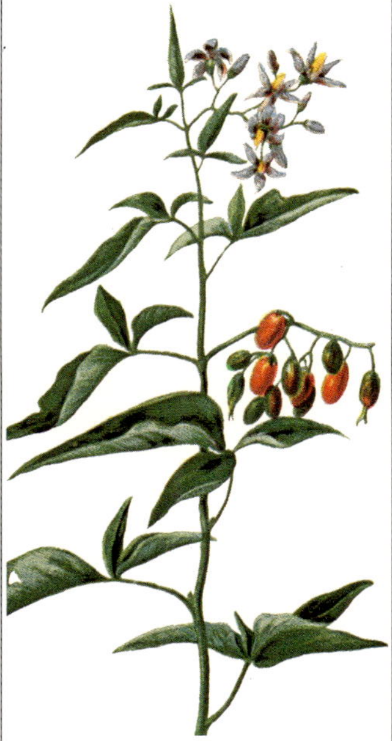

This plant is found on the banks of streams, in damp waste places, and near woods. The creeping root produces a woody stem which often creeps or clambers up branches. The alternate leaves do not adhere to rigid principles of form. The lower leaves are egg-shaped, pointed, thin, and dark-green; the higher they are, the narrower and more pointed they become. At the height of summer, deep purple flowers appear which have 5 downward-turning, pointed petals and bright golden-yellow anthers. Later the glossy oval berries, which are green at first, turn a bright red and sit prettily in their reddish-brown calyces. The herb and the berries are poisonous and taste bitter and rather rough at first, then unpleasantly sweet; hence its name. The bittersweet needs to be treated with respect since its stems and berries contain different principles from those of other *Solanaceae* (e.g., belladonna).

SOLIDAGO VIRGAUREA

GOLDENROD

Asteraceae / Compositae

218 Eur, N Asia, N Am

The goldenrod seems to give expression to its medicinal powers not only in its beautiful name but also in its handsome form. The name *Solidago* (Latin *solido* = to make whole) indicates its use as a wound-healing herb. *Virga aurea* is the Latin for goldenrod, named for the stem with its golden-yellow flowers. The cylindrical root finds the depth of soil it needs for a firm hold everywhere in the dry earth of woodlands, among bushes in waste places, on dunes and rocks, right up to the mountain regions. The round stem branches only at the top and grows 20–50 cm high, but may occasionally reach 100 cm. The alternate leaves on the lower part of the stem are large, pointed, and elliptical with toothed margins. In the flowering region they are narrow and lance-shaped, with margins entire. Numerous stalked golden-yellow flower heads form branched spikes at the top of the stem, the lower ones opening first, so that the plant flowers continuously from July into autumn. Insects and butterflies of all kinds are frequent visitors. When the flowering is over, the calyx holds a crown of hairs *(pappus)*, which later carry the small fruits on the wind. The flowering tips of the branches are used in teas and pharmaceutical preparations. The active principles—saponins, floral pigments, and tannins—are used in the treatment of kidney and intestinal inflammations. Another species, the Canadian goldenrod, is taller (60–200 cm), has 1-sided spikes, in a branched cluster, of numerous yellow flower heads (3–5 mm), and spreads widely in Europe.

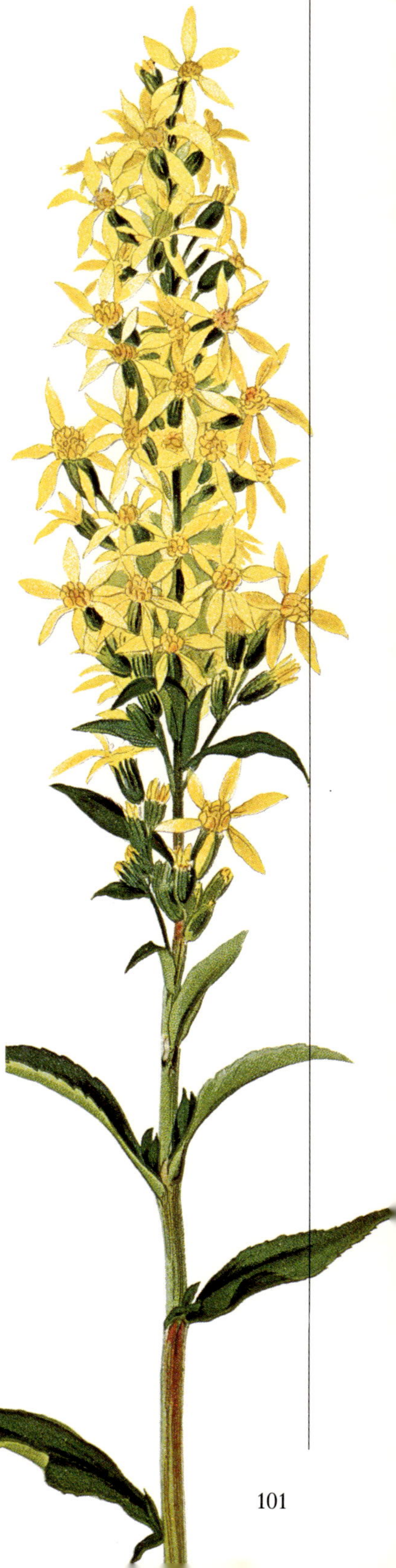

SOPHORA JAPONICA

CHINESE PAGODA TREE, SOPHORE

Fabaceae (=Leguminosae)

219 E Asia

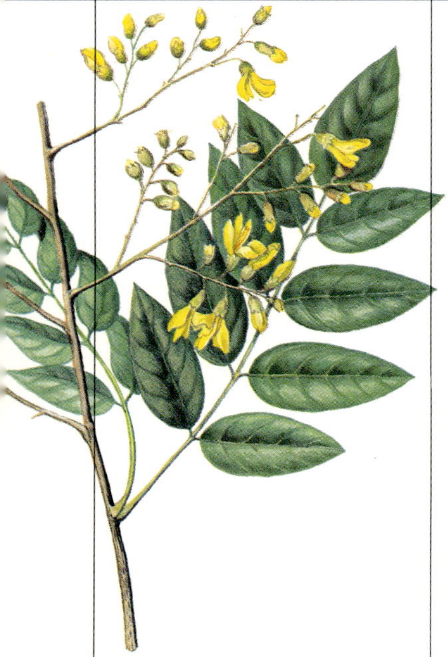

Originally this tree, growing up to 20 m high, was only cultivated in temple precincts in Japan, but later it came to be used as an ornamental plant in many other countries. The fruits are seed pods constricted between the seeds, like strings of beads, and contain black bean-shaped seeds. The leaves are alternate, up to 25 cm in length, divided into pairs of leaflets with an odd one at the tip. The upper surface is dark green, the underside grayish-green. The leaflets are oval or lance-shaped, terminating in a prickly tip, and have short stalks. The yellowish-white flowers grow in loose terminal clusters. The flower buds of the plant contain up to 30 percent of flavonoids. In Siberia and the Far East, preparations of Sophora are used in popular medicine to treat fevers, seizures, and hemorrhages.

STROPHANTHUS KOMBÉ

STROPHANTHUS

Apocynaceae

220 C Af
E Asia

The genus *Strophanthus* (DC.) includes a number of species yielding active principles of considerable value in cardiology. *Strophanthus kombé* is indigenous to eastern tropical Africa. The natives use an extract prepared from the roots or seeds as an arrow poison. Active principles for pharmaceutical use are obtained from the seeds. *Strophanthus kombé* climbs to a height of 30 or 40 m. Its branches are roughly hairy, as are the short-stemmed opposite leaves. The leaves are broadly oval, 15–20 cm wide, pointed or slightly incurving at the tip, and have a crinkly surface. Small bunches of stalked flowers grow from the terminal leaf axils. A calyx of pointed sepals holds 5 yellowish-white petals fused into a funnel-shape. These terminate in long drooping tails, 10–20 cm in length. The fruits are 2 narrow pods, 20–30 cm long, which burst open when ripe and eject numerous tufted seeds. These are 10–20 mm long, flat, rounded, and covered with a silky, greenish-yellow pelt of hair. Some species of *Strophanthus* yield small amounts of steroidal saponins, which are chemically related to cortisone. Scientists went to Africa in the 1950s to seek such plants for cortisone production, but found insufficient quantities of saponins.

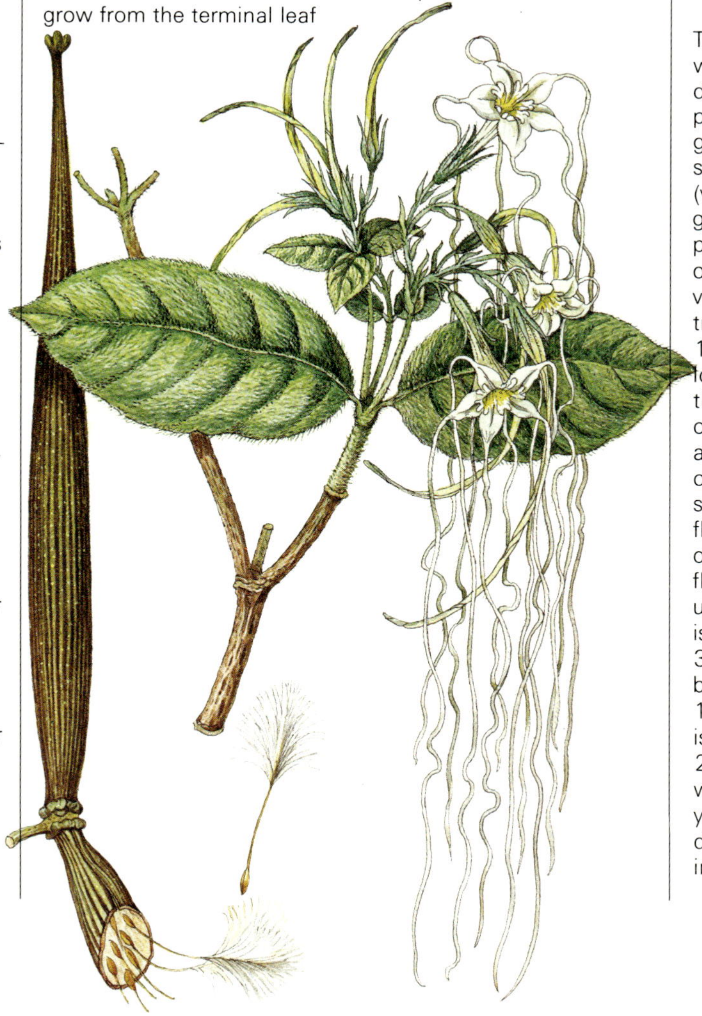

STRYCHNOS NUX-VOMICA

NUX-VOMICA

Loganiaceae

221 S Asia
Af, Aus

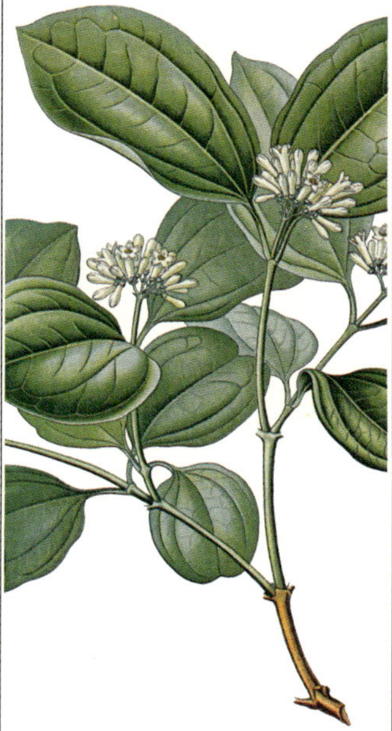

The seeds of *S. nux-vomica* were first brought to Europe during the fifteenth century, probably as poison bait for game and rodents. The specific name "nux-vomica" (vomiting nut) was probably given in error; the active principles are highly poisonous but do not cause vomiting. Growing wild, the trees reach a height of 10–12 m; they are kept at a lower height in the plantations. The branches bear opposite pairs, each at right angles to the preceding pair, of broadly egg-shaped, stalked, smooth leaves. The flowers are reddish, the tops of their petals spread in a flat disk. They grow in umbel-like clusters. The fruit is an orange red berry 3–6 cm in diameter, with a brittle membranous skin 1–3 mm thick. The fruit flesh is white and very bitter, with 2–4 seeds placed upright within it. The seeds are yellowish-green, very hard, disk-shaped, and 10–30 mm in diameter.

SWERTIA CHIRATA

CHIRATA

Gentianaceae

222 Himalayas
C Af, S Asia

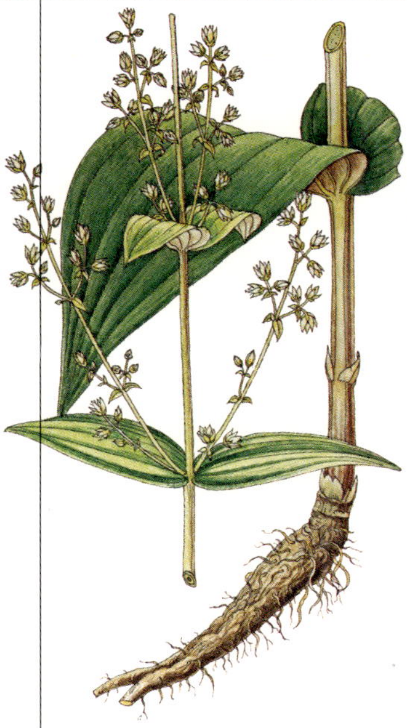

Like most other members of the Gentian Family, this is an alpine plant. Its original home is in the area around the Himalayas, in Tibet, Nepal, and farther east. In folk medicine it is used in the same way as the gentian root, and the Hindus have always valued it highly as a stomachic and febrifuge. The specific name is thought to derive from the Sanskrit word *Kirata*. The plant is annual or perennial. It grows to a height of 10–20 cm, with an erect angular stem bearing opposite pointed lance-shaped leaves of a rich green color. Those nearer the base are often long-stemmed. The steel-blue flowers grow in tight terminal spikes. Inside the tubular corolla, the stamens are set at different levels. The egg-shaped or round seeds are winged. The gentian bitters are of medicinal value. In India the drug is sold as chiretta herb. It is used in the preparation of tonics and aperitifs.

SYMPHYTUM OFFICINALE

COMFREY, COMMON COMFREY

Boraginaceae

223 Eur, Asia
N Am

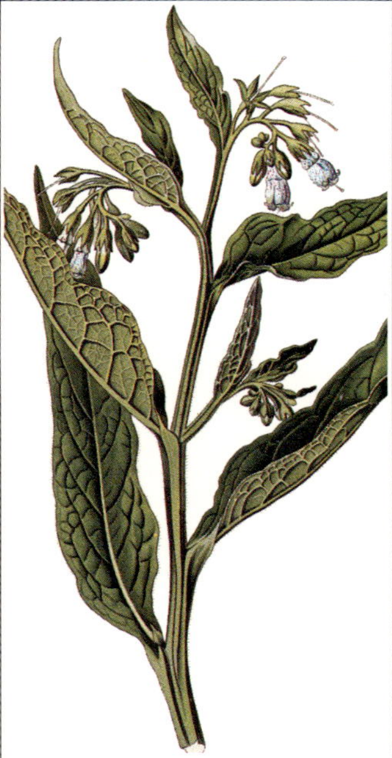

Comfrey is a corruption of the Latin *confirmare:* to heal or unite. Comfrey has a preference for damp places by streams and ditches, in meadows, and on the edges of ponds where its beet-shaped root, black on the outside, is able to penetrate the soft earth. The plant produces erect fleshy stems, 30–90 cm high, and branching only near the top. The elongated alternate leaves growing on the stem are oval and lance-shaped and continue downward into wings on the stem. Both stems and leaves are covered with rough hairs. From the axils of the smaller leaves, higher on the stem, grow reddish stalks bearing mauve, or sometimes white, bell-shaped flowers which form in dense clusters curving down toward the ground. The root, which is a creamy white inside, is used either fresh or dried. It contains medicinal principles which are used in pharmaceutical preparations.

TARAXACUM OFFICINALE

DANDELION

Asteraceae, Compositae

224 Temperate Zones

The dandelion is one of the familiar plants seen everywhere in meadows. By either having their flowers open or closed, they tell us if the weather is fair or foul. The name dandelion (lion's tooth) refers to the way the leaves are formed into pointed teeth. In the rich green of springtime meadows, the golden-yellow flowers often form carpets of blazing color. The short rootstock, with its fleshy taproot, produces a basal rosette of leaves. These are a light green with irregularly toothed margins. The shape of the leaves varies with the site and climate. In mountain regions, they are much smaller, while the root is relatively large. The hollow flowering stems contain milky juice, as do the root and the leaves. They are leafless, grow to a height of about 20–25 cm, and bear the thick calyx of numerous green sepals which holds the many golden- yellow strap florets. While the flowers are wide open when the sun is shining, they close up at night and in rainy weather. The spherical ovary is covered closely with small dark fruits, each with a beak about 10 mm long, and a parachute of hairs *(the pappus)* on which the ripe seeds are borne away by the wind. The active principles are found in the young spring shoots, which contain vitamins, and the root.

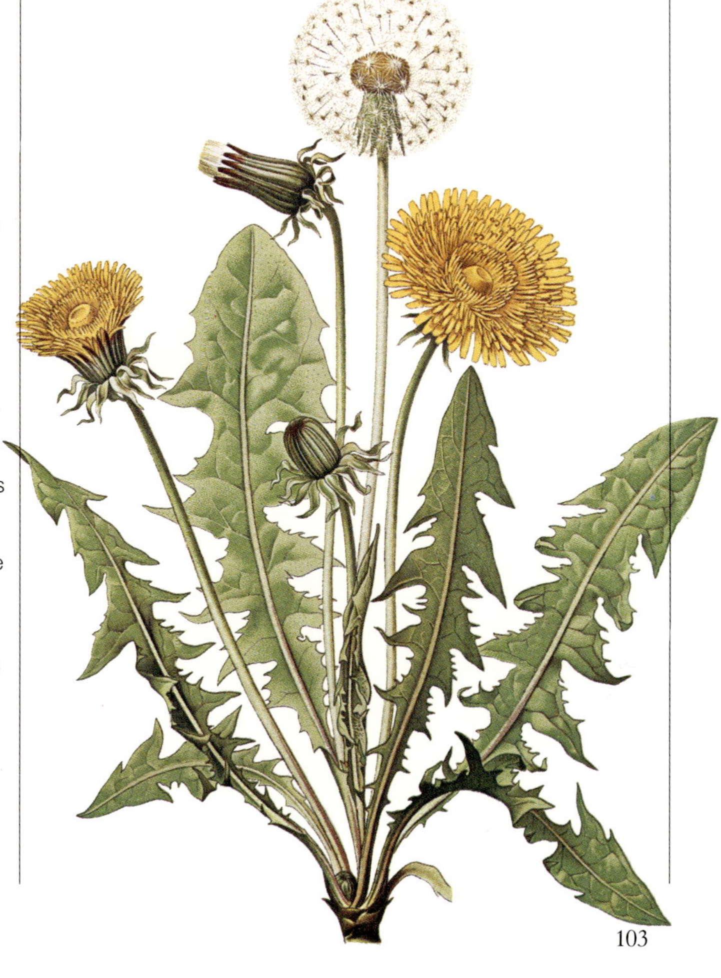

TEUCRIUM CHAMAEDRYS

GERMANDER

Lamiaceae, Labiatae

225 C+R Eur, NW Af, SW Asia

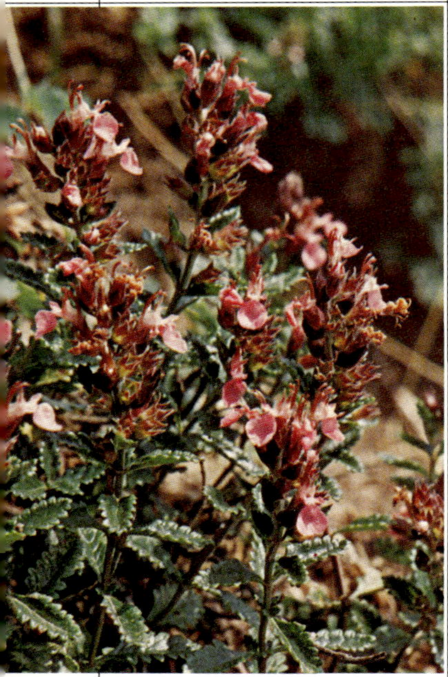

The germander prefers to grow on limestone, in dry meadows, and on rocky slopes. The roots, with their far-ranging underground runners, produce round, partly woody stems, which grow to a height of about 15–25 cm, often having a purplish tinge. The small opposite leaves are an elongated oval with toothed margins. Both stems and leaves are hairy. An extended spike of flowers dominates the otherwise rather small plant. The rose-red flowers, held in calyces with pointed lobes, sit in the upper leaf axils. Their stamens stand out above them. The germander is faintly aromatic. The flowering herb is collected and contains tannins and a small amount of volatile oil. In open woodlands, the wood sage *(Teucrium scorodonia)* may be found. This species grows to a height of 40–70 cm, has heart-shaped leaves, and one-sided spikes of yellowish flowers. It is a very bitter, aromatic herb.

THYMUS VULGARIS

THYME

Lamiaceae, Labiatae

226 S Eur
Warm Temperate Zones

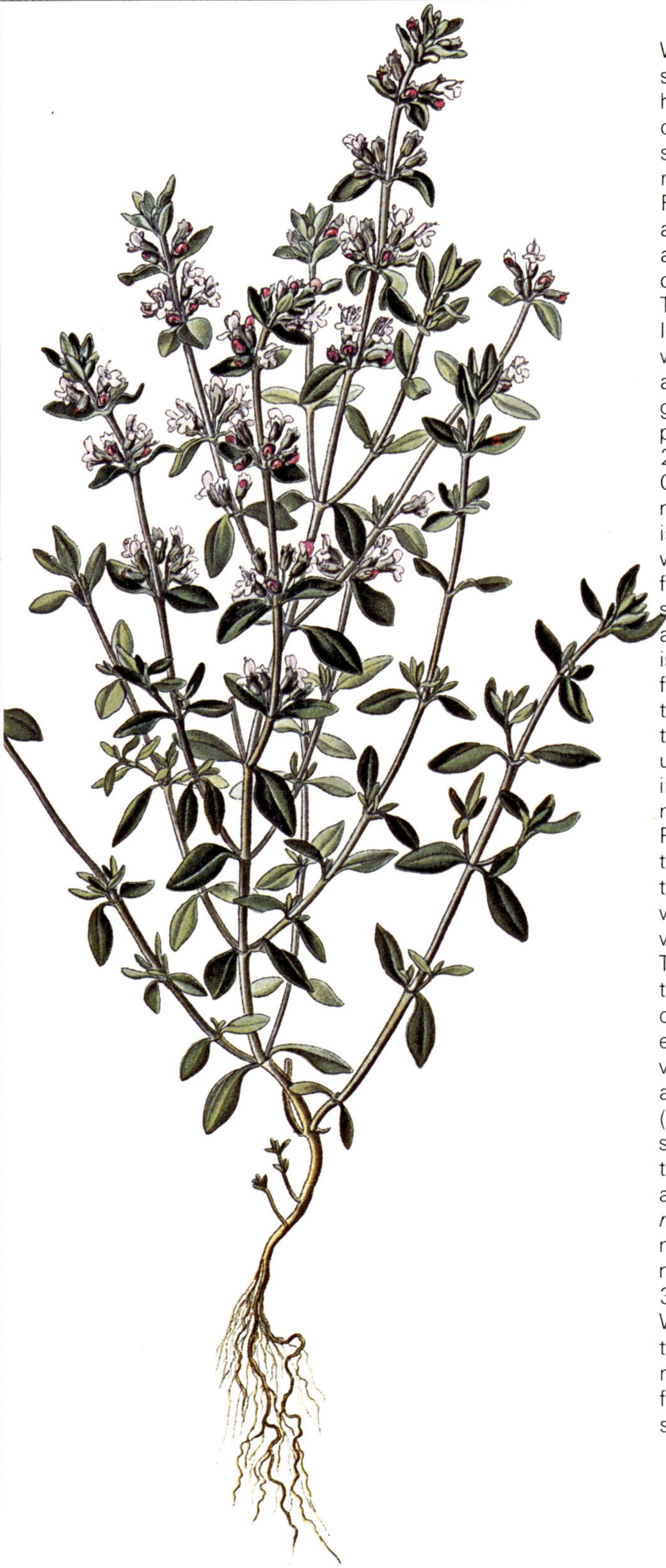

With branching, often woody stems, thyme grows as a half-shrub reaching a height of 30–40 cm. In dry sunny sites around the Mediterranean and in the south of France, it covers quite large areas. Being a popular herb and medicinal plant, it frequently is grown in gardens. The small, straight, narrow leaves are covered with a woolly pelt on the underside and may curl in at the margins. They grow in opposite pairs on short stalks with 2 small leaflets at the base. On the upper leaf axils, numerous small 2-lipped pinkish flowers grow in false whorls. The larger bisexual flowers have protruding stamens; the female flowers are smaller. The whole plant is pleasantly aromatic. The fresh young shoots are used to season salads and tomatoes; the dried leaves are used as a culinary seasoning, either individually or in mixtures (e.g., "Herbes de Provence"). Apart from bitters and tannins, thyme contains, above all, a volatile oil with thymol, a principle which acts as an antiseptic. The aromatic strength and the amount of thymol vary considerably between different types of wild and cultivated thyme. A variety adapted to northern regions (German or winter thyme) is sufficiently hardy to survive the winter, but also is less aromatic. Wild thyme *(Thymus serpyllum* is found in northern areas, in the mountains at altitudes to 3000 m, and in the Arctic. With its stems creeping over the ground, it forms permanent carpets which tend to flower throughout the summer.

TILIA PLATYPHYLLOS
TILIA CORDATA

BIGLEAF LINDEN, BROAD-LEAVED LIME

Tiliaceae

227 a) Eur
b) C+S Eur
N Am

Limes are deciduous trees belonging to the temperate regions. The small-leaved lime *(T. cordata)* tends to have a relatively short trunk and its smooth brown bark becomes rough and fissured with age. It prefers a good depth of friable soil on the edges of woods and also is planted in avenues. The broad-leaved lime *(T. platyphyllos)* is familiar as a shade-provider in continental village squares. It may attain a height of 33 m and 1000 years in age (historical linden trees). Numerous varieties of limes are known. The leaves of the broad-leaved lime are heart-shaped, with toothed margins, and have a whitish down on the underside, particularly at the angles of the veins. The leaves of *T. cordata* are tougher, less broad, and have rust-colored hairs at the angles of the veins on the underside. The flowers are born on a long stalk in clusters of 3–5 *(T. platyphyllos)* or 5 *(T. cordata)*. The stalk is partly fused with a papery, wine-yellow bract. During flowering time, the rich sweet scent of the volatile oil fills the air for a considerable distance. The flowers of both species are used medicinally (but not those of *T. tomentosa* Moench, a species with an overly rich scent), as well as the inner bark (bast).

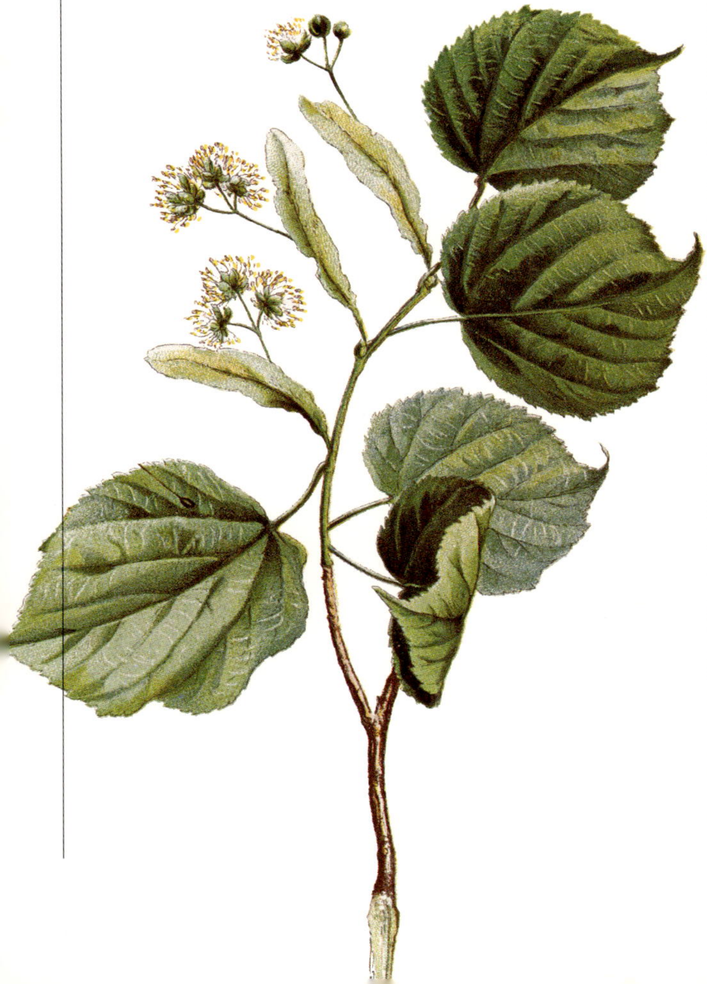

TRIGONELLA FOENUM-GRAECUM

FENUGREEK, GREEK HAYSEED

Fabaceae, Papilionaceae

228 SW Asia
Warm Temperate Zones

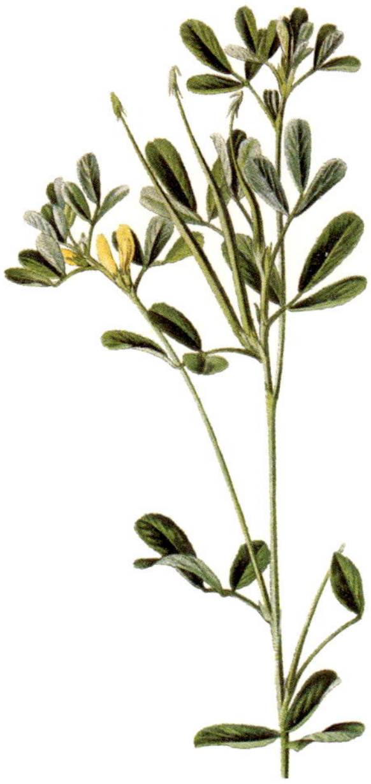

This plant, cultivated since ancient times, was known to the Egyptians. The Latin name *Foenum graecum* (Greek hay) indicates that it was used in antiquity. The annual, clover-like herb grows to a height of about 50 cm with erect or prostrate smooth, round stems which only branch a little. The stalked leaves are trefoil, the leaflets being of an inverted egg-shape. The unstalked yellowish-white pea-type flowers sit in the axils of the upper leaves. The pods are sickle-shaped and grow to a length of 20 cm, with an extended tip. They contain 5–20 hard, irregularly shaped seeds. The whole plant has a sharp aromatic scent. The dry pods are thrashed and the seeds, whole or ground, are used in concentrated cattle foods. The seeds contain fatty and volatile oils, protein, and saponins but are not much used now because of the strong smell. One variety of *Trigonella* is used to season cheeses.

TRILLIUM ERECTUM

PURPLE TRILLIUM, BIRTHWORT

Liliaceae

229 E-N Am

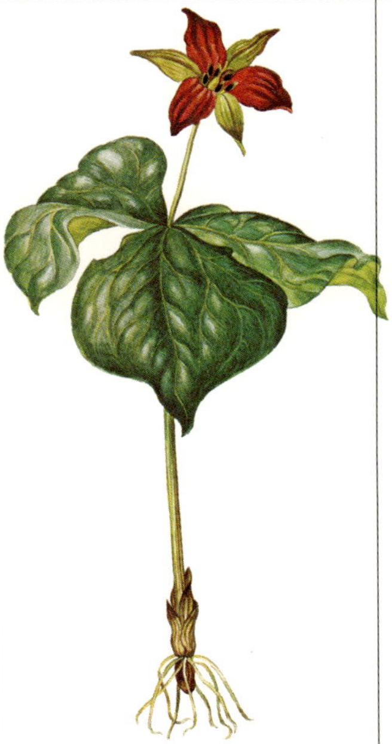

This attractive member of the Lily Family was used by the North American Indians to facilitate the course of childbirth. The early settlers learned of this and spread the use of the root for female troubles. Other *Trillium* species are found in other continents, but tend to be rare. The color of their flowers varies from reddish-brown to white, pink, or greenish. The compact knotty rootstock produces a slim, straight tubular stem 20–40 cm high. This bears a whorl of 3 wavy pointed oval leaves, 10–15 cm in length, with margins entire and prominent veins. From the leaf axil rises the flowering stem, 5–10 cm in length, bearing a single reddish-brown, crimson, yellow, or greenish flower with an unpleasant odor. It has 3 persistent lance-shaped sepals and 3 petals of inverted egg-shape. The fruits are dark red tripartite angular berries.

TROPAEOLUM MAJUS

COMMON NASTURTIUM, GARDEN NASTURTIUM

Tropaeolaceae

230 S Am
Torrid + Temperate Zones

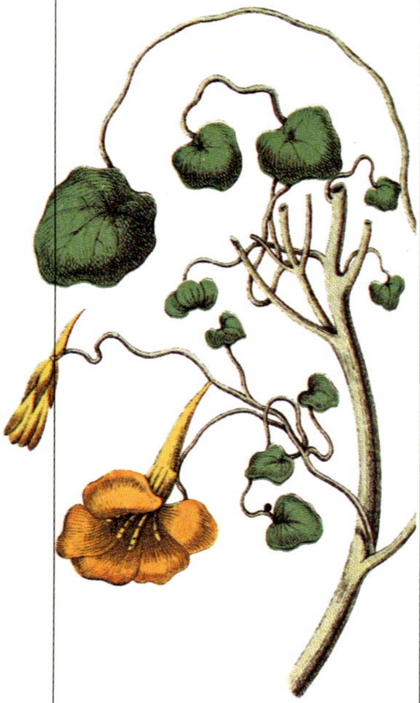

The nasturtium or Indian cress is indigenous to Peru, where it has for long been used in popular medicine to disinfect and heal wounds. The plant was brought to Europe in the seventeenth century and has become one of our best-loved garden flowers. The creeping rootstock produces angular green stems with round, kidney-shaped stalked leaves. The flowers are large and trumpet-shaped; they are bred in many colors, the most common being orange, yellow, and white, with the posterior sepal ending in a spur. Low-growing *(T. minus)* and climbing varieties are available. If chewed, the leaves have a sharp, mustard-like flavor. They contain appreciable amounts of vitamin C, as well as compounds with antibiotic properties. Pickled in vinegar, the flower buds may be used like capers. The flowers are added to salads, as a stimulant.

TURNERA DIFFUSA

DAMIANA

Turneraceae

231 C-S Am
C Am, N-S Am

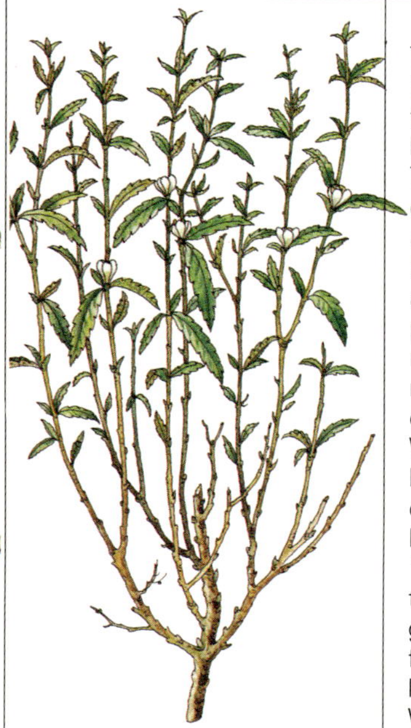

This shrub grows both wild and in cultivation in the hot, humid climate of the area around the Gulf of Mexico and in some South American countries. It branches a great deal and reaches a height of 2 m; in the plantations it is kept cut back to about 1 m. The smooth straight branches are yellow or reddish-brown. The small leaves are alternate or in small bunches. Their upper surface is olive green, the underside lightly covered with whitish hairs, and they have toothed margins. Small yellow flowers grow in the upper leaf axils. The fruits are small capsules, tripartite and slightly curved, with a rough skin. The leaves are occasionally used as a substitute for tea. Their aromatic, slightly bitter flavor makes them well suited to the purpose. They contain a volatile oil and also substances with disinfectant properties. The plant's traditional reputation is as an aphrodisiac.

TUSSILAGO FARFARA

COLTSFOOT

Asteraceae, Compositae

232 Eur, W Asia
N Am

Tussilago derives from the Latin *tussis* = (cough), and is the name given to this plant by herbalists in antiquity. The coltsfoot is one of the earliest spring flowers and adorns damp waysides, the banks of brooks and rivers, and sandy and clayey waste places from lowlands to medium-high mountain regions. The rootstock produces creeping shoots. When the snow has melted; hairy flowering stems, covered with brown scaly leaves, grow to a height of 10–12 cm. These bear the terminal flowerheads, with golden-yellow tubular disk florets surrounded by lighter-colored ray florets. When the flowering is finished, the stems grow to 20–25 cm. They now bear a sphere of white down, the flying equipment for the seeds. Meanwhile the long-stemmed basal leaves have appeared. These are rounded, heart-shaped, and grow to 20 cm in length, with their margins incurving and, at intervals, toothed. Smooth and rich green on top, they are covered with a whitish down on the underside. The fresh leaves are used as a wound dressing (first washed and crushed), and the dried flowers and leaves are used in cough remedies, since they contain much mucilage, tannins, and floral pigments.

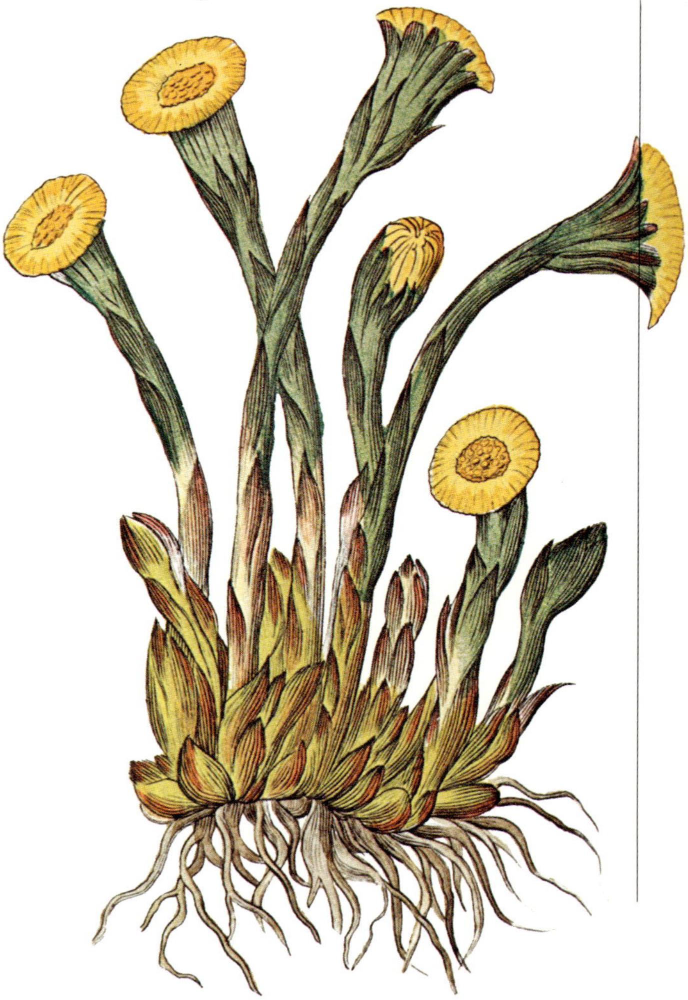

ULMUS MINOR (ULMUS GLABRA)

SMALL-LEAF ELM, SMOOTH ELM

Ulmaceae

233 a) C+S Eur, NW Af, SW Asia
b) Eur, SW Asia
N Am

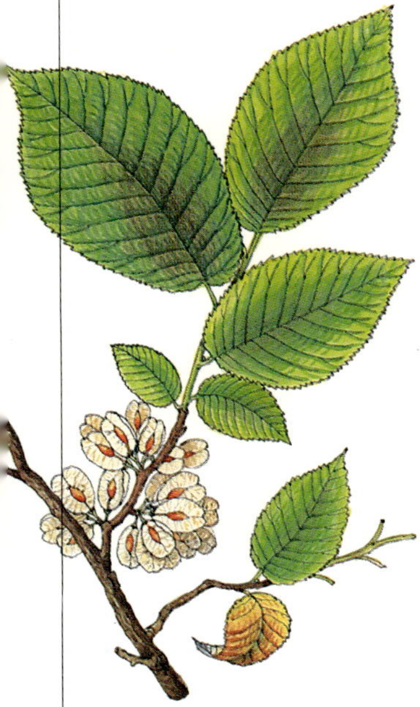

The elm is a handsome foliage tree requiring warmth with plenty of light and a good depth of soil rich in minerals. The slender trunk has a smooth brown bark which later becomes rough and fissured. It grows to a height of up to 40 m and may become several hundred years old. The more robust wych or Scots elm *(U. glabra)* does not need such a warm climate and is often planted in parks and avenues. The flowers appear before the leaves in early spring. They are bisexual and grow in small, short-stalked red or yellow tufts. The alternate leaves are strong, irregularly oval, pointed, a glossy dark green on top and lighter colored on the underside, and have toothed margins. The fruits are unstalked smooth nutlets at the center of a wing disk. The bark of young branches is used in homeopathy and, less commonly, by herbalists. It contains tannins and mucilage.

URGINEA MARITIMA

SEA ONION, RED SQUILL

Liliaceae

234 S Eur, N Af
Warm Temperate Zones

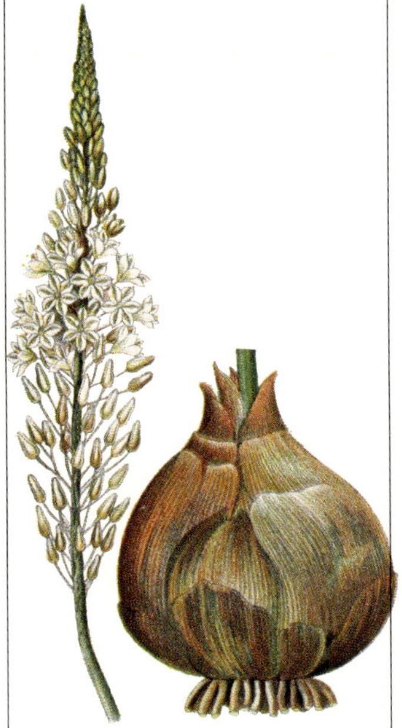

The sea onion is found in sandy soil and on sea coasts around the Mediterranean, mostly growing wild, but occasionally also cultivated (Algeria, Morocco). The base of the "onion" is a flat disk with fibrous roots. Its bulb consists of numerous fleshy scale leaves, the outer ones being near white or red. The bulb may weigh 1–3 kg (the red Algerian may even weigh 6 kg) and grows to the size of a small cabbage. The broadly lance-shaped leaves grow from the top of the bulb when the flowering is over; they dry out in early summer. From July to September, a leafless flowering stem grows to a height of 1–2 m. On its upper third this bears a spike of numerous flowers, white and occasionally with a tinge of red, opening in succession from below upward. The bulbs are harvested before the leaves appear. Only the inner scales of the white variety are used medicinally. They contain principles with an action similar to Digitalis.

URTICA DIOICA/ URTICA URENS

STINGING NETTLE, SMALL NETTLE

Urticaceae

235 Eur, Asia
Temperate Zones

The nettles are ruderal plants, meaning they like to grow in soil rich in nitrogen, which usually is close to houses or stables. They are unusual not only because their leaves and stems are covered with stinging hairs, but also for their high content in chlorophyll and a relatively high concentration of iron. The young shoots are rich in vitamin C. One only has to touch a nettle to discover the extraordinary power of its poison sting. The smallest quantity of this is enough to cause an instant burning sensation. When the sting pierces the skin, it produces a burning, itching weal with reddening of the surrounding skin area. This skin irritant effect is used for pharmaceutic purposes. Branching underground stems produce numerous shoots (self-propagation) which grow into erect, unbranched, square stems. The stalked alternate leaves are heart-shaped with elongated points and have strongly toothed margins. They are a rich green and covered with hairs on both surfaces. In the stinging nettle, male and female flowers appear on separate plants (*dioica*=two houses), in the leaf axils. The male grow in erect greenish catkins; the female in more extended, hanging catkins. Nettles are most active during the flowering season. *Urtica dioica* grows to a height of 50–150 cm. *Urtica urens* reaches only 30–60 cm, has smaller leaves, and male and female flowers are on the same plant.

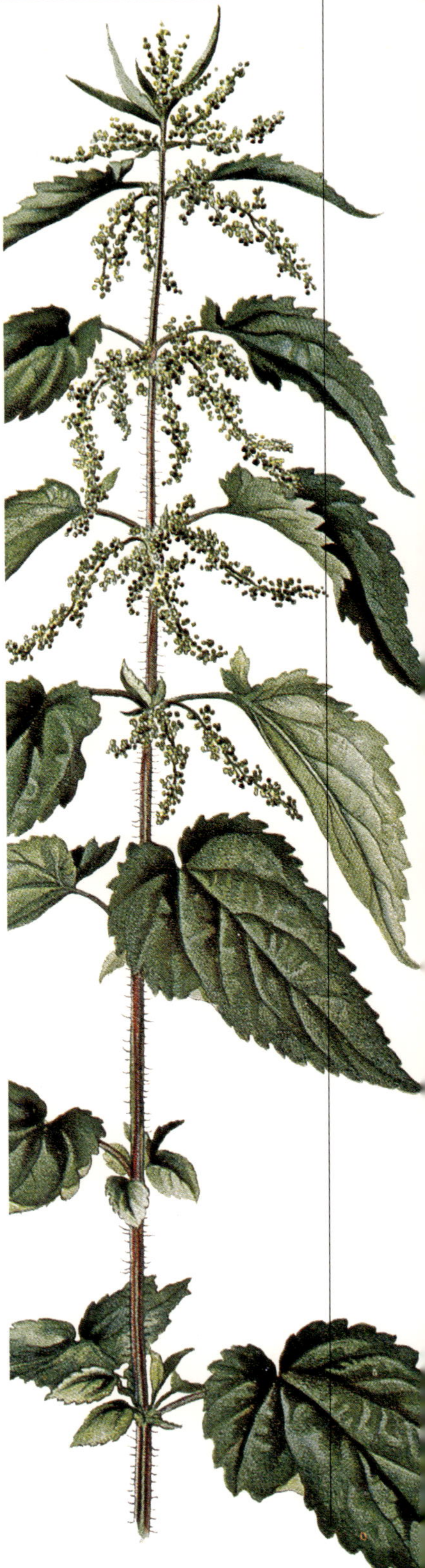

USNEA BARBATA

OLD MAN'S BEARD, BEARDED USNEA

Usneaceae

236 Temperate Zones

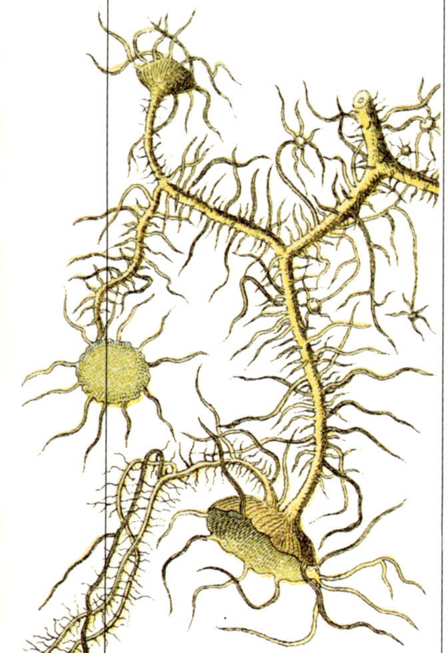

Bearded lichens are the beard-like greenish-gray growths hanging from the branches of fir trees growing in damp woods. They are plant-like structures formed by an association of algae and fungi living in symbiosis. The outer body usually consists of a network of fungal components, with the algae embedded within it. Lichens are able to withstand extreme environmental conditions. They are found on stones and rocks, and on dead and living wood. There are about 18,000 species, classified in 200 genera. Like most species of pharmaceutical interest, the bearded lichens are fruticose (shrubby or bushy). The Cetraria lichens *(Lichen islandicus)* yield valuable mucilage. *Usnea barbata* contains usnic acid, which has some antibiotic activity. Use is made of it in the preparation of products designed to improve resistance to disease.

VACCINIUM MYRTILLUS

BILBERRY, WHORTLEBERRY

Ericaceae

237 Eur, W Asia

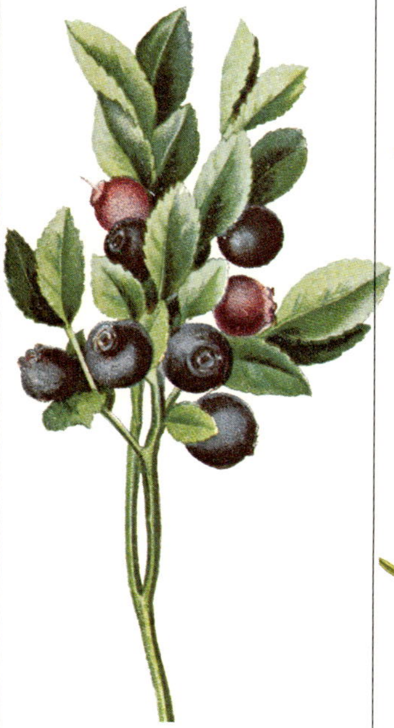

The *Ericaceae* (heath family) are a prominent feature not only of heathlands in northern countries and mountain regions, but also in South Africa. Bilberry is a small half-shrub found mainly on moors, in humus-rich soil, and in open woods from lowlands to mountains. The creeping rootstock branches below ground and produces extensive colonies. The runners produce green, partly woody, angular stems which grow to a height of 20–50 cm. These bear alternate short-stemmed leaves that are egg-shaped and bright green with finely toothed margins. In early summer, charming small yellowish-green or reddish bell-shaped flowers appear on the leaf axils. The globular, flat-topped, blue-black berries begin ripening in August. Their juice has a high vitamin content. The skin of the berry contains tannin and a blue pigment which is effective in the treatment of diarrhea.

VALERIANA OFFICINALIS

VALERIAN, GARDEN HELIOTROPE

Valerianaceae

238 Eur, Asia
Temperate Zones

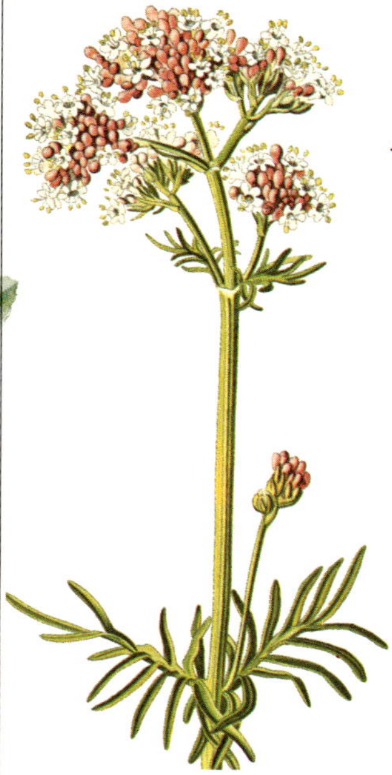

The valerian likes damp places on the banks of streams and rivers and marshy meadows. It is cultivated for its root in several central and northeastern parts of Europe. Other varieties of valerian also grow on limestone *(V. montana)* and in mountain woods. The stout rootstock produces many secondary roots and a round, fluted stem which grows to a height of 80–120 cm with opposite pairs of branches at the top only. The large, juicy green leaves are divided into 9–21 leaflets. These are dark green on the upper surface, a lighter color below and their margins are toothed at intervals. The stems terminate in umbel-like clusters of small, pale pink flowers. While in a true umbel, the flower stems rise in one point, in this case they are produced by repeated branching. The fresh plant has no scent. The typical odor of valerian is perceivable only faintly in the fresh root.

VERATRUM VIRIDE

FALSE HELLEBORE, AMERICAN HELLEBORE

Liliaceae

239 E-N Am

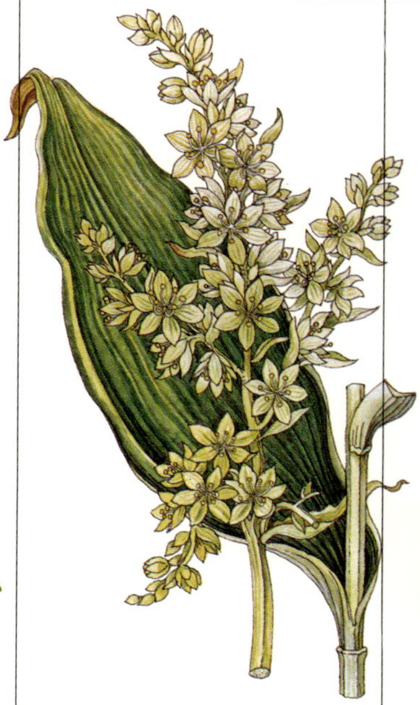

The white hellebore *(Veratrum album)* is found chiefly in the hills and montains of Europe. False hellebore, on the other hand, is indigenous to North America. There is practically no difference between the two as regards their active principles. Both are highly poisonous and irritate the skin or mucous membranes. Damp meadows and swamps provide a suitable habitat for the thick cylindrical rootstock with its numerous roots. This produces a tubular nonflowering stem up to 1.5 m in height. The large leaves, pleated lengthwise and with prominent veins, are alternate around the stem, their sheath extending down to the rootstock. The lower leaves are 20–25 cm long, elliptical and terminating in a point, while those higher up are shorter and narrower. The flowering stem appears less often, not usually every year. It terminates in a tall spike of small green or white star-shaped flowers.

VERBASCUM PHLOMOIDES/ VERBASCUM DENSIFLORUM

MULLEIN

Scrophulariaceae

240 Eur, W Asia

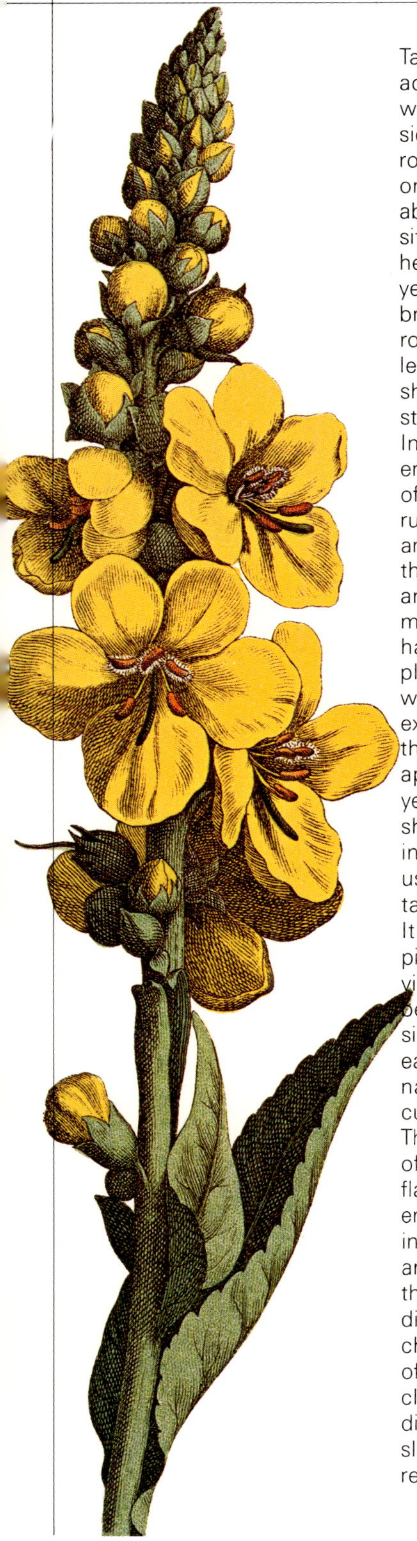

Tall and stately, the mullein adorns slopes of rubble, railway embankments, and waysides. With its deep-reaching root and dense cover of hair on its leaves and stems, it is able to flourish in quite arid sites and stand up to the heat of the sun. In the first year, the spindle-shaped, branching root produces a rosette of large elongated leaves which are lance-shaped, end in a point, and stay close to the ground.
In the second year, the flowering stem rises to a height of more than 2 m with leaves running down into the stem and growing smaller toward the top. The stem and leaves are covered with a dense mass of yellowish-white hairs – a typical feature of plants containing mucilage which protects them from excessive evaporation. On the upper part of the stem appear numerous golden-yellow flowers with 5 egg-shaped petals opening out into a wheel. The flowers are used medicinally. They contain mucilage and saponins. It is possible that the floral pigment also has medicinal virtues. The flowers need to be dried with great care since they can turn dark easily and lose their medicinal action. The mullein is cultivated in many countries. The particular combination of mucilage, saponins, and flavonoids found in the flowers is of considerable medicinal interest and the flowers are used in modern phytotherapy to treat respiratory diseases, particularly bronchitis. Many different uses of the plant have been claimed, for ailments as diverse as tumors and sleeplessness, but they remain unconfirmed.

VIBURNUM PRUNIFOLIUM

BLACK HAW, STAGBUSH

Caprifoliaceae

241 E-N Am

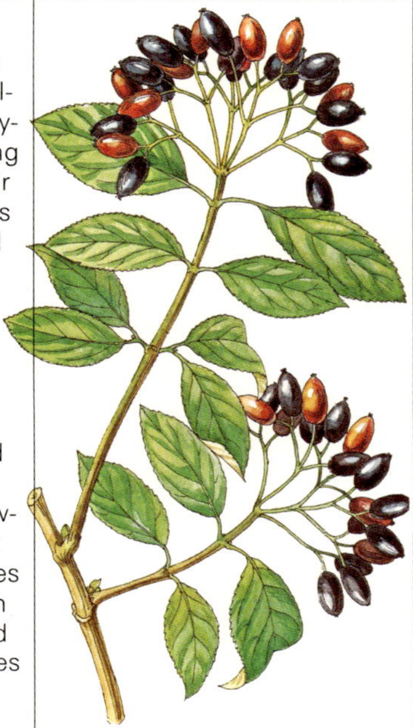

This is a handsome shrub or tree, up to 5 m high, growing in woods, on the edges of woods, in clearings and by the roadside, in dry or damp soil. The trunk and branches are dark gray to brown on the outside and much branched to produce a bushy growth at the top. The stalked opposite leaves are 5–8 cm long, elliptical, and pointed. They have toothed margins. The upper surface is a dark yellowish-green, with the underside a lighter color. The small white flowers grow in umbrella-shaped umbel-like terminal clusters, like white snowballs among the green foliage. The fruits are blue-black berries of an elongated egg-shape, each containing a flat seed. Properly ripened berries are said to be edible after the first frost, but even then they taste very sour. The bark of the trunk and branches is gray to gray-brown on the outside and yellowish-brown inside. An extract is prepared from it.

VIOLA ODORATA

ENGLISH VIOLET, SWEET VIOLET

Violaceae

242 S Eur *Temperate Zones*

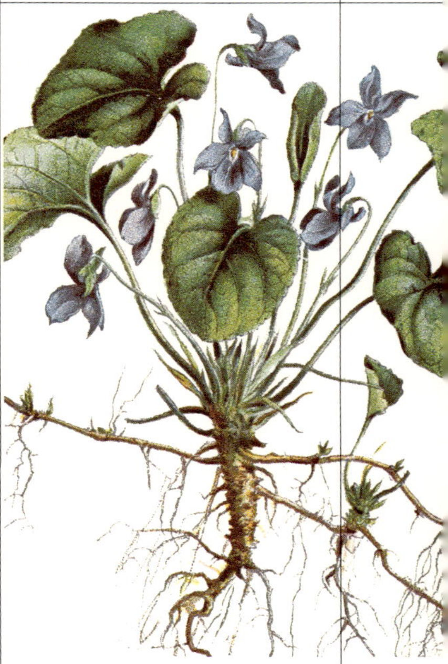

The violet family has numerous species. For centuries they have been popular as ornamental plants and cultivated in the Mediterranean regions for the perfume industry. The method used by most species to propagate themselves is by rooting runners. The sweet violet prefers shady places and friable soil among bushes, on sloping meadows, and along old walls. A short, thick rootstock, which is partly above ground, produces a rosette of stalked, dark green, heart-shaped leaves with lightly toothed margins. The long-stemmed, bluish-violet scented flowers appear at the same time. Later, larger leaves develop and smaller, less conspicuous flowering shoots appear with almost colorless, but fertile, flowers. The seeds are distributed by ants. The dried plant is used medicinally, sometimes with the root. Other species of violet also are collected. Important active principles are saponins and salicylic compounds.

VIOLA TRICOLOR

PANSY, HEARTSEASE

Violaceae

243 Eur, N Af, W Asia
Temperate Zones

The wild pansy, or heartsease, with its three-colored *(tricolor)* flowers may be regarded as the original ancestor of the garden pansy. It is one of the adventive plants which are the first to appear on fallow ground. Fields, sandy hills, dunes, and both dry and damp mountain pastures provide the most suitable conditions for this annual or biennial herb. The angular stems, which branch at straight angles, may be creeping or erect and bear small opposite elongated oval leaves with lightly toothed margins and divided leaflets (stipules) at the base of the stalk. From the very distinct leaf axils grow slender leafless flowering stalks bearing the beautifully formed, generally 3-colored flowers. Two petals (usually violet) stand upright, 2 are bent back sideways, and the lowest and largest petal (usually yellow or blue) continues into a spur filled with nectar. The field pansy appears in many subspecies which differ primarily in the color of the flowers and shape of the leaves. Various species are used medicinally, with the whole herb dried and cut. They contain saponins, flavonoids, and salicylic compounds.

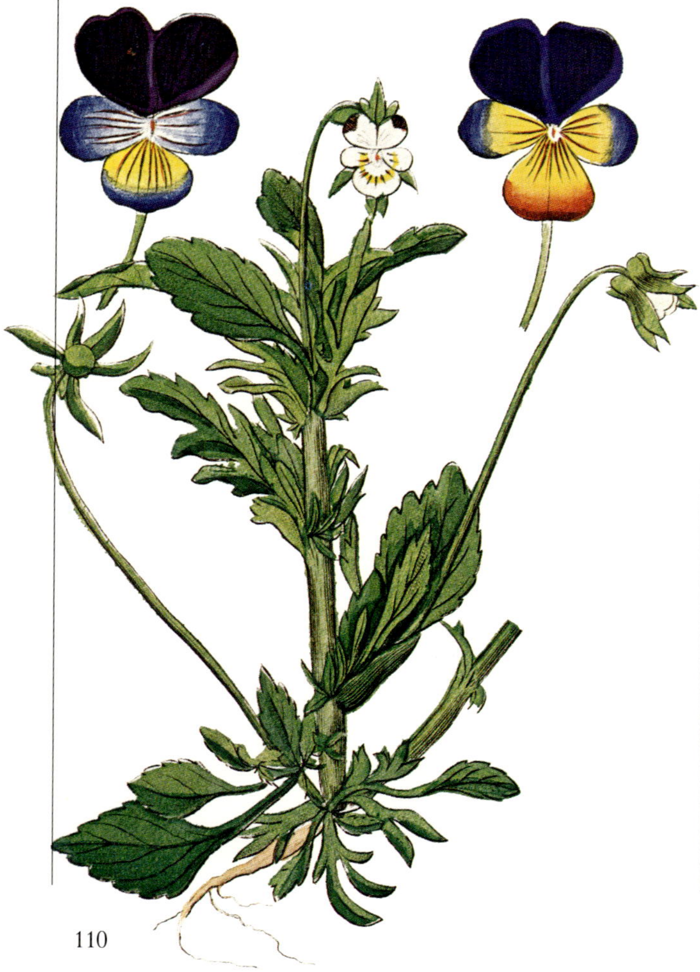

VISCUM ALBUM

EUROPEAN MISTLETOE

Loranthaceae

244 Eur, N Af, Asia

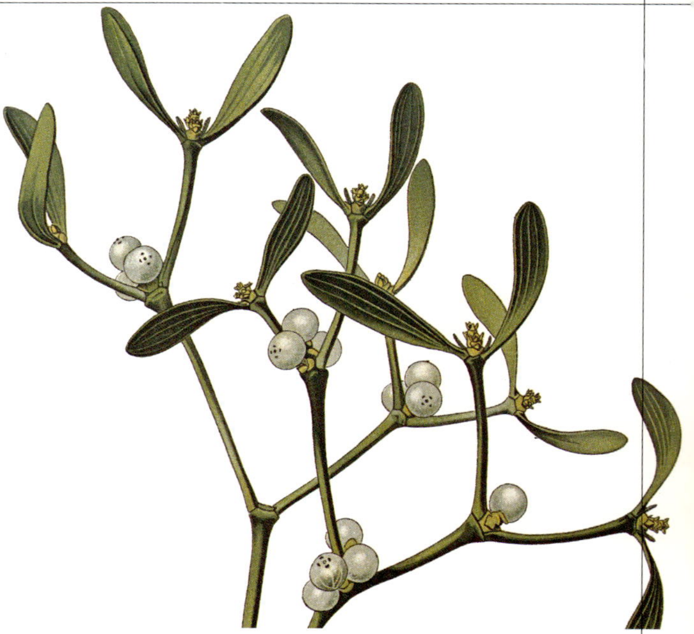

Mistletoe is a semiparasitic plant which draws water and minerals from its host. For medicinal use, mistletoe grown on deciduous trees, usually on lateral branches in the upper part of the crown, is preferred. It is generally harvested in winter. The bush consists of regular greenish-brown branches growing from a short trunk. The pale green leathery leaves look like small propellers at the ends of their stems. They have parallel veins and remain green throughout the winter, dropping only after 2 years. In spring, small, scarcely visible, male or female flowers (on different plants) appear at the branching points. They develop into white spherical berries full of mucilage. The berries are inedible, though birds do eat them and thus transfer the seeds to other trees. The leaves contain some interesting active principles which as yet have not been fully explored. They slightly reduce the blood pressure and promote the flow of urine, but are best used in the form of pharmaceutical preparations. Clinical trials are now in progress on the anticancer actions of certain constituents of mistletoe.

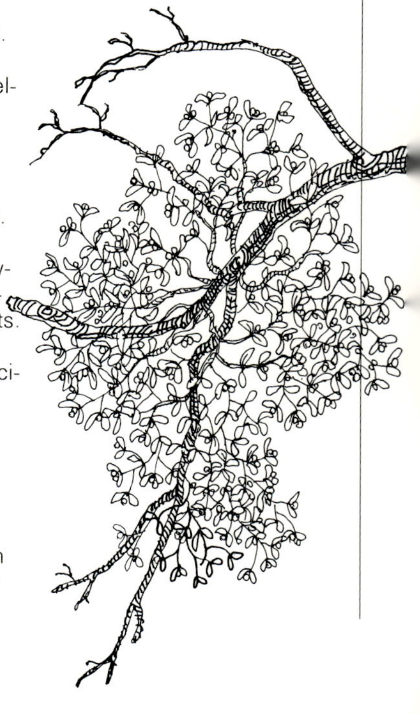

VITEX AGNUS-CASTUS

CHASTE TREE, HEMP TREE

Verbenaceae

245 S Eur, W Asia
S-N Am

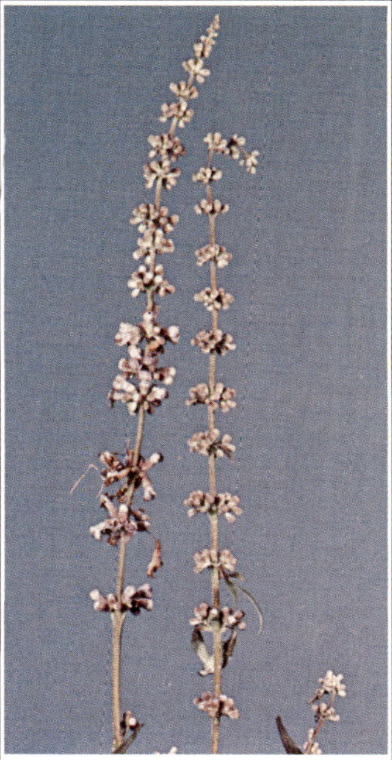

This shrub native to the Orient has rather unusual leaves. In antiquity it was regarded as a symbol of chastity. During the Middle Ages, extracts of the fruits were used to suppress sexual excitability, as the popular names given to the plant still indicate. It now seems probable that *Agnus-castus* extracts may act on certain hormone-producing glands. The shrub grows 3–5 m high, its dense branches dividing frequently at the top. The large dark green leaves are composed of 5–9 narrow segments radiating from a long, hairy leafstalk. The shoots terminate in a slender spike, about 30 cm in length, composed of whorls of violet flowers. The fruits are black spherical berries, 5 mm in size, with 4 seeds. They contain the active principles—a volatile oil, glycosides, and flavonoids as tips of the flowering shoots. Comparable principles are obtained from other species of *Vitex* in the tropics.

VITIS VINIFERA

GRAPE, VINE

Vitaceae

246 SE Eur, SW Asia
Warm Temperate Zones

The grape vine is one of the oldest cultivated plants. In its native habitat, in the Caucasus, the Crimea, and Asia, it grows wild in the woods of the great river valleys, its roots penetrating deeply and its stems clambering up to 20 m high. The numerous cultivated varieties are kept short, letting them grow to about 2 m, to encourage fruiting. During the first few years, the plant develops a root which may reach several meters in length, and above ground a stocky, gnarled stem, the actual vine. This produces numerous shoots which are carefully pruned and trained. The shoots bear handsome short-stemmed alternate leaves, each the size of a hand, with 5 lobes and bluntly toothed margins. The plant holds on to stakes and trellises with tendrils growing opposite to the leaves. The insignificant greenish-yellow flowers grow in pendant clusters and develop by autumn into the familiar grapes of many berries. Grape juice has a high content of dextrose and also contains vitamins and mineral salts. Large quantities of it are fermented to produce wine. The leaves contain tannin, organic acids, flavonoids, and mineral salts. Medicinally the "grape vine" has of recent years taken a new lease on life.

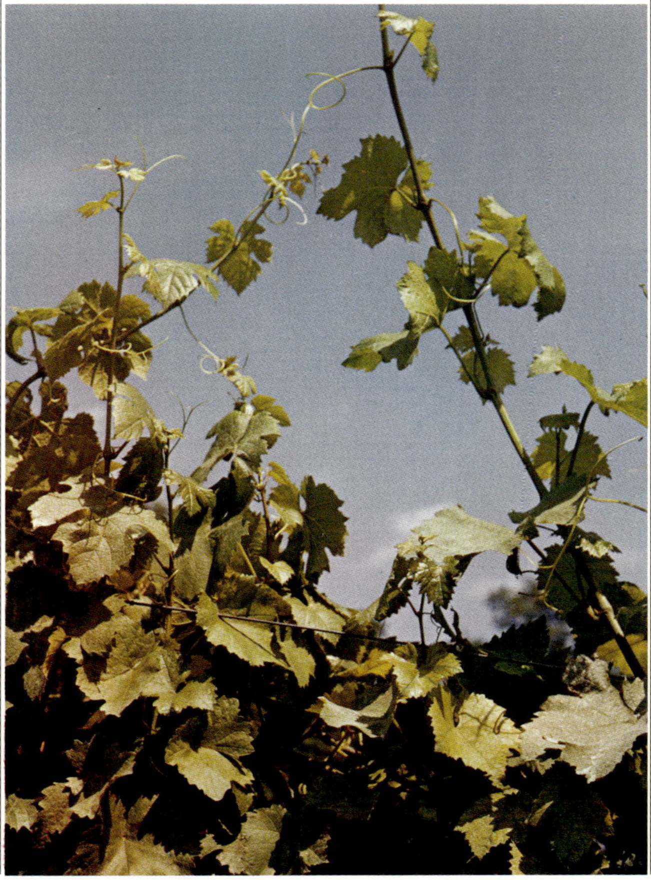

ZINGIBER OFFICINALE

GINGER

Zingiberaceae

247 S Asia
Torrid Zones

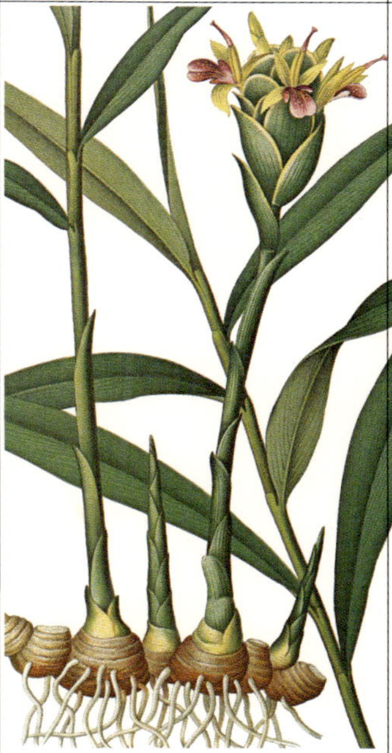

Ginger has been cultivated for centuries, its popularity as a spice gradually spreading from China and India to the West, until today it is probably one of the most universally popular spices. From the tuberous, creeping rootstock grow short tuberous joints, usually laterally compressed. These produce leafy stems about 1.5 m in length with narrow lance-shaped leaves about 20 cm long and 1.5–2.5 cm wide. The closely packed spikes of flowers grow on separate, shorter stems. The flowers are purple and yellow spotted and have large green bracts with yellow margins. The roots are dug when the leaves have died down. They are scraped, washed, and dried in the sun after removing the outer bark. The dried plant drug consists of yellowish-white and frequently slightly reddish pieces of root, sold in cuts according to requirements. Pharmaceutical interest attaches to the volatile oil.

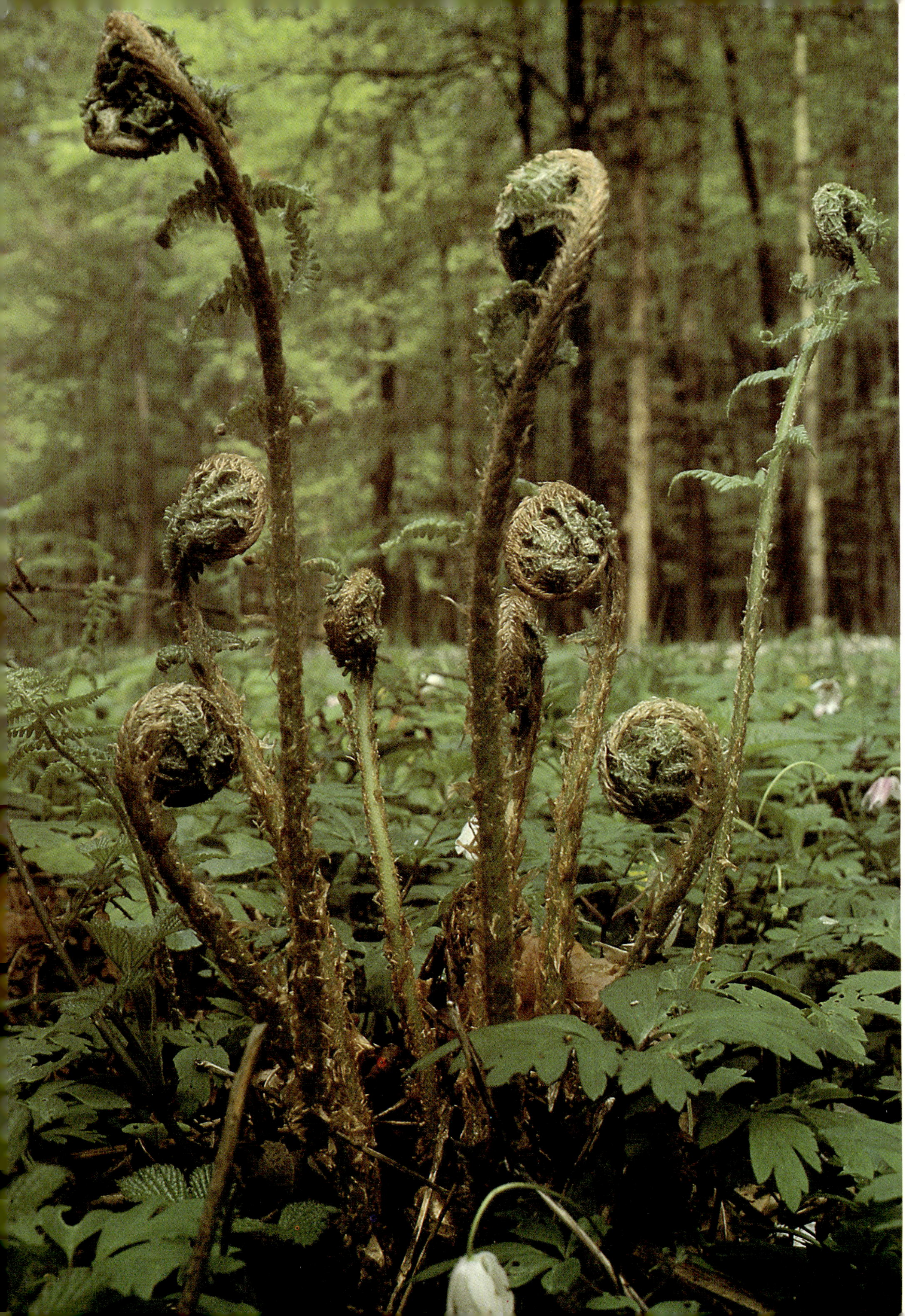

Complaints and Illnesses

Reference Section II

In this section some of the commoner complaints for which herbal remedies may be used are listed alphabetically, along with notes on the form in which the plant is used. Further instructions on how to prepare the plant, for example as tea, tincture, or the like, will be found beginning on page 151.

Until very recent times, a doctor was an expensive luxury which only a small section of the community could afford. It was Mother or Grandmother who made the diagnosis and prescribed, prepared, and administered the appropriate remedy. On occasion, she might consult the itinerant "quack" on market day or, in more recent times, the local pharmacist. In the Middle Ages the lady of the manor assumed that it was part of her duty to help those of her husband's tenants who were ill, and therefore she maintained a herb garden where she grew, harvested, and prepared the appropriate plants for treating her family, staff, and tenants. The Church, too, cared for the bodies, as well as the souls, of mankind, their herb gardens being among some of the most famous in Europe.

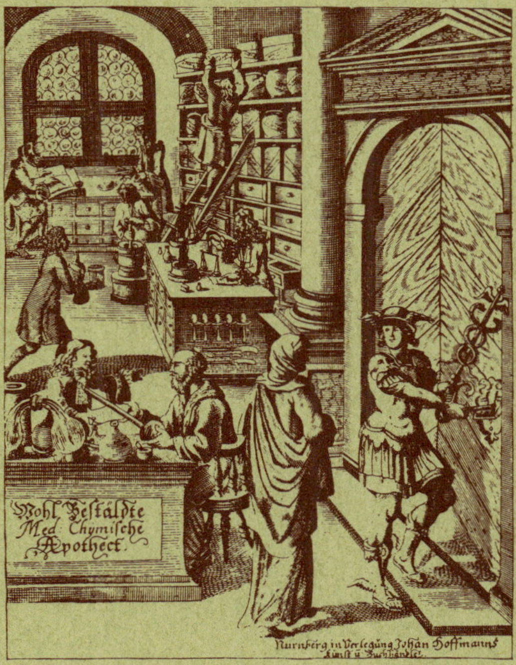

Woodcut illustration of a seventeenth-century apothecary shop: a sign of the rise of chemical procedures in medicine, and the deemphasis of herbal remedies. From the 1685 German edition of the *Pharmacopoea medico-chymica* by the prominent physician Johann Schröder.

Today, doctors are being so overwhelmed by patients that they do not have the opportunity to give adequate time and attention to those sufferers who require more than a cursory consultation. What is necessary, therefore, is that the pendulum should be allowed to swing back toward the happy medium. People should be prepared and able to diagnose those minor ailments to which we are all heir and treat them ourselves. For many ailments (e.g., the common cold, rheumatic aches and pains) there is, unfortunately, no specific remedy and all that can be done is to give Nature an opportunity of rectifying matters. This, fortunately, she usually does. Much, however, can often be done to aid the natural healing process, and the patient, if an adult, or the mother, in case of a child, can do as much as the doctor. To rush off to the doctor to seek advice in these circumstances is not necessary. Indeed, it is not justified because it takes the doctor's valuable time and thereby penalizes those patients for whom a skilled medical opinion is necessary, or even lifesaving.

On the other hand, this self-diagnosis and self-treatment must be practiced with discretion. This is particularly true concerning babies. Indeed, during the first year of life, there is much to be said for the rule of never giving any medication without medical advice. The sound rule is for the mother to heed all the advice she is given, during her first pregnancy, at the pre-natal clinic and from her mother. With this and a modicum of common sense, she should have little difficulty in coping with the minor ailments of her firstborn. As her family grows, so does her skill.

In the case of the adult the golden rule is not to persist with self-medication if the condition being treated does not show signs of improving. The other obvious rule to obey is to seek medical advice immediately when any acute condition develops (e.g., acute abdominal pain). Any appreciable rise in temperature indicates that a doctor's opinion should be sought.

For many of our minor ailments, however, self-medication is fully justified, and this section is presented as a guide to help in making the right choice of herb.

WILLIAM A.R. THOMSON, M.D.

Opposite:
Male Fern
(Dryopteris filix-mas)

Complaint	Plant	Form of application	Preparation and dose	Notes
APPETITE LOSS	150 Buckbean	Tea	Place 1 teaspoon dried or fresh leaves in 1 cup cold water, bring to a boil, remove. Let stand 5–10 minutes. Take 1 cup 15–30 minutes before each meal.	All remedies for a failing appetite are to be taken approximately ½ hour before meals.
	50 Centaury	Tea	Pour 1 cup boiling water over 1 teaspoon dried or fresh chopped herb. Let stand 5–10 minutes. Take 1 cup, 15–30 minutes before main meals.	
		Wine	Pour 1.5 liters (1.5 quarts) white wine over 60 g (2 oz) centaury, 40 g (1.5 oz) chamomile blossoms, 40 g (1.5 oz) finely chopped orange peel, and the juice of 2 oranges. Let stand, corked, at least 1 week in the sun or in a warm place. Filter. Take ½ wine glass 2–3 times daily before meals.	
	3 Sweet flag	Tea	Pour 1 cup boiling water over 2 teaspoons shredded root (with root bark removed). Let stand at least 15 minutes. Drink lukewarm.	
	105 Yellow gentian	Tea	Boil ½ teaspoon shredded root in 1 cup water for 2 minutes. Let stand 5–10 minutes. *Or:* Pour 1 cup hot water over ½ teaspoon shredded root. Let stand 4–5 hours. Take 1 cup, 15–30 minutes before each meal.	
		Tincture	Mix 20–40 drops in ½ glass water before meals.	
ARTERIO-SCLEROSIS	74 Artichoke	Tea	Pour 1 cup cold water over 1–2 teaspoons dried leaves. Bring to the boil, let boil 1 minute. Let stand 5–10 minutes. Take 1 cup 2–3 times daily for 1 week or longer.	
		Extract	Can be bought in specially prepared form. Use as directed.	
	10 Bear's garlic	Fresh plant	Just before serving, shred several fresh leaves. Add to salad, cooked soup, or vegetables. Take daily throughout spring season.	
		Tea	Pour 1 cup hot water over 1–2 teaspoons dried leaves. Let stand 5–10 minutes. Take 1 cup twice daily.	
	244 European mistletoe	Tea	Pour 1 cup cold water over 2–3 teaspoons fresh or dried shredded mistletoe branches. Let stand 8 hours. Take 1 cup morning and evening for several weeks or even longer.	
	9 Garlic	Fresh plant	Finely chop or crush 1 clove fresh garlic. Spread on bread, or mix in lukewarm milk. Take 1 clove several times daily for several weeks or even longer.	
ASTHMA	130 Elecampane	Tea	Pour 1 cup cold water over 1–2 teaspoons shredded root. Let stand 8–10 hours. Reheat. Take very hot, in small sips, sweetened with honey; 1 cup twice daily.	

	83 Ephedra	Tea	Pour 1 cup boiling water over 1 teaspoon dried herb. Let stand 5–10 minutes. Take 1 cup 2–3 times daily.	
		Tincture	Take 15–20 drops in water, 2–3 times daily.	Can also be taken in an acute asthma attack, on doctor's advice.
	80 Sundew	Tea	Pour 1 cup boiling water over ½–1 teaspoon dried herb. Let stand 5–10 minutes. Take 1 cup twice daily, sweetened with honey to taste.	Sundew dyes the urine a dark color (a harmless side effect).
		Tincture	Pour 50–70 percent alcohol (5 parts) over 1 handful (1 part) fresh chopped herb. Let stand in a well-sealed container for 8–10 days in the sun or in a warm place. Shake often. Strain. Take 10 drops diluted with water, 2–3 times daily.	
	77 Thornapple	Powder	Pour out 1 teaspoon dried leaves onto a plate. Ignite with match, inhale the smoke. Use as needed.	Posisonous plant. Use only with a doctor's prescription.
		Asthma cigarettes	Mix 2 parts loose tobacco with 1 part dried thornapple leaves (which may be treated first in a solution of ammonium nitrate). Roll the mixture in a cigarette paper. In case of an attack, smoke the cigarette slowly and with care.	
		Tincture	Doctor's prescription.	
BILIARY DISORDERS: *(see Liver Ailments)*				
BLADDER STONES	224 Dandelion	Tea	Place 1–2 teaspoons fresh or dried root (or mixture of root and leaves) in 1 cup water. Bring to boil, remove from heat. Let stand 20 minutes. Take 1 cup 3 times daily for 4–6 weeks. Repeat several times per year.	
		Combined tea	Combine equal parts of dandelion root, juniper berries, parsley seeds, and rupturewort to make 1 tablespoon total. Pour ½ liter (1 pint) boiling water over the mixture, let stand 20 minutes. Take 2 cups each morning.	
	14 Khella	Commercial preparation	Khella is available only in commercial preparations.	
	197 Madder	Tea	Pour 1 cup cold water over ½–1 teaspoon shredded root. Let stand 8 hours. Take 1 cup twice daily.	Madder dyes the urine red (a harmless side effect).
		Powder	Stir 1 g (3/100 oz) pulverized root into 1–2 tablespoons water or honey (to taste). Take 3 times daily.	
	120 Rupturewort	Tea	Pour 1 cup hot water over 1 teaspoon chopped herb (fresh or dried). Let stand ½ hour. Take 1 cup 3 times daily. *Or:* Pour 1 cup cold water over 1 teaspoon chopped herb. Let stand 8 hours. Take 1 cup, reheated, 3 times daily.	Also useful for kidney stones.

Complaint	Plant	Form of application	Preparation and dose	Notes
BLOOD PRESSURE, HIGH	244 European mistletoe	Tea	Pour 1 cup cold water over 2–3 teaspoons chopped herb (fresh or dried). Let stand 8 hours. Take 1 cup mornings and evenings for several weeks or months.	
	9 Garlic	Fresh plant	Finely slice or crush 1 fresh garlic clove. Spread on bread or mix in lukewarm milk. Take 1 clove 2–3 times daily for several months.	Garlic is effective only after prolonged, regular use.
		Juice	Press 2–3 fresh garlic cloves. Drink mixed in warm milk or in honey. Take 2–3 times daily for several months.	
	70 Hawthorn	Tea	Pour 1 cup boiling water over 2 teaspoons blossoms (or blossoms and leaves, 1 teaspoon each). Let stand 20 minutes. Take 1 cup 2–3 times daily.	
	189 Indian snakeroot	Powder extract	Dosage according to doctor's prescription.	Use only on doctor's orders.
	154 Olive	Tea	Place 2 teaspoons leaves in 1 cup cold water, bring to boil, remove. Let stand 15–20 minutes. Take 1 cup after meals 2–3 times daily.	Olive leaves can irritate the stomach. Take only after meals.
BLOOD PRESSURE, LOW	158 American and Asiatic ginseng	Tea	Place ½ teaspoon shredded root in 1 cup water. Boil for 1 minute. Let stand 15 minutes. Take 1 cup twice daily.	
		Powder	Mix 1 pinch (1 g or 3/100 oz) pulverized root in 1–2 tablespoons water or other liquid. Take 2–3 times daily.	
	196 Rosemary	Tea	Pour 1 cup boiling water over 1 teaspoon fresh or dried leaves. Let stand 5–10 minutes. Take twice daily.	
		Bath	Pour ½ liter (1 pint) water over 1 handful (50 g) leaves. Let stand 20 minutes. Strain the liquid and add it to bath water Bathe at 34–36 °C (93–97 °F) for 10 minutes.	Has a stimulating, invigorating effect. Not for evening bath. Rest at least ½ hour after bath.
	4 Spring adonis	Tincture, extract	Dosage according to doctor's prescription.	Contains poisonous glycosides which affect heart. Use only on doctor's orders.
BRONCHITIS	232 Coltsfoot	Tea	Pour 1 cup boiling water over 1–2 teaspoons blossoms and/or leaves. Let stand 5–10 minutes. Take 1 cup 3–4 times daily, sweetened with honey, as hot as possible.	
	182 Cowslip	Tea	Place 1 teaspoon root in cup cold water. Boil 2–3 minutes. Let stand 10 minutes. Take 1 cup 3 times daily, rather hot, sweetened with honey. *Or:* Place 1–2 teaspoons blossoms with calyx in 1 cup cold water. Bring to simmer. Let stand 5–10 minutes. Take 1 cup 3 times daily, as hot as possible, sweetened with honey.	

		Combined tea	Combine equal parts of cowslip root (or blossoms), coltsfoot blossoms, and anise seeds to make total of 2 teaspoons. Place in 1 cup cold water. Bring to simmer. Let stand 15–20 minutes. Reheat. Take 1 cup 2–3 times daily, as hot as possible, sweetened with honey.	
	88 Eucalyptus	Tea	Pour 1 cup boiling water over 1–2 teaspoons dried leaves. Let stand 5–10 minutes. Take 1 cup sweetened with honey 2–3 times daily.	
		Bath	Combine equal parts eucalyptus and thyme leaves to make total of 4–5 tablespoons. Pour 1 liter (1 quart) boiling water over the mixture. Let stand 30 minutes. Strain. Add liquid to bath water. Bathe at 38 °C (100 °F) for 10–15 minutes.	
		Rub	Dilute 1 part Eucalyptol (from pharmacy) with 5 parts water. Rub on chest and back several times daily, especially in the evening.	
	55 Irish Moss	Tea	Place 1 teaspoon shredded moss in 1 cup cold water. Boil 3 minutes. Let stand 10 minutes. Take 1 cup mornings and evenings.	
	243 Pansy	Tea	Place 1 teaspoon root in 1 cup cold water. Boil 2–3 minutes. Let stand 10 minutes. *Or:* Pour 1 cup boiling water over 2 teaspoons fresh or dried leaves and blossoms. Let stand 5–10 minutes. Take 1 cup twice daily, as hot as possible, sweetened with honey.	
BRUISES, CONTUSIONS	27 Arnica	Compress	Mix 1 tablespoon arnica tincture in ½ liter (1 pint) cool water. Make compress. Apply frequently. *Preparation of the tincture:* Pour ½ liter (1 pint) 70 percent alcohol over 1 handful (50 g) freshly picked arnica blossoms. Seal tightly in clear glass container and let stand at least 1 week in the sun. Filter.	
	40 Marigold	Compress	Pour ½ liter (1 pint) boiling water over 1–2 teaspoons of chopped herb. Let stand 15 minutes. Make cool compress. Apply frequently. *Or:* Use marigold tincture-compress (see Eczema, below).	
	113 Witch hazel	Compress	Place 1–2 tablespoons leaves and/or bark in ½ liter (1 pint) cold water. Boil 15 minutes, let stand until cool. Make cool compress. Apply frequently. Do not allow compress to dry out.	
	147 Yellow sweetclover	Compress	Place 2 tablespoons chopped herb (fresh or dried) in ½ liter cold water. Heat; let boil 1 minute. Let stand 20 minutes. Make cool compress. Apply frequently.	
BURNS	13 Marsh mallow	Compress	Pour ½ liter (1 pint) cold water over 1–2 tablespoons shredded root (or 2 tablespoons leaves). Let stand 6–8 hours. Make loose compress. Repeat often.	Only for mild burns.
	73 Quince	Compress	Pour ½ liter (1 pint) cold water over 2 tablespoons seeds. Let stand several hours. Collect the slime from seeds and place it on a linen towel. Apply to burned areas. Several times daily.	Only for mild burns.

Complaint	Plant	Form of application	Preparation and dose	Notes
CIRCULATORY DISORDERS	108 Ginkgo	Tea	Pour 1 cup boiling water over 2–3 teaspoons leaves. Let stand 15 minutes. Take 1 cup twice daily.	
		Commercial preparation	Dosage according to instructions on package, or doctor's prescription.	The more effective commercial preparations are those made from fresh leaves.
	70 Hawthorn	Tea	Pour 1 cup boiling water over 2 teaspoons blossoms or leaves (or equal combination of both). Let stand 20 minutes. Take 1 cup hot, sweetened with honey, 2–3 times daily for several weeks or months.	Effective only after prolonged use.
	84 Horsetail	Bath	Heat 5 tablespoons dried chopped herb in 1 liter (1 quart) water. Boil 1 minute. Let stand 20 minutes. Strain the liquid and add to bath water. Bathe at 35°–37 °C (95°–98.5 °F) for 10 minutes.	
		Hand and foot bath	Place 2–3 tablespoons dried chopped herb in ½ liter (1 pint) water. Place the mixture in bath water. Bathe hand or foot at moderate heat.	
	136 Lavender	Combined tea	Combine equal parts of lavender blossoms and rosemary leaves. Pour 1 cup boiling water over 1 teaspoon of the mixture. Let stand, covered, 10–15 minutes. Take 1 cup mornings and evenings for several weeks.	
		Bath	Pour 1 liter (1 quart) boiling water over 100 g (3½ oz) blossoms. Let stand, covered, 20–30 minutes. Strain the liquid and add it to bath water. Bathe at 34°–36° (93°–97 °F) for 10 minutes 3 times weekly.	Bath has invigorating, stimulating effect. Do not bathe in evening.
	68 Lily-of-the-valley	Tea tincture	Dosage according to doctor's prescription	Poisonous plant. To be used only on doctor's orders.
	196 Rosemary	Tea	Pour 1 cup boiling water over 1 teaspoon leaves. Let stand, covered, 10 minutes. Take 1 cup twice daily (in daytime) for several weeks.	
		Bath	Pour 1 liter (1 quart) boiling water over 2 handfuls (about 100 g or 3½ oz) leaves. Let stand, covered, 20 minutes. Strain the liquid and add to bath water. Bathe at 34°–36 °C (93°–97 °F) for 10 minutes 3 times weekly.	Rest at least ½ hour after bath. Do not bathe in evening.
	171 Scotch pine	Bath	Place 100 g (3 oz) fresh or dried pine needles or twig ends in ½ liter (1 pint) water. Boil 1 minute. Let stand 20 minutes. Add to the bath water. Bathe at 34°–36° C (93–97° F) for 10 minutes.	
CLIMACTERIC, DISORDERS OF	8 Lady's mantle	Tea	Place 1–2 teaspoons leaves or herbs in 1 cup cold water. Bring to boil. Let stand 10 minutes. Take 1 cup mornings and evenings for several weeks.	
	137 Motherwort	Tea	Pour 1 cup boiling water over 1 teaspoon herb. Let stand 10 minutes. Take 1 cup mornings and evenings for several weeks.	

	127 Saint John's wort	Tea	Place 2 teaspoons chopped herb or fresh or dried blossoms in 1 cup cold water. Bring to a simmer. Let stand 15 minutes. Take 1 cup mornings and evenings for several weeks or months.	
COMMON COLD	236 Bearded usnea	Tea	Boil 1 handful of fresh or dried moss in ½ liter (1 pint) water for 2–3 minutes. Let stand 5–10 minutes. Take 1 cup twice daily.	
	227 Bigleaf linden	Tea	Pour 1 cup boiling water over 1 teaspoon fresh or dried blossoms. Let stand 10 minutes. Drink quite hot in small sips, 1 cup 2–3 times daily.	
		Combined tea	Combine equal parts bigleaf linden, European elder, and chamomile blossoms to make 1 teaspoon mixture. Pour 1 cup boiling water over the mixture. Let stand 5–10 minutes. Drink very hot in sips, 1 cup twice daily.	
	195 Dog Rose	Tea	Place 2 teaspoons shredded dried rose hips (with or without pits) in ½ liter (1 pint) cold water. Boil 10 minutes. Take 1 cup twice daily.	
	204 European elder	Tea	Pour 1 cup boiling water over 2 teaspoons dried or fresh blossoms. Let stand 10 minutes. Drink hot, 1 cup twice daily.	At the onset of a cold, after a hot bath take 2 cups elder blossom tea, or 2 glasses diluted elder juice, very hot in small sips.
		Juice	Boil fresh berries in water for 2–3 minutes, then express their juice. To preserve, bring juice to the boil with honey or sugar (1 part to 10 parts juice). Take 1 glass diluted with hot water (water should be as hot as possible) twice daily.	
	128 European holly	Tea	Boil 2 teaspoons dried leaves in 1 cup water for 2–3 minutes. Let stand 5–10 minutes. Take 1 cup twice daily.	Helps reduce fever.
	89 Hemp agrimony	Tea	Pour 1 cup boiling water over 1–2 teaspoons chopped herb. Let stand 5–10 minutes. Take 1 cup 2–3 times daily.	
	82 Purple coneflower	Tincture	Mix 10–20 drops in a little water, several times daily.	To be taken when infections begin, every 2 hours.
	92 Queen-of-the-meadow	Tea	Pour 1 cup boiling water over 2 teaspoons blossoms. Let stand 5–10 minutes. Take 1 cup twice daily.	Helps reduce fever.
	122 Sea buckthorn	Juice	Press ripe berries, with skins and pits, into a juice. For conservation, parboil with sugar or honey (1 part sugar or honey to 3 parts juice). Take 1 teaspoon, diluted with water if desired, 3 times daily.	Helps reduce fever.
	201 White willow	Tea	Boil 1 teaspoon dried bark in 1 cup water for 1 minute. Let stand 15 minutes. Take 1 cup twice daily.	Helps reduce fever.
	28 Wormwood	Tea	Pour 1 cup boiling water over 1 teaspoon chopped herb (fresh or dried). Let stand 5–10 minutes. Drink hot, 1 cup 3 times daily.	
	59 Yellowbark cinchona	Tea	Boil gently ½ teaspoon shredded bark in 1 cup water for 5 minutes. Let stand 5–10 minutes. Take 1 cup twice daily.	

Complaint	Plant	Form of application	Preparation and dose	Notes
CONSTIPATION	190 Alder buckthorn	Tea	Place 1 teaspoon stored, dried bark or berries in 1 cup cold water, bring to boil, boil 1 minute. Let stand 10–15 minutes. Take 1 cup in evening.	
	191 Cascara sagrada	Tea	Place 1 teaspoon aged, dried bark in 1 cup cold water. Bring to boil, boil 1 minute. Let stand 15 minutes. Take 1 cup evenings.	
	139 Flax	Porridge	Mix up 1–2 tablespoons whole or freshly ground flax seeds with a little water to make a porridge. Eat 1–2 times daily.	Recommended for long-term use.
	47 Senna	Tea	Pour 1 cup cold water over 1–2 teaspoons leaves or 5 pods. Let stand 6–8 hours. Take 1 cup evenings.	
		Combined tea	Combine equal parts of senna leaves, cascara sagrada bark, fennel seeds, and chamomile blossoms. Pour 1 cup boiling water over 1–2 teaspoons of this mixture. Let stand, covered, 10–15 minutes. Take 1 cup evenings.	
COUGHS	169 Anise	Tea	Gently crush 1–2 teaspoons seeds. Pour 1 cup boiling water over the seeds. Let stand, covered, 15 minutes. Reheat. Drink as hot as possible, 1 cup 2–3 times daily.	
	174 English plantain	Tea	Pour 1 cup boiling water over 2 teaspoons leaves or chopped herb. Let stand, covered, 10–15 minutes. Take 1 cup hot, sweetened with honey, 2–3 times daily.	
		Syrup	Shred the fresh herb or leaves and press out juice. Combine juice with equal amount of honey or brown sugar. Heat, boil 20 minutes. Take 1 tablespoon of the syrup 2–3 times daily.	Recommended for children.
	109 Licorice	Tea	Boil 1–2 teaspoons shredded root in 1 cup water for 1 minute. Let stand 10 minutes. Take 1 cup twice daily.	
	240 Mullein	Tea	Pour 1 cup hot water over 1–2 teaspoons dried blossoms. Let stand 10 minutes. Take 1 cup hot, sweetened with honey, 2–3 times daily.	
	226 Thyme	Tea	Pour 1 cup boiling water over 1–2 teaspoons leaves or chopped herb (fresh or dried). Let stand, covered, 10 minutes. Take 1 cup 3 times daily.	For spasmodic or dry coughs.
		Bath	Pour 1 liter (1 quart) boiling water over 4 tablespoons chopped leaves or herb (fresh or dried). Let stand 20 minutes. Strain the liquid and add to bath water. Bathe at 38°C (100°F) for 10–15 minutes. Inhale the rising steam deeply.	
CUTS: *(see Wounds)*				

CYSTITIS	23	Bearberry	Tea	Pour 1 cup boiling water over 1–2 teaspoons dried leaves. Let stand 6–12 hours, according to desired strength. Take 1 cup, reheated, twice daily.	Not indicated for long-term use. Not recommended for sensitive stomachs (high tannin content).
	36	Birch	Tea	Pour 1 cup boiling water over 1 tablespoon fresh or dried leaves. Let stand 5–10 minutes. Take 1 cup 3 times daily.	
	132	Juniper	Tea	Pour 1 cup boiling water over 1 tablespoon lightly crushed berries. Let stand 20 minutes. Take 1 cup morning and evening.	Not to be taken in cases of kidney inflammation, or by pregnant women.
	138	Lovage	Tea	Place ½ tablespoon fresh root, or 1 teaspoon dried root, in 1 cup water. Bring to boil, remove. Let stand 5–10 minutes. Take 1 cup 2–3 times daily.	
	155	Prickly restharrow	Tea	Pour 1 cup boiling water over 1–2 teaspoons shredded root or chopped herb. Let stand 15–20 minutes. Take 1 cup 2–3 times daily.	
	120	Rupturewort	Tea	Pour 1 cup cold water over 1 teaspoon fresh or dried herb. Let stand 8 hours. Reheat and drink. *Or:* Pour 1 cup hot water over 1 teaspoon herb. Let stand ½ hour. Take 1 cup 3 times daily.	Fresh rupturewort is more effective.
DIARRHEA	107	Avens	Tea	Place 1 teaspoon root in 1 cup cold water. Bring to simmer. Let stand 5–10 minutes. Take 1 cup 2–3 times daily.	
	237	Bilberry	Tea	Pour ½ liter (1 pint) water over 3 tablespoons dried bilberries. Let soak 5–10 minutes. Boil 5 minutes. *Or:* Without prior soaking, boil 10 minutes. Take 1 wine glass 3–4 times daily.	
			Juice	Press juice from fresh berries. Take 1 glass unsweetened 3–4 times daily.	
	193	Black currant	Juice	Press juice from fresh berries. Take 1 glass unsweetened 3–4 times daily.	
	75	Hound's tongue	Tea	Pour 1 cup boiling water over 1 teaspoon branches. Let stand 5–10 minutes. Take 1 cup twice daily. *Or:* Place 1 teaspoon fresh or dried root in 1 cup water. Boil 2–3 minutes. Let stand 5–10 minutes. Take 1 cup twice daily.	
	8	Lady's mantle	Tea	Place 1–2 teaspoons leaves or branches in 1 cup water. Boil 2 minutes. Let stand 5–10 minutes. Take 1 cup 3 times daily.	
	181	Tormentil	Tea	Place 2–3 teaspoons root in 1 cup water. Boil 5–10 minutes. Take 1 cup several times daily.	
			Powder	Mix 1–2 pinches (1–2 g or 1/20 oz) pulverized root in 1 cup water, red wine, or peppermint tea. Take 1 cup 3–5 times daily.	

Complaint	Plant	Form of application	Preparation and dose	Notes
DROPSY	165 Bean	Tea	Place 1 tablespoon dried bean shells in 1 cup cold water, heat, and boil 2–3 minutes. Let stand 15 minutes. Take 1 cup twice daily.	
	76 Broom	Tea	Pour 1 cup boiling water over 1 teaspoon blossoms. Let stand 15 minutes. Take 1 cup twice daily.	
	162 Parsley	Tea	Place 1 teaspoon seeds or shredded root in 1 cup cold water, bring to a simmer, remove. Let stand, covered, 15 minutes. Take 2 cups during the day.	Attention: do not use during pregnancy.
		Combined tea	Combine equal parts parsley seeds, prickly restharrow root, chopped horsetail herb. Pour 1 cup boiling water over 1–2 teaspoons of the mixture. Let stand, covered, 10–15 minutes. Take 1 cup twice daily.	
	155 Prickly restharrow	Tea	Pour 1 cup boiling water over 2 teaspoons shredded root or chopped herb. Let stand 15–20 minutes. Take 1 cup 2–3 times daily.	
DYSMENORRHEA: *(see Menstrual disorders)*				
DYSPEPSIA: *(see Indigestion)*				
ECZEMA	223 Comfrey	Compress	Place 3–4 tablespoons shelled fresh or dried root in ½ liter (1 pint) water. Boil 5 minutes. Let stand 20 minutes. Moisten a linen cloth, gauze, or muslin compress in the cooled liquid. Apply a damp, loose compress for 1–2 hours several times daily.	Moisten compress again as soon as it begins to dry (that is, every 15–20 minutes).
		Poultice	Mix in warm water 2–4 tablespoons finely crumbled fresh root or pulverized dried root, and make into a paste. Place on a linen towel, apply while warm. Leave in place at least 1 hour. Repeat several times daily.	Recommended for ulcers of the lower leg.
	131 English walnut	Tea	Bring to a simmer 2 teaspoons dried leaves in 1 cup water. Remove and let stand 5–10 minutes. Take 1 cup twice daily for a period of several weeks.	
		Compress	Bring to boil 2 tablespoons leaves in ½ liter (1 pint) water. Let boil 1 minute. Let stand 20 minutes. Make damp, loose compress with the cooled liquid. Apply for 1–2 hours 3 times daily.	
	25 European snakeroot	Compress	Bring to a boil 2 tablespoons herb or 1 tablespoon root in 1 liter (1 quart) water. Let boil a few seconds. Remove and let stand 20–30 minutes. Make a moist, warm compress with the liquid. Remoisten when the compress begins to dry out. Apply compress several times daily.	

139 Flax	Poultice	Place enough unground flax seeds in a small linen or muslin sack to fill it halfway. Let the sack stand in very hot or lightly boiling water for 5–10 minutes, until the sack has filled completely with the swollen seeds. Wring out and apply while still hot. Repeat several times daily.	
146 German chamomile	Compress	Pour ½ liter (1 pint) boiling water over 1–2 tablespoons blossoms. Let stand 20 minutes. Make a moist, warm compress.	
22 Great burdock	Tea	Place 1 teaspoon fresh or dried root in 1 cup cold water. Let stand 8 hours. Boil for 1 minute. Take 1 cup twice daily.	
	Compress	Boil 1 teaspoon shredded root in ½ liter (1 pint) water for 1 minute. Let stand 30 minutes. Make a damp, loose compress (see Comfrey).	
	Salve	Press sap from fresh root, and mix thoroughly in Vaseline or other petroleum jelly. Spread on the irritated skin area several times daily.	
143 High mallow	Compress	Boil 2–3 tablespoons leaves or blossoms in 1 liter (1 quart) water for 1 minute. Let stand 20 minutes. Make a damp compress with the cooled liquid (see Comfrey).	
75 Hound's tongue	Compress	Boil 3 tablespoons fresh peeled bark, in ½ liter (1 pint) water for 5–10 minutes. Let cool slightly. Make warm, damp compress. Apply for 1 hour several times daily, remoistening it at intervals.	
	Poultice	Mix 2–4 tablespoons crumbled fresh root, or pulverized dried root, with a little warm water to make a paste. Spread on a linen or gauze cloth and apply to skin while warm. Leave in place at least 1 hour. Repeat several times daily.	
40 Marigold	Compress	Pour ½ liter (1 pint) boiling water over 2 tablespoons fresh or dried blossoms or blossoms mixed with leaves. Let stand 20 minutes. Make compress with the liquid. *Or:* Pour ½ liter (1 pint) 70 percent alcohol over 1 handful freshly picked blossoms. Let stand at least 2 weeks in the sun or in a warm place. Filter. Dilute to make compress (1–2 tablespoons liquid in ½ liter or 1 pint water). Make moist compress. Leave in place for about 1 hour. Use 2–3 times daily.	
188 Oak	Compress	Boil 1–2 teaspoons shredded bark in ½ liter (1 pint) water for 10–15 minutes. Let cool. Make a loose compress (see Comfrey).	
243 Pansy	Tea	Pour 1 cup boiling water over 2 teaspoons dried chopped herb. Let stand 5–10 minutes. Take 1 cup mornings and evenings for several weeks.	
	Compress	Pour ½ liter (1 pint) boiling water over 1–2 tablespoons chopped herb. Let stand 15 minutes. Make damp compress with the cooled liquid (see Comfrey).	

Complaint	Plant	Form of application	Preparation and dose	Notes
EYE DISORDERS	90 Eyebright	Tea	Boil 1 teaspoon dried herb in 1 cup wate for 2 minutes. Let stand 5–10 minutes. Take 1 cup 3 times daily.	
		Compress	Place 1 tablespoon dried herb in ½ liter (1 pint) water, boil 10 minutes, let cool slightly. Moisten a compress (cotton wool, gauze, or muslin) in the lukewarm liquid, wring out slightly, place over the eyes. Leave compress in place for 15 minutes. Repeat several times daily.	For inflamed eyelids.
	93 Fennel	Compress	Crush gently 1 tablespoon fennel seeds. Pour ½ liter (1 pint) boiling water over the seeds. Let stand for 15 minutes. Place luke warm compress (cotton wool or gauze) over the eyes for 10–15 minutes.	For inflamed eyelids.
	146 German chamomile	Compress	Pour ½ liter (1 pint) boiling water over 1 tablespoon blossoms. Let stand 15 minutes. Place lukewarm compress (cotton wool or gauze) over the eyes for 10–15 minutes. Repeat several times daily.	For inflamed eyelids. For styes, use hot compresses.
	188 Oak	Compress	Place 1 tablespoon shredded bark in ½ liter (1 pint) water, boil for 15 minutes, let cool. Place lukewarm compress (cotton wool or gauze) over the eyes for 10–15 minutes. Repeat several times daily.	For inflamed eyelids.
	187 Pasque flower	Tea	Pour 1 cup boiling water over ½ teaspoon dried herb. Let stand 5–10 minutes. Take 1 cup twice daily.	Not to be taken during pregnancy.
FEVER: *(see Common cold)*				
FLATULENCE	16 Angelica	Tea	Place 1 teaspoon root in 1 cup cold water. Boil 1 minute, remove. Let stand 15 minutes. Take 1 cup twice daily.	
	169 Anise	Tea	Gently crush 1–2 teaspoons anise seeds. Pour 1 cup boiling water over the seeds. Let stand 5–10 minutes. Take 1 cup twice daily.	Anise, dill, fennel, and caraway seeds are to be partly crushed before the tea is prepared, so that the essential oil is freed. Teas to treat flatulence should be taken warm, in sips, before meals.
	46 Caraway	Tea	Gently crush 1 teaspoon caraway seeds. Pour 1 cup boiling water over the seeds. Take 1 cup twice daily.	
		Mixture	Combine equal parts caraway seeds, fennel seeds, and peppermint leaves to make 1–2 teaspoons altogether. Pour 1 cup boiling water over the mixture. Let stand 5–10 minutes. Take 1 cup twice daily.	
	15 Dill	Tea	Gently crush 1–2 teaspoons dill seeds. Pour 1 cup boiling water over the seeds. Let stand 5–10 minutes. Take 1 cup twice daily.	
	93 Fennel	Tea	Gently crush 1–2 teaspoons fennel seeds. Pour 1 cup boiling water over the seeds. Let stand 5–10 minutes. Take 1 cup twice daily.	
FLU: *(see Common cold)*				

GALL BLADDER DISORDERS	6 Agrimony	Tea	Pour 1 cup boiling water over 1 teaspoon leaves or herb. Let stand 10 minutes. Take 1 cup twice daily.	All teas for the treatment of gall bladder ailments are to be drunk unsweetened, as hot as possible, in small sips.
	63 Blessed thistle	Tea	Pour 1 cup boiling water over 1 tablespoon chopped herb. Let stand 15–20 minutes. Reheat. Take 1 cup 2–3 times daily.	
	97 Fumitory	Tea	Pour 1 cup boiling water over 1–2 teaspoons herb. Let stand, covered, 15 minutes. Take 1 cup twice daily for 4–6 weeks.	
	144 Horehound	Tea	Place 2 teaspoons herb in 1 cup cold water. Bring to the boil. Let stand 10–15 minutes. Take 1 cup 2–3 times daily.	
	149 Peppermint	Tea	Pour 1 cup boiling water over 1–2 teaspoons fresh or dried leaves. Let stand, covered, 10–15 minutes. Take 1 cup 2–3 times daily.	
	38 Wormwood	Tea	Pour 1 cup boiling water over 1 teaspoon fresh or dried herb. Let stand, covered, 10 minutes. Take 1 cup after meals 3 times daily.	
GALLSTONES	74 Artichoke	Tea	Place 1–2 teaspoons dried leaves in 1 cup cold water. Bring to boil, remove. Let stand, covered, 10 minutes. Take 1 cup 2–3 times daily for 4–6 weeks.	
	161 Butterbur	Tea	Place ½–1 teaspoon shredded root in 1 cup cold water. Boil 1 minute. Let stand 15 minutes. Take 1 cup twice daily for several weeks.	Recommended for attacks of gall-stone colic.
	53 Celandine	Tea	Place 1–2 teaspoons dried herb or ½–1 teaspoon shredded root in 1 cup cold water. Bring to boil. Let stand, covered, 10–15 minutes. Take 1 cup 3 times daily between meals for 3 weeks.	
	57 Chicory	Tea	Boil 2 teaspoons shredded root in 1 cup water for 2–3 minutes. Let stand, covered, 10 minutes. Take 1 cup twice daily. *Or:* Place 2 teaspoons dried herb in 1 cup cold water. Bring to boil. Let stand, covered, 15 minutes. Take 1 cup twice daily.	
	224 Dandelion	Tea	Place 1–2 teaspoons shredded root (or equal mixture of root and leaves) in 1 cup cold water. Heat, let boil 1 minute. Let stand, covered, 15 minutes. Take 1 cup morning and evening for 4–6 weeks.	
GINGIVITIS	27 Arnica	Mouthwash	Use tincture, prepared as follows: Pour ½ liter (1 pint) 70 percent alcohol over 1 handful (50 g or 2 oz) freshly picked arnica blossoms. Seal tightly in clear glass container and let stand at least 1 week in the sun. Filter. Mix 1 teaspoon tincture in 1 cup warm water. Rinse the mouth for 10–15 minutes 3–4 times daily or more often.	Take small sips. Keep mouthwash in mouth for several minutes, rinsing carefully and thoroughly.
		Gum tincture	Use undiluted tincture to coat individual inflamed areas.	For aphthae and gum ulcers.
	237 Bilberry	Mouthwash	Place 1 tablespoon dried berries in 1 cup cold water, heat, and boil 10 minutes. Rinse mouth with the hot liquid (see Arnica).	

Complaint	Plant	Form of application	Preparation and dose	Notes
GINGIVITIS *(Continued)*	146 German chamomile	Mouthwash	Pour 1 cup boiling water over 1–2 teaspoons chamomile blossoms. Let stand 10 minutes. Rinse mouth thoroughly with lukewarm liquid.	
	143 High mallow	Mouthwash	Place 2–3 teaspoons dried or fresh leaves in 1 cup cold water, heat, and boil 1 minute. Let stand 5–10 minutes. Rinse (see Arnica).	
	181 Tormentil	Mouthwash	Place 2 teaspoons shredded root in 1 cup cold water, heat, and boil 5 minutes. Let stand 10 minutes. Rinse mouth with the hot liquid (see Arnica).	
GUMS, BLEEDING OF	213 Alpine ragwort	Tea	Place 1 teaspoon chopped herb in 1 cup cold water. Bring to simmer, remove. Let stand 15 minutes. Take 1 cup 2–3 times daily.	Also useful for slight bleeding after extraction of a tooth.
HAIR LOSS	36 Birch	Lotion	Mix 300 milliliters (1 cup) freshly collected birch sap with 100 ml (3 oz) 96 percent alcohol. (One may also add a preservative, obtainable from pharmacy.) Dilute with 100 ml (3 oz) distilled water. Massage scalp with 1–2 tablespoons daily for several weeks. *Or:* Pour 300 ml (1 cup) 70 percent alcohol over 2 handfuls fresh or dried birch leaves. Add enough distilled water to cover the leaves. Let stand 3 days. Filter. Massage scalp with 1–2 tablespoons daily for several weeks.	Consult physician to determine whether organic disturbance exists. Medicinal herbs can help only in mild cases of hair loss, such as following an illness or pregnancy.
	22 Great burdock	Lotion	Pour 400 ml (1⅓ cup) 70 percent alcohol over 3 tablespoons dried or fresh shredded burdock root. Let stand 5 days. Dilute with 100 ml (3 oz) distilled water. Filter. Massage scalp with 1–2 tablespoons daily.	
	235 Stinging nettle	Lotion	Pour 300 ml (1 cup) 70 percent alcohol over 2 handfuls fresh or dried nettle leaves. Add enough distilled water to cover the leaves. Let stand 3–5 days. Filter. Massage scalp with 1–2 tablespoons daily.	
HEADACHE	148 Balm	Rub	Spirits of balm: Pour ½ liter (1 pint) 90 percent alcohol over 1 handful (50 g or 2 oz) fresh leaves or branch tips. Place in clear glass container and let stand in the sun at least 8 days. Shake often during this period. Filter the liquid. Rub undiluted spirits on brow and temples.	
		Tea	Pour 1 cup boiling water over 2 teaspoons fresh or dried leaves. Let stand 10 minutes. Drink 1 cup hot, sweetened, twice daily.	For nervous headaches.
	182 Cowslip	Tea	Pour 1 cup boiling water over 2 teaspoons blossoms without calyx. Let stand 15 minutes. Take 1 cup 1–2 times daily.	
	136 Lavender	Tea	Pour 1 cup boiling water over 1 teaspoon blossoms. Let stand, covered, 10–15 minutes. Take 1 cup mornings and evenings regularly for 2–3 weeks.	
	92 Queen-of-the-meadow	Tea	Pour 1 cup boiling water over 2 teaspoons blossoms. Let stand 15 minutes. Take 1 cup twice daily.	

	238	Valerian	Tea	Pour 1 cup cold water over 2 teaspoons shredded root. Let stand 8 hours. Take 1 cup evenings and as needed.	
	201	White willow	Tea	Place 1 teaspoon shredded bark in 1 cup cold water. Boil 1 minute. Let stand 10 minutes. Take 1 cup twice daily.	
HEART DISORDERS, NERVOUS	70	Hawthorn	Tea	Pour 1 cup boiling water over 2 teaspoons blossoms or leaves, or equal combination of the two. Let stand 20 minutes. Sweeten with honey to taste. Take 1 cup 2–3 times daily for several weeks.	
	123	Hops	Tea	Pour 1 cup boiling water over 1 tablespoon hops. Let stand, covered, 10–15 minutes. Take 1 cup evenings, and also during day if needed.	
	136	Lavender	Tea	Pour 1 cup boiling water over 1 teaspoon blossoms. Let stand, covered, 10 minutes. Take 1 cup mornings and evenings.	
	137	Motherwort	Tea	Pour 1 cup boiling water over 1 teaspoon herb. Let stand 10 minutes. Take 1 cup mornings and evenings.	
	238	Valerian	Tea	Pour 1 cup cold water over 2 teaspoons shredded root. Let stand 8 hours. Reheat and drink. Take 1 cup evenings, and also during day if necessary.	
			Tincture	Take 1 teaspoon tincture (from pharmacy) in some water each evening, and also during day if necessary.	
HEMORRHOIDS	146	German chamomile	Steam bath	Place 1–2 handfuls chamomile blossoms in a bidet or toilet. Pour 2–3 liters (2–3 quarts) boiling water over the herbs. Sit over the steam and cover up with a blanket. Let the steam work for 10 minutes. Repeat several times daily if necessary.	For inflamed hemorrhoids.
	180	Silverweed	Compress	Bring to a boil 1–2 tablespoons chopped herb in ½ liter (1 pint) water. Let stand 20 minutes. Mak a moist compress with the lukewarm liquid. Moisten again as soon as the compress begins to dry.	
	177	Smartweed	Tea	Place 2–3 teaspoons fresh or dried herb in 1 cup cold water. Heat to simmering. Let stand covered 15 minutes. Take 1 cup mornings and evenings.	For bleeding hemorrhoids.
	113	Witch hazel	Tea	Boil 1 teaspoon leaves or bark in 1 cup water for 2–3 minutes. Let stand 10 minutes. Take 1 cup mornings and evenings.	For bleeding and inflamed hemorrhoids.
			Compress	Boil 2 tablespoons leaves or bark in ½ liter (1 pint) water for 5 minutes. Let stand 10 minutes, strain, let cool. Soak linen towel or face cloth in the liquid and lightly wring out to make cool, moist compress. Apply for 1 hour 2–3 times daily. Re-moisten compress before it dries.	
	1	Yarrow	Sitz bath	Pour 1 liter (1 quart) boiling water over 1–2 handfuls blossoms. Let stand 20–30 minutes. Strain the liquid and add it to bath water. Bathe at 34°–36 °C (93°–97 °F) for 10–15 minutes, 2–3 times weekly.	

Complaint	Plant	Form of application	Preparation and dose	Notes
INDIGESTION	148 Balm	Tea	Pour 1 cup boiling water over 2–3 teaspoons leaves. Let stand, covered, 15 minutes. Take 1 cup twice daily.	All plants listed under Appetite Loss and Flatulence can be used.
		Combined tea	Combine 1 teaspoon balm leaves and 1 teaspoon peppermint leaves. Pour 1 cup boiling water over the mixture. Let stand, covered, 10–15 minutes. Take 1 cup twice daily.	For acute stomach pain.
	61 Bitter orange	Tea	Pour 1 cup boiling water over 1–2 teaspoons blossoms, leaves, or shredded orange skin. Let stand, covered, 10–15 minutes. Take 1 cup twice daily.	
	53 Celandine	Tea	Place 2 teaspoons herb or 1 teaspoon root in 1 cup cold water. Bring to a simmer, remove. Let stand 10 minutes. Take 1 cup twice daily.	For acute stomach pain.
	93 Fennel	Tea	Lightly crush 1 teaspoon fennel seeds. Pour 1 cup boiling water over the seeds. Let stand, covered, 10–15 minutes. Drink 1 cup, hot, 2–3 times daily.	Especially suitable for small children.
	123 Hop	Tea	Pour 1 cup boiling water over 1 tablespoon hops. Let stand 10–15 minutes. Take 1 cup 1–2 times daily before main meals.	
	163 Masterwort	Tea	Place 1–2 teaspoons shredded root in 1 cup cold water. Bring to simmer. Let stand, covered, 15 minutes. Take 3 times daily after meals.	
	149 Peppermint	Tea	Pour 1 cup boiling water over 1–2 teaspoons leaves. Let stand, covered, 10 minutes. Take 1 cup 2–3 times daily after meals.	
	28 Wormwood	Tea	Pour 1 cup boiling water over 1 teaspoon herb. Let stand, covered, 10 minutes. Take 1 cup 2–3 times daily after meals.	
	1 Yarrow	Tea	Pour 1 cup boiling water over 1–2 teaspoons blossoms or herb. Let stand, covered, 10 minutes. Take 1 cup 2–3 times daily after meals.	
INFLUENZA: *(see Common cold)*				
INSOMNIA: *(see Sleeplessness)*				
KIDNEY DISEASES	203 Dwarf elder	Tea	Boil ½ teaspoon shredded root in 1 cup water for 1–2 minutes. Let stand 10 minutes. Take 1 cup twice daily.	Plants listed under Bladder Stones can also be used.
	218 Goldenrod	Tea	Place 2–3 teaspoons chopped herb in 1 cup cold water. Bring to simmer, remove. Let stand 10–15 minutes. Take 1 cup 2–4 times daily.	
	157 Java tea	Tea	Pour 1 cup boiling water over 2 teaspoons leaves. Let stand 15 minutes. Take 1 cup 2–3 times daily.	

	162 Parsley	Tea	Pour 1 cup boiling water over 1 teaspoon parsley fruits. Let stand, covered, 15 minutes. Take 1 cup twice daily, but not in evening.	Not for pregnant women. Do not exceed given dosage.
KIDNEY STONES: *(see Kidney diseases)*				
LACTATION, DEFECTIVE	46 Caraway	Combined tea	Combine 2 parts caraway seeds, 1 part fennel seeds, 1 part anise seeds, to make 1–2 teaspoons. Gently crush the seeds and place in 1 cup cold water. Bring to simmer, remove. Let stand, covered, 10 minutes. Take 1 cup 3 times daily.	
	228 Fenugreek	Combined tea	Combine 2 parts fenugreek seeds and 1 part anise seeds to make 2 teaspoons. Place seeds in 1 cup cold water. Bring to simmer, remove. Let stand 10 minutes. Take 1 cup 3 times daily.	
	98 Goat's rue	Tea	Boil 1–2 teaspoons herb in 1 cup water for 2–3 minutes. Let stand 10 minutes. Take 1 cup 3 times daily.	
LARYNGITIS	170 Black caraway	Tea	Place 1–2 teaspoons shredded root in 1 cup cold water. Bring to simmer. Let stand 15–20 minutes. Take 1 cup twice daily.	
		Mouthwash	Gargle 5–10 minutes with hot tea (prepared as above), several times daily.	
	202 Garden sage	Mouthwash	Bring to a simmer 2 tablespoons leaves in ½ liter (1 pint) water. Let stand, covered, 15 minutes. Gargle deeply with the hot tea for 5–10 minutes several times daily.	
	143 High mallow	Mouthwash	Boil 1–2 tablespoons blossoms or leaves (or equal mixture of both) in ½ liter (1 pint) water for 1 minute. Let stand 10 minutes. Gargle deeply with the hot tea for 5–10 minutes several times daily.	
	30 Wild ginger	Tea	Place 1 teaspoon shredded root in 1 cup cold water. Bring to a simmer. Let stand 15 minutes. Take 1 cup twice daily.	
LIVER AILMENTS	63 Blessed thistle	Tea	Pour 1 cup boiling water over 1 teaspoon herb. Let stand 15–20 minutes. Take 1 cup 2–3 times daily.	
	246 Grape	Tea	Place 2–4 teaspoons fresh or dried leaves in 1 cup cold water. Bring to a simmer, remove. Let stand 15 minutes. Take 1 cup 3 times daily for several weeks.	
	89 Hemp agrimony	Tea	Pour 1 cup boiling water over 1–2 teaspoons herb. Let stand, covered, 10–15 minutes. Take 1 cup 2–3 times daily. *Or:* Place 1 teaspoon shredded root in 1 cup cold water. Bring to boil, let boil 1 minute. Let stand 15 minutes. Take 1 cup 2–3 times daily.	
	215 Milk thistle	Tea	Pour 1 cup boiling water over 1 teaspoon fruit (seeds). Let stand 15–20 minutes. Drink 1 cup, very hot, 3 times daily: ½ hour before breakfast and lunch, and before bedtime. Continue for 4 weeks.	

Complaint	Plant	Form of application	Preparation and dose	Notes
MENSTRUAL DISORDERS	213 Alpine ragwort	Tea	Place 1–2 teaspoons herb in 1 cup cold water. Bring to a simmer, remove. Let stand 15–20 minutes. Take 1 cup 2–3 times daily.	
	8 Lady's mantle	Tea	Place 1–2 teaspoons leaves or herb in 1 cup cold water, heat. Boil 1 minute. Let stand 10–15 minutes. Take 1 cup mornings and evenings.	
	127 Saint John's wort	Tea	Place 2 teaspoons herb in 1 cup cold water. Bring to a simmer, remove. Let stand 15 minutes. Take 1 cup mornings and evenings over a long period.	
	41 Shepherd's purse	Tea	Place 2 teaspoons dried or 3–4 teaspoons fresh herb in 1 cup cold water. Bring to boil, let boil 1 minute. Let stand 15 minutes. Take 1 cup 2–4 times daily.	For excessive menstruation.
	134 White deadnettle	Tea	Pour 1 cup boiling water over 2 teaspoons blossoms or herb. Let stand 10 minutes. Take 1 cup twice daily.	
		Combined tea	Combine 1 teaspoon each yarrow blossoms (or herb) and white deadnettle blossoms. Pour 1 cup boiling water over the herbs. Let stand, covered, 10 minutes. Take 1 cup twice daily, regularly over a period of 3–4 weeks.	
	1 Yarrow	Tea	Pour 1 cup boiling water over 1–2 teaspoons herb or blossoms. Let stand, covered, 10 minutes. Take 1 cup twice daily.	For painful menstruation.
		Bath	*For sitz bath:* Pour ½ liter (1 pint) boiling water over 1 handful (50 g or 2 oz) blossoms or herb. Let stand 20–30 minutes. Strain the liquid and add to bath water. Bathe at 35°–37°C (95°–98.5°F) for 10–15 minutes, 3 times weekly, regularly over long period. *For full bath:* Double measurements.	
METABOLIC DISTURBANCES	224 Dandelion	Tea	Place 1–2 teaspoons shredded root (or mixed root and leaves) in 1 cup cold water, heat, and boil 1 minute. Let stand 15 minutes. Take 1 cup twice daily for 4–6 weeks.	
	7 Quack grass	Tea	Place 2 teaspoons shredded root in 1 cup cold water, heat, and boil 2–3 minutes. Let stand 15 minutes. Take 1 cup twice daily for several weeks.	
	18 Sweet vernal grass	Bath	Place 400 g (¾ pound) hayflowers in 4 liters (4 quarts) cold water, heat, and boil 1 minute. Let stand, covered, 15 minutes. Strain the liquid and add to bath water. Bathe at 38°C (100°F) for 10 minutes twice weekly for 1–2 months.	
MIGRAINE: *(see Headache)*				

NASAL CATARRH	88 Eucalyptus	Inhalation	Pour 1–2 liters (1–2 quarts) boiling water over 2–3 tablespoons leaves in a basin. Inhale the steam deeply. Keep head and basin covered with a towel to prevent steam from escaping. After 10 minutes more boiling water can be added. Use 1–2 times daily.	After steam bath, wash face with cool water. Do not go outside immediately after inhalation.
	146 German chamomile	Inhalation	Pour 1–2 liters (1–2 quarts) boiling water over 2–3 tablespoons blossoms in a basin. Inhale steam deeply (see Eucalyptus) for 10 minutes 1–2 times daily.	
	171 Scotch pine	Inhalation	Pour 1–2 liters (1–2 quarts) boiling water over 1–2 handfuls (50–100 g or 2–3 oz) fresh or dried pine needles or tips. Inhale steam deeply (see Eucalyptus) for 10 minutes 1–2 times daily.	
NAUSEA	74 Artichoke	Tea	Place 1–2 teaspoons leaves in 1 cup cold water, bring to simmer, and remove. Let stand 15 minutes. Take hot, 1–2 cups as needed.	
	107 Avens	Tea	Pour 1 cup boiling water over 1 teaspoon shredded root. Let stand, covered, 15 minutes. Take 1–2 cups as hot as possible.	
	149 Peppermint	Tea	Pour 1 cup boiling water over 1–2 teaspoons leaves. Let stand, covered, 10 minutes. Take 1–2 cups as hot as possible.	
		Combined tea	Combine equal parts of peppermint leaves, chamomile blossoms, and balm leaves, to make 1–2 teaspoons. Pour 1 cup coiling water over the mixture. Let stand, covered, 10 minutes. Take 1–2 cups in sips, as hot as possible.	
NERVOUS EXHAUSTION	158 American ginseng	Tea	Boil ½ teaspoon shredded root in 1 cup water for 1 minute. Let stand 15 minutes. Take 1 cup 2–3 times daily.	
		Powder	Mix 1 small pinch (1 g or 1/30 oz) pulverized root in a few teaspoons water. Take 2–3 times daily.	
	136 Lavender	Bath	Pour 1 liter (1 quart) boiling water over 2 handfuls (100 g or 3 oz) blossoms. Let stand 20–30 minutes. Strain the liquid and add to bath water. Bathe at 35°–37°C (95°–98.5°F) for 10–15 minutes.	Bath has a stimulating effect. Do not bathe in the evening.
		Combined tea	Mix ½ teaspoon lavender blossoms and ½ teaspoon rosemary leaves. Pour 1 cup boiling water over the mixture. Let stand, covered, 10 minutes. Take 1 cup twice daily.	
	196 Rosemary	Bath	See under Circulatory Disorders, above.	Do not bathe in evening.
		Tea	Pour 1 cup boiling water over 1 teaspoon leaves. Let stand, covered, 10 minutes. Take 1 cup twice daily.	
		Wine	See Old Age, disorders of. Take 1 small wine glass twice daily.	
	3 Sweet flag	Bath	Boil 100 g (3 oz) root (with or without root bark) in 1 liter (1 quart) water for 10 minutes. Follow directions for Lavender bath, above.	Do not bathe in the evening.

Complaint	Plant	Form of application	Preparation and dose	Notes
NERVOUS TENSION	148 Balm	Tea	Pour 1 cup boiling water over 2–3 teaspoons dried leaves. Let stand, covered, 10 minutes. Take 1 cup mornings and evenings.	All plants listed for Sleeplessness can also be used here. Dosage: 2 cups daily.
		Bath	Pour 1 liter (1 quart) water over 2–3 handfuls dried leaves (100–150 g or 3–5 oz). Let stand 20–30 minutes. Strain the liquid and add to bath water. Bathe at 34°–36°C (93°–97°F) for 10–15 minutes 3–4 times weekly.	
	61 Bitter orange	Tea	Pour 1 cup boiling water over 1–2 teaspoons blossoms, leaves, or shredded orange peel. Let stand, covered, 10–15 minutes. Take 1 cup mornings and evenings.	
	100 Sweet woodruff	Tea	Pour 1 cup boiling water over 2 teaspoons dried or fresh chopped herb. Let stand 10–15 minutes. Take 1 cup mornings and evenings.	
NEURALGIA	136 Lavender	Liniment	Prepare spirits of lavender: Pour ½ liter (1 pint) 90–96 percent alcohol over 1 handful (50 g or 2 oz) fresh or dried blossoms. Let stand tightly sealed at least 1 week in a bright, warm place. Shake often during this period. Filter. Rub painful areas with undiluted spirits of lavender several times daily.	
	33 Oats	Bath	Boil 500 g (1 pound) shredded oat straw in 2 liters (2 quarts) water for ½ hour. Strain liquid and add to bath water. Bathe at 36°–38°C (97°–100°F) for 10–15 minutes.	
	196 Rosemary	Liniment	Prepare spirits of rosemary, using 1 handful (50 g or 2 oz) fresh or dried leaves and ½ liter (1 pint) 90–96 percent alcohol (see Lavender). Rub painful areas with undiluted spirits of rosemary several times daily.	
	127 Saint John's wort	Liniment	Prepare oil: Crush 1 handful (50 g or 2 oz) freshly picked blossoms, or mixture of blossoms and leaves, with about 1 teaspoon olive oil or sunflower oil. Place in a tall glass container, cover seeds with 3 or 4 times as much oil. Let stand in sun 14 days. Shake several times daily during this period. Filter. Pour off thin liquid floating on surface. Store in a dark place. Rub undiluted oil on painful areas, or moisten muslin cloth in oil to make compress. Use several times daily.	
	201 White willow	Tea	Place 1 teaspoon shredded bark in 1 cup cold water, heat, and boil 2 minutes. Let stand 15 minutes. Take 1 cup twice daily.	
		Combined tea	Combine 2 parts white willow bark, 1 part queen-of-the-meadow blossoms, and 1 part European elder blossoms, to make 1–2 teaspoons. Place in 1 cup cold water, heat, let boil 1 minute. Let stand 15 minutes. Take 1 cup twice daily.	

OLD AGE, DISORDERS OF	158 American ginseng	Tea	Boil ½ teaspoon shredded root in 1 cup water for 1 minute. Let stand 15 minutes. Take 1 cup, 2–3 times daily.	Healing plants cannot reverse or cancel any of the aging processes. Ginseng relieves aches and pains.
		Powder	Use 1 pinch of pulverized root. Take 2 to 3 times daily, in water, fruit juice, or other liquid if desired.	
	9 Garlic	Fresh plant (whole herb)	Finely chop or crush 1eclove fresh garlic. Spread the garlic on bread, or mix in lukewarm milk. Take 1 clove several times daily, regularly for several weeks or even months.	For sensitive stomachs, garlic in capsule form is preferable.
	196 Rosemary	Tea	Pour 1 cup boiling water over 1 teaspoon fresh or dried leaves, or leaves and blossoms. Let stand 5–10 minutes. Take 1 cup twice daily.	Eases aches and pains.
		Wine	Pour 1 liter sherry or port wine over 6–7 fresh or dried branches (or 1 handful of leaves). Allow to stand in a bottle, tightly corked, at least 1 week, then pour through a strainer or filter. Take 1 small glass twice daily, before meals.	For aches and pains.
PEPTIC ULCER	139 Flax	Tea	Pour 1 cup cold water over 1 teaspoon flax seeds. Let stand 8 hours. Drink 1 cup, lukewarm, 1–3 times daily (before breakfast, and ½ hour before main meals).	
	146 German chamomile	Tea	Pour 1 cup boiling water over 1–2 teaspoons fresh or dried blossoms. Let stand, covered, 10–15 minutes. Take 1 cup, as hot as possible, in small sips, 3 times daily (between meals) for several weeks.	
	109 Licorice	Extract	Shred 20–25 g (¾ oz) licorice sticks and dissolve in 2–3 cups warm water or chamomile tea. Drink 2–3 cups daily in small doses after each meal, for 3–4 weeks.	Side effects such as swelling of face and joints, slight dizziness, or headaches will disappear when the treatment ends. A salt-free diet is recommended.
	38 Winter cabbage	Juice	Cut up fresh head of cabbage and press out juice (a small amount of water can be added for taste). Drink ½–1 liter (1 pint–1 quart) of the juice daily in small installments. Continue for 3–4 weeks.	Cabbage juice must be prepared fresh each day. Do not take on empty stomach.
PHLEBITIS	27 Arnica	Compress	Prepare as indicated under Bruises.	
	223 Comfrey	Compress	Prepare as for Eczema, above.	
		Poultice	Mix 4–5 tablespoons finely crumbled fresh root, or pulverized dry root, with water to make a paste. Place the paste on a cloth strip or a gauze and apply it to the affected part of the body. Leave in place for ½–1 hour.	
	200 Rue	Tea	Pour 1 cup boiling water over 2 teaspoons chopped herb. Let stand, covered, 15 minutes. Take 1 cup 3 times daily.	
	147 Yellow sweetclover	Tea	Pour 1 cup boiling water over 2 teaspoons chopped herb. Let stand 10 minutes. Take 1 cup 3–4 times daily.	

Complaint	Plant	Form of application	Preparation and dose	Notes
PILES: *(see Hemorrhoids)*				
PSORIASIS: *(see Skin ailments)*				
RHEUMATISM	37 Black mustard	Poultice	Mix 100 g (3 oz) freshly ground mustard seeds with fairly hot water (45 °C or 113 °F maximum), to form a thick paste or dough. Place on a piece of cloth the size of the painful body area. Apply the cloth. Remove after 1 minute. A dampened gauze laid on the skin will prevent the mustard mixture from sticking. Reddened parts of the skin can be lightly coated with powder, or dabbed with olive oil, after poultice is used.	This is a potent preparation and must not be used on tender skins.
	224 Dandelion	Tea	Place 1–2 teaspoons shredded root (or mixture of root and leaves) in 1 cup cold water, heat, and boil 1 minute. Let stand 15 minutes. Take 1 cup mornings and evenings for 4–8 weeks in spring and fall.	
	115 Grapple plant	Tea	Bring to the boil 1 teaspoon shredded root in ½ liter (1 pint) water. Let boil 1 minute, remove. Let stand 8 hours. Drink in installments during the day (before meals), ½ liter (1 pint) daily. Continue taking tea for 3–6 weeks.	Plants listed for neuralgia can also be used for rheumatism.
	132 Juniper	Tea	Pour 1 cup boiling water over 1 teaspoon lightly crushed berries. Let stand, covered, 20 minutes. Take 1 cup mornings and evenings for 4–6 weeks.	Recommended for chronic rheumatism, twice yearly (spring and fall).
	235 Stinging nettle	Tea	Place 1–2 teaspoons dried leaves in 1 cup cold water, heat, boil 1 minute. Let stand 15 minutes. Take 1 cup twice daily for 4–6 weeks, 2–3 times per year.	
	18 Sweet vernal grass	Poultice	Fill a small cloth sack loosely with hayflowers and close it tightly. Place in 2–3 liters (quarts) water, bring to boil, let boil 1 minute. Let sack stand in liquid 15 minutes and then wring out well. Apply to painful body area as hot as possible.	
		Bath	Place 400–500 g (¾–1 pound) hayflowers in 4 liters (4 quarts) water, bring to boil, boil 1 minute. Let stand 15 minutes. Strain the liquid and add to bath water. Bathe at 38°C (100°F) for 10–15 minutes, 2–3 times weekly.	Rest ½–1 hour after bathing.
SKIN AILMENTS	84 Horsetail	Tea	Pour 1 cup boiling water over 2 teaspoons herb. Let stand 15 minutes. Take 1 cup morning and evenings for several weeks.	
	243 Pansy	Tea	Pour 1 cup boiling water over 2 teaspoons herb. Let stand, covered, 15 minutes. Take 1 cup mornings and evenings for a period of several weeks.	

		Bath	Mix 2 parts pansy, 1 part soapwort root, 1 part English walnut leaves, and 1 part witch hazel leaves, to make total of 4 tablespoons. Heat in 1 liter (1 quart) water and boil 1 minute. Let stand 20–30 minutes, strain, and add liquid to bath water. Bathe at 34°–36 °C (93°–97 °F) for 10–15 minutes, 2–3 times weekly.	
	7 Quack grass	Tea	Place 2 teaspoons shredded root in 1 cup cold water. Boil 1 minute. Let stand 15–20 minutes. Take 1 cup mornings and evenings. These teas should be taken for several weeks.	
	207 Soapwort	Tea	Pour 1 cup cold water over 1 teaspoon shredded root. Let stand 6–8 hours. Heat and drink, 1 cup mornings and evenings.	
	235 Stinging nettle	Tea	Pour 1 cup boiling water over 1–2 teaspoons leaves or herb. Let stand 10 minutes. Take 1 cup mornings and evenings for several weeks.	
		Juice	Press juice from fresh young plants. Take 1 tablespoon 2–3 times daily for several weeks.	
SLEEPLESSNESS	87 California poppy	Tea	Pour 1 cup boiling water over 1–2 teaspoons herb. Let stand 15 minutes. Take 1 cup evenings.	
	123 Hops	Tea	Pour 1 cup boiling water over 1 tablespoon hops. Let stand 10–15 minutes. Take 1 cup evenings.	
	238 Valerian	Tea	Pour 1 cup cold water over 2 teaspoons shredded root. Let stand 8 hours. Warm and drink in the evening.	
		Bath	Pour 1 liter (1 quart) boiling water over 1–2 handfuls (50–100 g or 2–3 oz) shredded root. Let stand 30 minutes. Strain liquid and add to bath water. Bathe at 35°–37 °C (95°–98.5 °F) for 10 minutes.	Bathe before bedtime.
	160 Wild passionflower	Tea	Pour 1 cup boiling water over 1 teaspoon chopped herb. Let stand 15 minutes. Drink 1 cup evenings.	
SORE THROAT	139 Flax	Mouthwash	Place 1 tablespoon flax seeds in 1 cup cold water. Let stand 8 hours. Heat. Gargle as often as possible.	
	202 Garden sage	Mouthwash	Heat 2 tablespoons leaves in ½ liter (1 pint) cold water to simmering point. Let stand, covered, 10 minutes. Reheat. Gargle often.	Recommended for inflammation of the tonsils.
	146 German chamomile	Mouthwash	Pour 1 cup boiling water over 1–2 teaspoons blossom. Let stand, covered, 10 minutes. Reheat. Gargle as often as possible.	
	156 Marjoram	Mouthwash	Pour ½ liter (1 pint) boiling water over 2 tablespoons chopped herb. Let stand, covered, 10 minutes. Reheat. Gargle for 5–10 minutes, 3–4 times daily or more.	
	13 Marsh mallow	Mouthwash	Place 2–3 teaspoons shredded root or leaves in 1 cup cold water. Let stand 6–8 hours. Reheat. Gargle as often as possible.	

Complaint	Plant	Form of application	Preparation and dose	Notes
VARICOSE VEINS	200 Rue	Tea	Pour 1 cup boiling water over 1–2 teaspoons herb. Let stand 15 minutes. Take 1 cup 2–3 times daily for several weeks.	
	147 Yellow sweetclover	Tea	Pour 1 cup cold water over 1 teaspoon herb. Let stand 8 hours. Take 1 cup 3 times daily for several weeks.	
WHOOPING COUGH	117 English ivy	Tea	Boil 1 teaspoon fresh or dried leaves in 1 cup water for 2–3 minutes. Let stand 10 minutes. Drink 1 cup, as hot as possible, 2–3 times daily.	
	48 Spanish chestnut	Tea	Pour 1 cup boiling water over 2 teaspoons dried leaves. Let stand 15 minutes. Drink hot, 1 cup 3 times daily.	
	80 Sundew	Tea	Pour 1 cup boiling water over ½–1 teaspoon herb. Let stand 10–15 minutes. Take 1 cup twice daily.	Sundew dyes the urine a dark color (a harmless side effect).
	226 Thyme	Tea	Pour 1 cup boiling water over 2 teaspoons leaves or chopped herb. Let stand, covered, 10 minutes. Take 1 cup 3–4 times daily.	
		Combined tea	Combine 2 parts thyme leaves with 1 part sundew herb, to make 2 teaspoons altogether. Pour 1 cup boiling water over the mixture. Let stand 10–15 minutes. Take 1 cup 2–3 times daily.	
WOUNDS, SLOWLY HEALING	27 Arnica	Compress	Use arnica tincture (see Gingivitis). Dilute 1–2 tablespoons of tincture with ½ liter (1 pint) water. Soak a piece of gauze, muslin, or linen in the liquid and place it loosely on the wound several times daily.	All these preparations can also be used as baths for wounds.
	25 European snakeroot	Compress	Bring to boil 2–3 tablespoons herb or 1–2 tablespoons root in 1 liter (1 quart) water. Boil 1 minute. Let stand 30 minutes. Make loose, moist compress with the cooled liquid (see Arnica).	
	146 German chamomile	Compress	Pour ½ liter (1 pint) boiling water over 1–2 tablespoons blossoms. Let stand 20 minutes. Make a loose compress when cooled (see Arnica). Apply several times daily.	
	40 Marigold	Salve	Press out 4–6 g (¼ oz) juice from freshly picked blossoms (or blossoms and leaves). Combine juice with 30 g (1 oz) Vaseline or other petroleum jelly; mix well. Apply salve to wound several times daily.	Marigold compress can also be used; see Eczema.
	206 Snakeroot	Compress	Bring to a simmer 2 tablespoons herb or leaves in ½ liter (1 pint) water. Let stand 20–30 minutes. Make moist, loose compress with the cooled liquid. Apply several times daily.	
	113 Witch hazel	Compress	Place 2 tablespoons leaves in ½ liter (1 pint) cold water, heat, and boil 2–3 minutes. Let stand 15 minutes. Make moist, loose compress with the cooled liquid. Apply several times daily.	

The Heritage of Folk Medicine

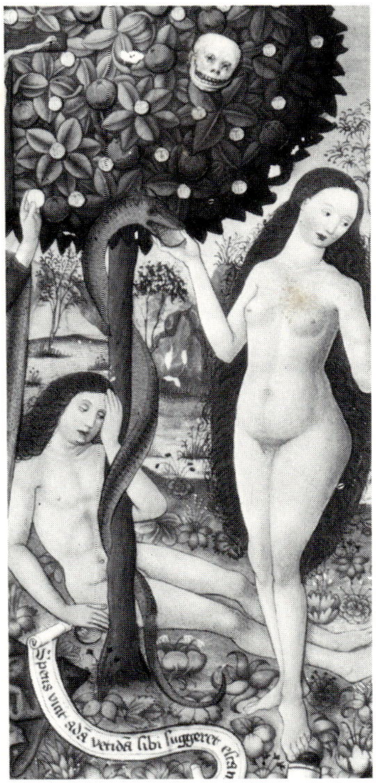

The tree of the knowledge of good and evil, a symbol of the strength and power of plants: "For in the day that thou eatest thereof thou shalt surely die" (Genesis 2:17).

Below: Healing plants used by the Neanderthals 60,000 years ago, according to archaeological evidence from Shanidar in Iraq.

Human beings have always had to rely on plants for their foods and many other necessities, including their medicines. Folk medicine based on plants, originally the only healing known to man, has never entirely disappeared. In rural outposts or among ethnic minorities of modern industrial society, it has persisted as a poorman's complement, or alternative, to the inaccessible physician. It flourishes, above all, in the pockets of surviving aboriginal cultures, where modern medical science has remained unknown and where plants still provide the only medicines.

We owe a great debt to folk medicine: it is the source of our knowledge of many, if not most, of the healing plants. The wealth of lore accumulated for millennia by folk medicine has developed into the modern discipline of ethnopharmacology, the critical study of native medicines, which has only recently come into its own. Although the identification of pharmacologically active plants and plant derivatives is far from complete, it is nevertheless very extensive. Science can continue to learn and profit from the practices of the folk healers—provided we do not allow this rich source of knowledge to dry up.

The aboriginal cultures still extant in the world today—in remote areas of Africa, Asia, Latin America, and elsewhere—are rapidly disappearing. There is a danger that much of the knowledge and practice of the alleviative properties of plants will vanish with these cultures. It is not too soon to pay serious attention to this popular healing tradition and to review some examples of the pharmacological contributions it has made in the past—and can go on making—to modern medicine and our knowledge of plants.

PREHISTORIC SOCIETIES

The scanty archaeological remains of plant materials that have come to light indicate that, after foods, construction, and clothing materials, healing plants were man's primary interest in the Plant Kingdom. There is evidence from several widely separated parts of the world.

Archaeological studies at Shanidar in Iraq indicate that the Neanderthals living there may have had a rudimentary pharmacopoeia. Of the eight species of plants identified through pollen grains from remains in this site, seven represent plants still prominent in ethnomedicine in this locality and elsewhere in Asia. Included in this 60,000-year-old burial site are Yarrow *(Achillea)*, Hollyhock *(Althaea)*, Groundsel *(Senecio)*, Grape Hyacinth *(Muscari)*, St. Barnaby's

YARROW
Achillea

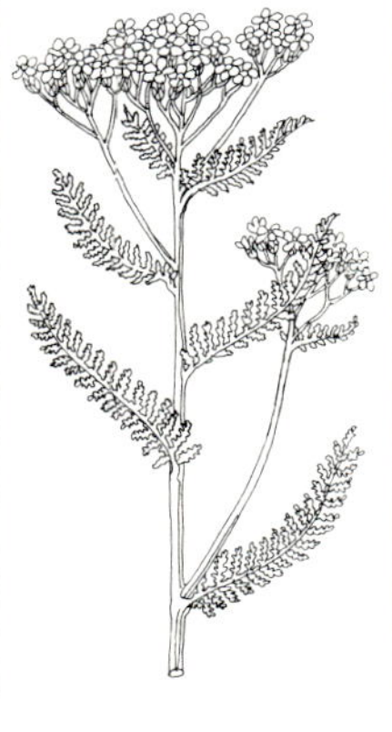

HOLLYHOCK
Althaea

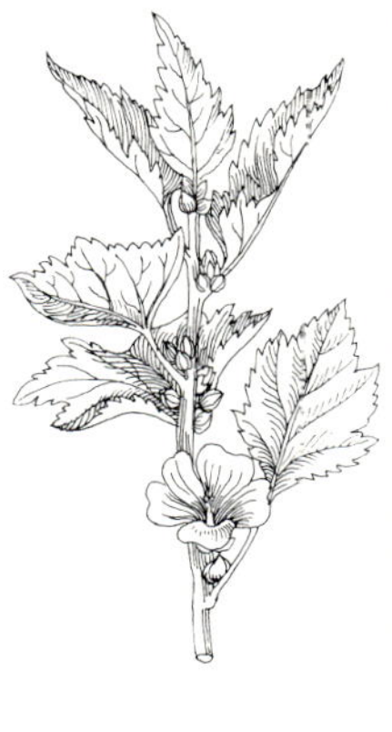

GROUNDSEL
Senecio

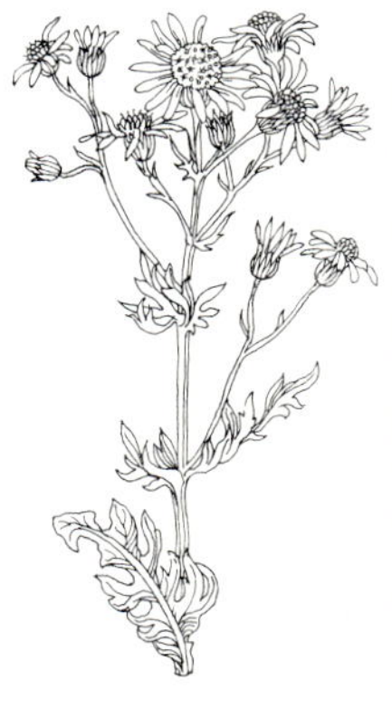

GRAPE HYACINTH
Muscari

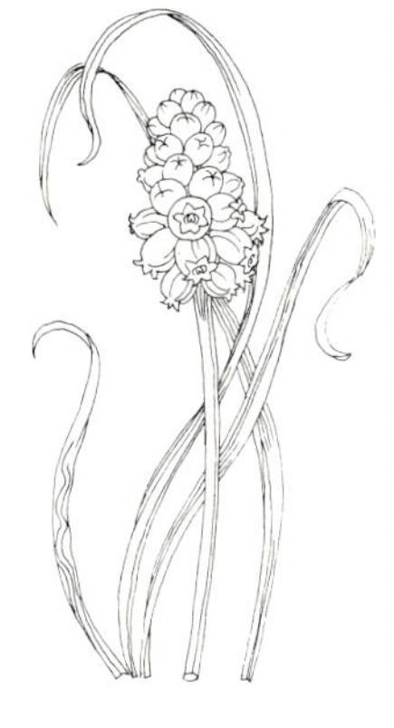

ST. BARNABY'S THISTLE
Centaurea

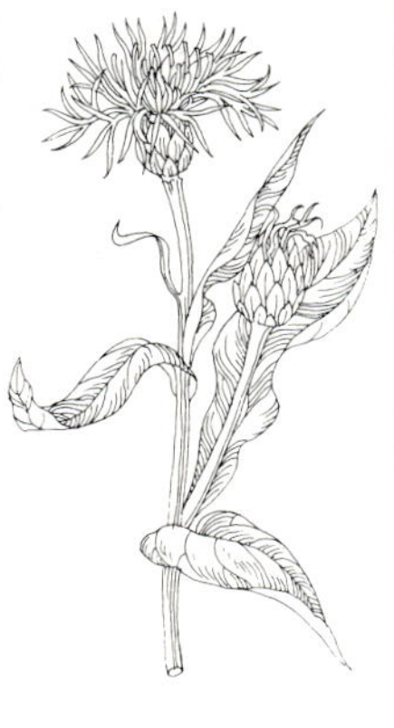

JOINT PINE
Ephedra

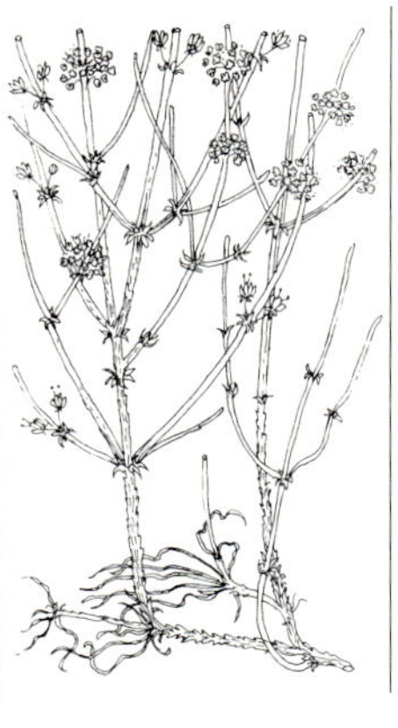

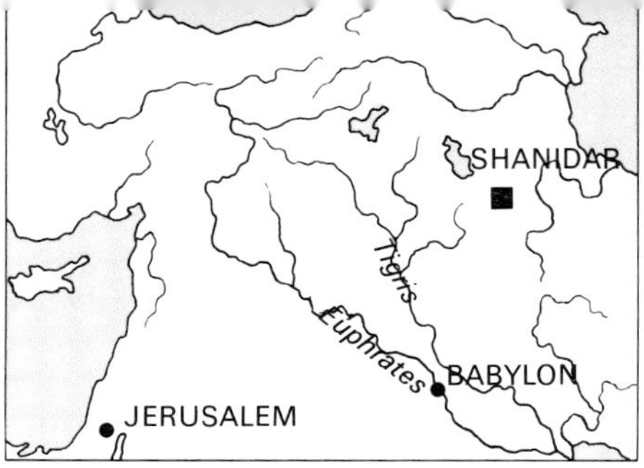

Excavations at Shanidar, Iraq, indicate that prehistoric peoples even 60,000 years ago may have had knowledge of medicinal plants. Such evidence could cause traditional estimates of the Neanderthals' intellectual capacity to be revised.

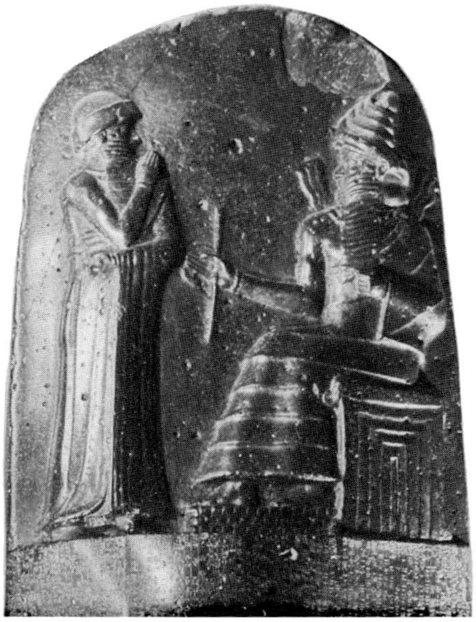

Healing plants are mentioned in the Code of Hammurabi (ca. 1700 B.C.), one of the earliest written historical sources.

Thistle *(Centaurea)*, and Joint Pine *(Ephedra)*. Ralph Solecki, the archaeologist who excavated this site, maintained that the finding of so many plants with known medicinal properties may well cause "speculation about the extent of the human spirit in Neanderthals" leading to the acceptance of the opinion that they indeed did possess an extensive knowledge of the effective medicinal properties of their flora.

In Peruvian graves 2000 years older than the height of the Inca Empire (which occurred some 2500 years ago), bags for Coca leaves and the *lliptu* or lime used with Coca-leaf chewing have been found. Coca leaves discovered in Inca mummy bundles and dated some 1500 years ago have been examined and chemically show the presence of alkaloids. While Coca chewing was practiced widely in pre-Hispanic times from northernmost Colombia down the Andes and in adjacent parts of the Amazon and the eastern slopes of the Argentinian Andes, its main hedonistic use was as a stimulant and narcotic—as it still is. It had, however, in olden times as today, a host of purely medicinal uses, and as in the case of many sacred hallucinogens and narcotics, it is difficult to separate narcotic from medicinal use (in the aboriginal sense of "medicine").

A series of shelters in Coahuila, Mexico, spanning some 8000 years of occupation, have yielded material of the peyote cactus, mescal beans, and Mexican buckeye seeds. All may have been employed as medicines by the early inhabitants, since all are known to possess active principles. Peyote, employed mainly as a hallucinogen today, may have had ceremonial use this far back in time; but it is still valued by Mexican Indians as a physical medicine to hasten the healing of bruises, cuts, and wounds, and it has recently been shown to possess antibiotic activity. Study of dried peyote dated A.D. 810–1070 from these sites—possibly the oldest material yet subjected to chemical analysis—has demonstrated the enduring presence of alkaloids.

OLD HIGH CULTURES

No matter where historical records are consulted—in Babylonia, Egypt, India, China, Greece, Rome—the earliest sources contain numerous references to healing plants.

The Sumerian Ideograms, dated at approximately 2500 B.C., enumerate various medicines of plant origin, including opium, which was known as the "plant of joy." The Assyrians had at least 250 species of plants in their pharmacopoeia.

Perhaps the earliest extensive and tangible records are those in the Code of Hammurabi, who was King of Babylonia from 1728 to 1686 B.C. He caused various records to be carved in stone, some of which are still extant. Now deciphered, they contain many references to the use of healing plants—cassia, henbane, licorice, mints—all of which are used in modern medicine.

Mesopotamian pharmacy was equally dependent on plant drugs, naming some 250, including poppy, belladonna, mandrake, henbane, hemp, saffron, thyme, garlic, onion, licorice, cassia, asafoetida, and myrrh.

In Egypt, the Temple of Karnak has carvings of medicinal plants brought back from as far away as Syria in 1500 B.C. by an expedition sent out for this purpose by Thothemes II. The earliest written records can be traced back to Egypt and are preserved on scrolls of papyrus, a kind of precursor of paper made from the pith of the bullrush of the Nile. The most famous scroll, the Ebers Papyrus dating from the sixteenth century B.C., is a compilation of earlier works. It has a large number of prescriptions and recipes—877 to be exact. Among the many drugs mentioned are cannabis, opium, frankincense, myrrh, aloe, juniper, linseed, castor oil, fennel, cassia, senna, thyme, and henna. Many of the prescriptions employed gums and resins of plant origin.

The Egyptians may have used antibiotics: mud—probably with soil-inhabiting acti-

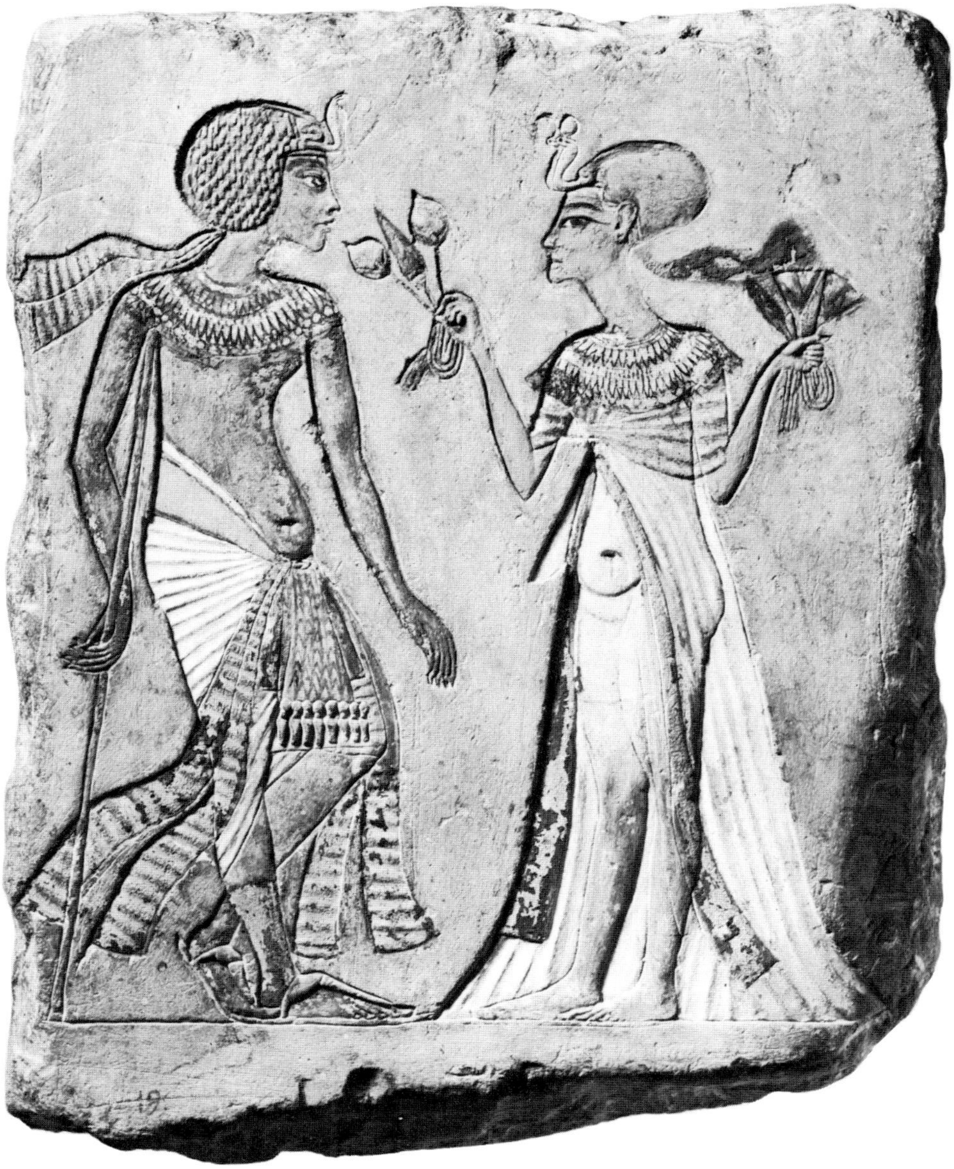

An Egyptian queen holds a mandrake flower, in this fourteenth-century B.C. relief from Echet-Aton. The mandrake *(Mandragora officinarum)* was believed to possess many medicinal qualities, but they have not been confirmed by modern research.

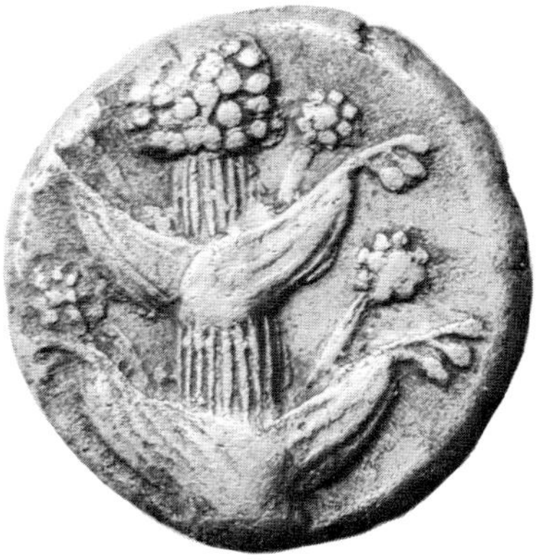

Valued by the ancient Greeks as a spice and a healing agent, the so-called *silphion* (shown on a coin of 480 B.C.) is now extinct. It was an Umbelliferae, possibly of the *genus Thapsia*.

nomycetes that produced antibiotic substances—was applied as a poultice to ulcerated sores. Moldy bread was another Egyptian healing agent, which owed its activity perhaps to fungi. Had modern medicine taken these early practices seriously, man might not have had to wait until the 1930s for the almost accidental discovery of the bactericidal properties of these life-saving substances.

In India, where naturalistic medicine coexisted with superstition and metaphysics, the oldest written records are comparatively recent, but they put us in touch with much older traditions, going back to 1400–1500 B.C. They were passed down orally from generation to generation and were finally formalized in sacred poems or *vedas*. The *Rig Veda,* for example, has more than poems dedicated solely to the supermedicine and god-narcotic *Soma* (only recently identified as the mushroom *Amanita muscaria*) which soothed pain, increased vital forces, and was hallucinogenic.

The *Charaka Samhita,* a later Indian herbal, mentions more than 500 plant remedies, richer in number than the Egyptian pharmacopoeias. Many of the drugs mentioned

FLY AGARIC
Amanita muscaria

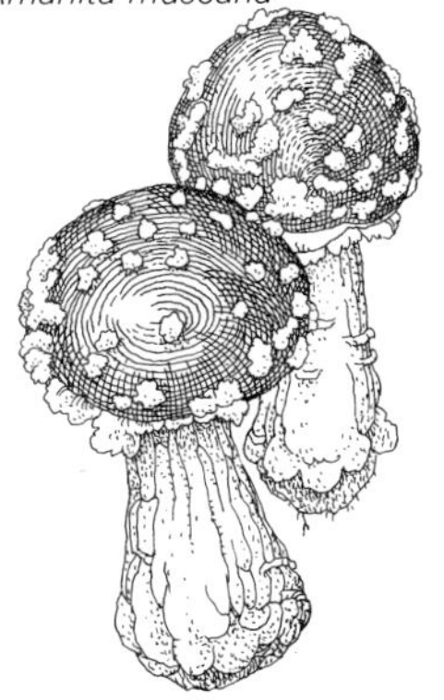

SNAKEROOT
Rauvolfia

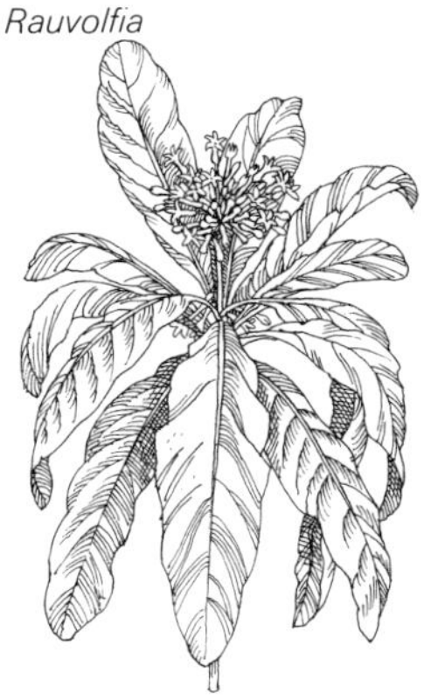

HEMP
Cannabis

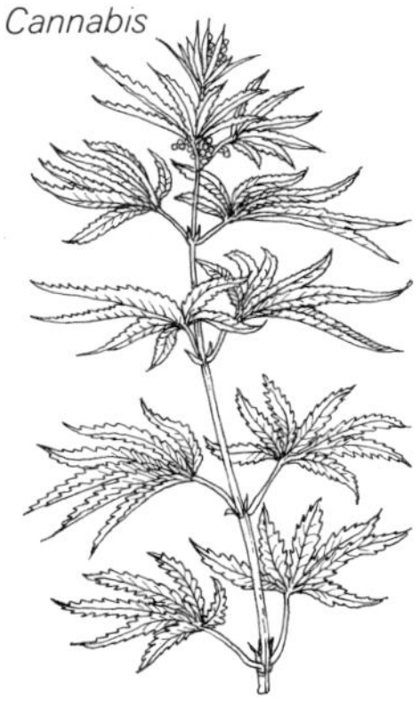

The medicinal plants illustrated above figure prominently in the ancient Indian sacred poems called the *Vedas,* and in other Indian as well as Chinese writings.

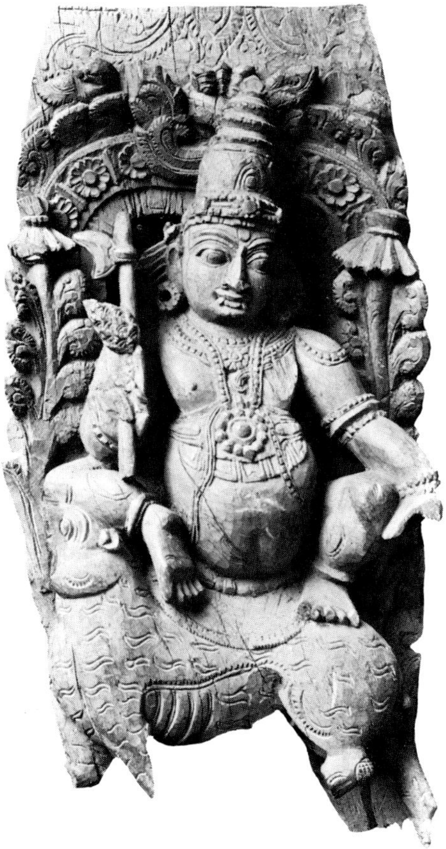

Indra, one of the major Vedic deities of ancient India, drew his extraordinary strength from the consumption of *Soma*. This drink, praised as a supermedicine and hallucinogen in the *Rig Veda*, is believed to have been an extract of the mushroom Fly agaric *(Amanita muscaria)*.

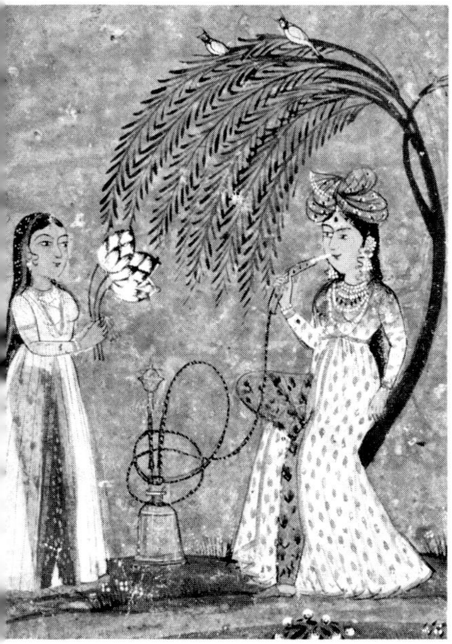

In this Persian miniature of the fourteenth century, a woman smokes hashish (from the Cannabis plant) in a hookah.

in this document eventually were adopted in Egypt, used later in Greece, and finally found their way into European folk medicine.

The number of references to healing plants in the *Vedas* is very great. One species mentioned there—the Snake Root or *Rauvolfia*—with 4000 years of use in India in treating snake bite, mental disorders, and epilepsy as well as a host of lesser ailments, has, during the past forty years, literally revolutionized western medicine as a tranquilizer and hypotensive agent. Largely as a result of the interest of Indian research workers in native ethnopharmacological lore, it was possible to isolate the principal alkaloid of Snake Root, reserpine.

While known now primarily as a narcotic, *Cannabis* or Hemp has had a long history in folk medicine, and all modern evidence points to the probability that some of its 50 cannabinolic constituents—or semisynthetic analogues of them—may become important in western medicine. One of man's oldest cultigens, Hemp is a five-purpose plant. Its use as a medicine goes back in Chinese tradition 4800 years, and to Indian writings dated about 3500 years ago. These sources reported the therapeutic value of Hemp in treating many ailments. Throughout the Middle Ages, in Europe, it was extolled as a medicine, and Hemp was official in the United States Pharmacopoeia as a tranquilizer until 1937.

Some 5000 years ago, the Chinese were probably utilizing a strange leafless desert vine known as *ma-huang* in treating pulmonary ills. The earliest Chinese medical work, the *Pen Tsao* of Shen Nung, written about 2900 B.C., represented the accumulation of centuries of earlier folk uses of plants. Listing a total of some 365 drugs, it recorded the virtues of *ma-huang:* a tea said to improve circulation, reduce fevers, aid in correcting urinary functions, calm coughing; but its main attributes related to its efficiency in relieving pulmonary or bronchial problems. Although chemical studies isolated the alkaloid ephedrine as early as the 1880s, it was not until the 1920s that

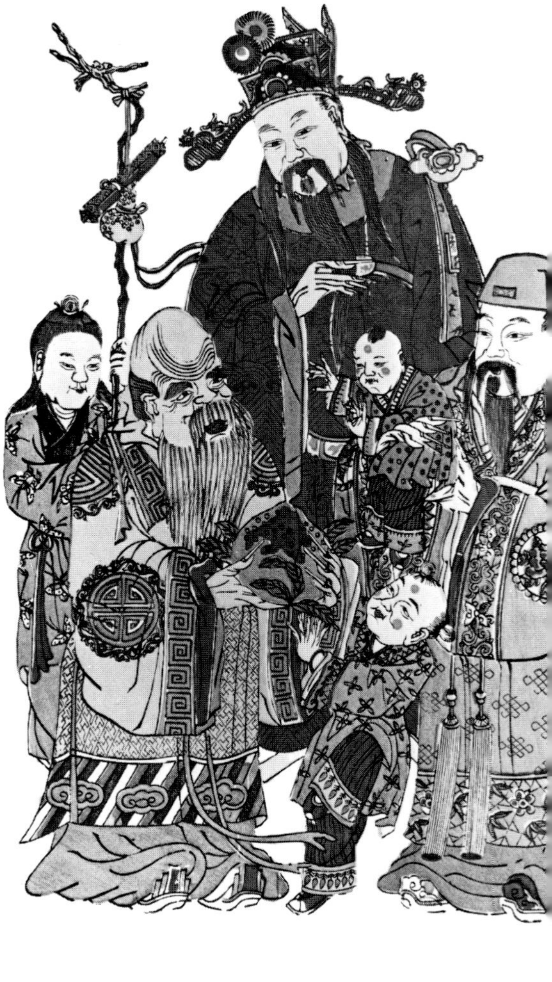

As early as 2500 B.C., the Chinese were using plant medicines to treat pulmonary complaints, poor circulation, fever, leprosy, and many other ills. The aged wise man shown in the foreground of the Chinese painting at the right is handing a fruit to a child. Behind him hangs a small gourd filled with medicine.

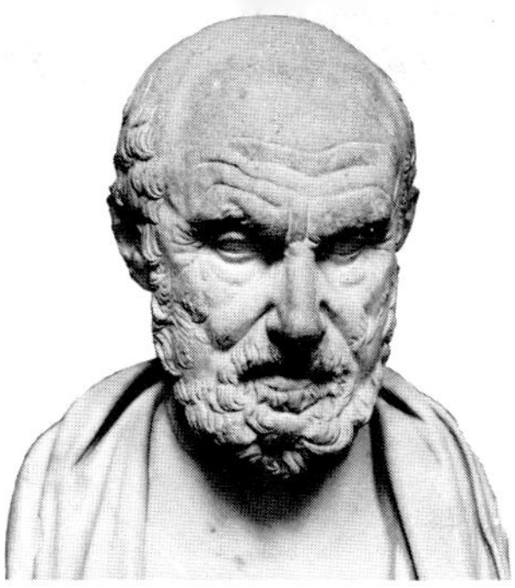

pharmacological investigations established its real value in relieving the discomforts of asthma, hay fever, and the common cold.

Other Chinese drugs of wide and early use were Rhubarb as a mild laxative and *Dichroa febrifuga* to reduce fevers. Castor Oil, Camphor, and Cannabis or *ta-ma* were major items in the Chinese pharmacopoeia. Although surgery was not generally practiced in early China, Hua To in the third century A.D. is said to have employed a mixture of Monkshood and Hemp to narcotize patients about to undergo the very painful trepanning operation.

Leprosy has been feared as a fatal disease from earliest times—a plague without cure. Yet the Chinese, as early as 2500 B.C., and the Indians somewhat later, reported the value of Chaulmoogra Oil in their folk pharmacopoeia. The source of the seed oil, however, was not known with certainty until the 1920s, when an American botanist, penetrating the interior of China, identified it as a product of several species of *Hydnocarpus.* Effective in curing incipient cases of leprosy, Chaulmoogra Oil was the first breakthrough in the fight against this ancient plague.

While not an ethnobotanical document, the Bible, both the Old and the New Testament, refers to the medicinal use of plants. The number of healing plants is, however, very reduced—approximately thirty being specifically mentioned, including garlic, onion, leek, oleander, cumin, oleaster, galbanum, bay, mandrake, mints, and nettles. It appears that the Jews may have utilized far fewer healing plants than neighboring peoples of the Near East, despite their long residence in Egypt and Babylonia.

Among the ancient Greeks four men contributed significantly to medical botany. Known as the Father of Modern Medicine, Hippocrates (in the late fifth–early fourth century B.C.) mentioned some 300 to 400 medicinal plants—fewer than those used in Egypt. He believed that the human body, to a large extent, is self-healing, needing but a little help from drugs and a proper diet to restore normal health. Hippocrates is notable, almost uniquely so, in not associating demonology with the healing properties of herbs. Aristotle (384–322 B.C.) ascribed to each plant the properties and virtues then known. Theophrastus (d. ca. 287 B.C.), primarily a botanist, described many Greek and foreign plants, with accounts of their use. His treatise *Enquiry into Plants* had a profound influence on the progress of botany and medicine for nearly twenty centuries. The most influential medico-botanical writer, however, was Dioscorides (first century A.D.) whose book *De Materia Medica* not only set the pattern for the great European herbals of the Middle Ages but became the prototype of our modern pharmacopoeias. The influence of Dioscorides was overpowering: up to the Renaissance, it was the infallible authority in both medicine and botany. The earliest version, transcribed about A.D. 512, is known as the Codex Juliana. Much of the plant lore of Europe stemmed directly from the writings of Dioscorides.

Rome, unlike Greece, produced little in medical botany. Pliny the Elder, in his *Natural History* (first century A.D.), offered no original ideas. The great value of his work is that it represents a compilation of about 2000 treatises written by some 326 Greeks and 146 Romans. Much of Pliny's folk medicine passed into the folklore of Europe and the New World.

"The Father of Modern Medicine," Hippocrates (460–377 B.C.) has left 87 treatises in which he mentions more than 300 healing plants.

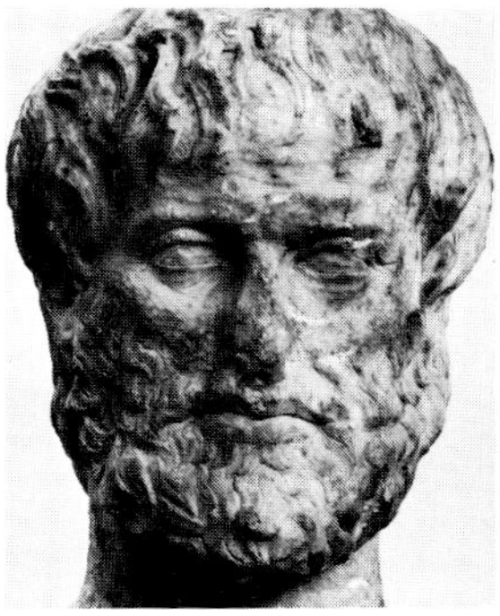

ARISTOTLE

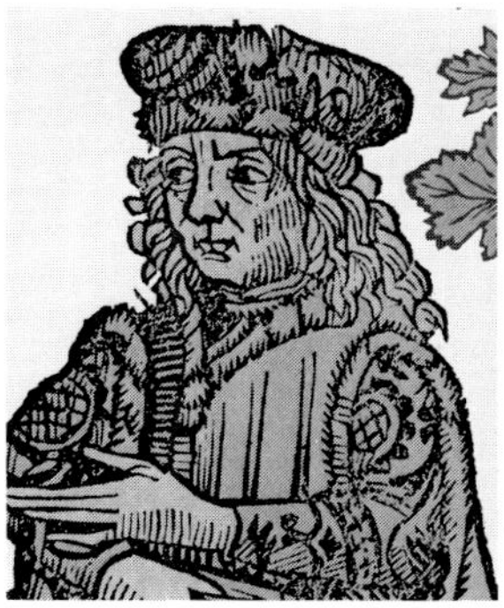

THEOPHRASTUS

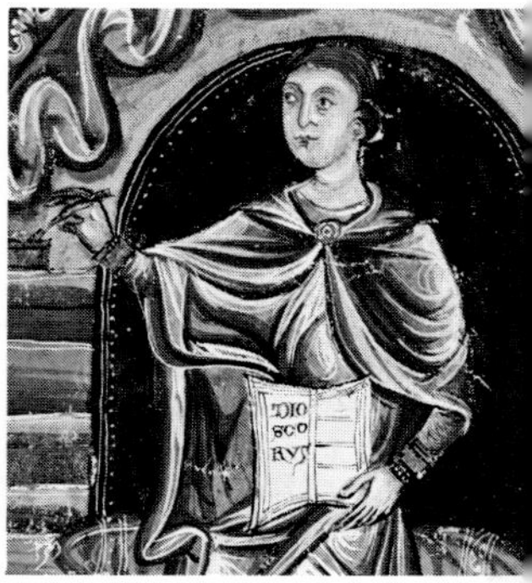

DIOSCORIDES

Aristotle, Theophrastus, and Dioscorides carried on the Greek medical tradition. Dioscorides (first century B.C.) had the greatest influence on European medicine up to the Renaissance.

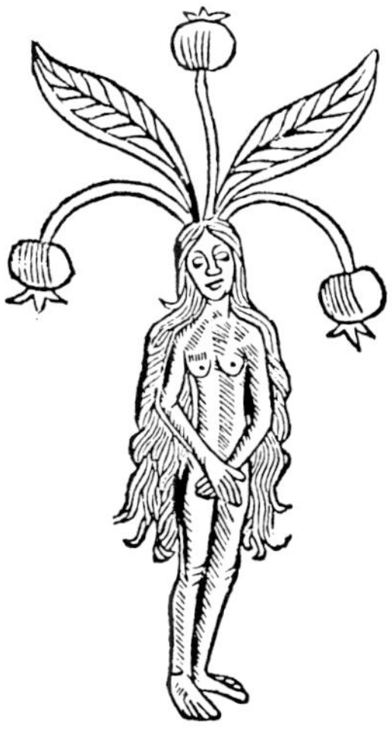

For the Middle Ages, a plant's appearance was decisive. The roots of the mandrake *(Mandragora officinarum)* resemble a human body, and the likeness was often exaggerated in drawings of the plant, such as this fantastical woodcut from an herbal of 1498.

The great herbalists from antiquity to the Middle Ages are shown assembled around the Greek Dioscorides, at center, in this illustration from an herbal of 1485. Seated in the foreground are the Roman Pliny (left) and an Arabic herbal doctor. The photographs at right show two of the most frequently used plants in medieval medicine, all with tropane alkaloid content.

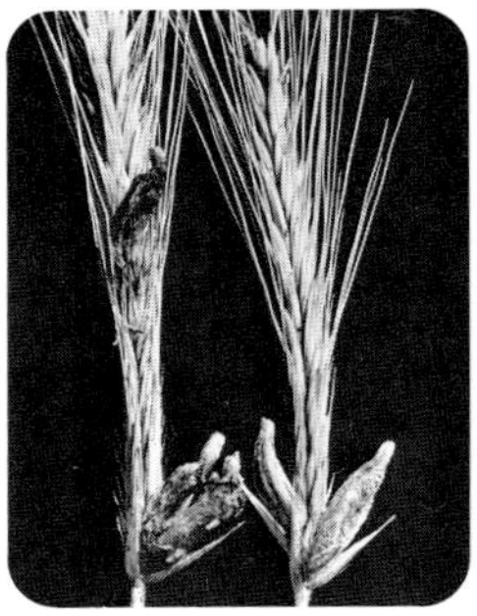

ERGOT
Claviceps purpurea

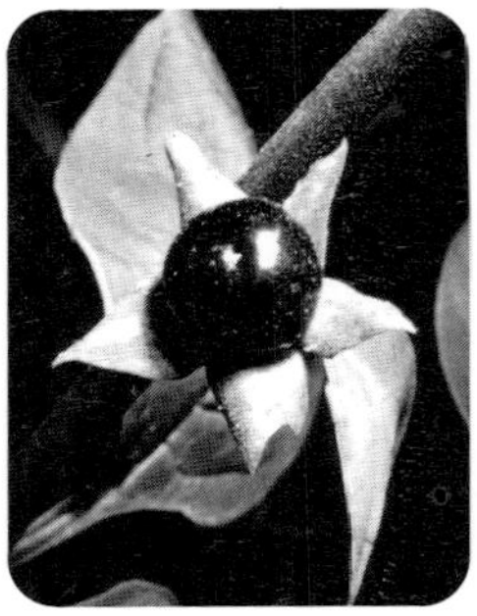

BELLADONNA
Atropa belladonna

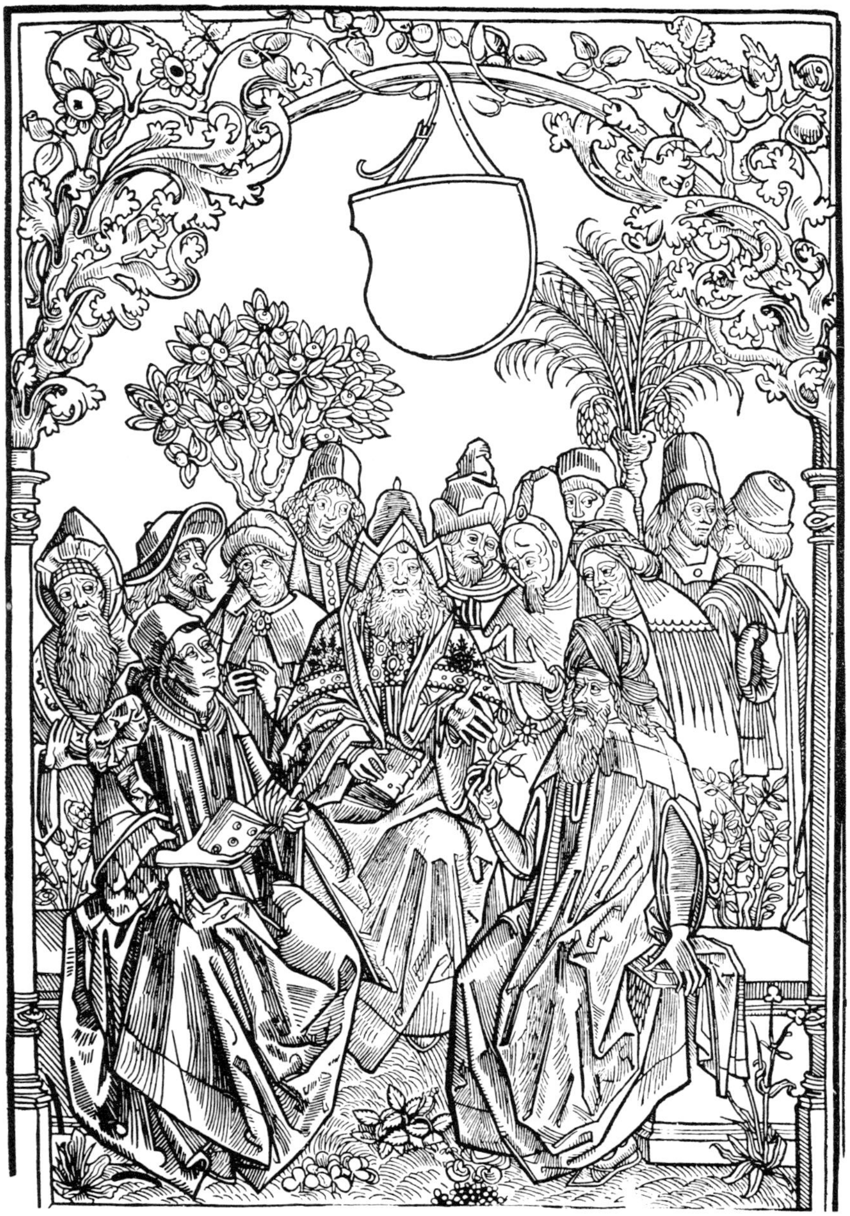

MEDIEVAL CULTURES

Early European knowledge of healing plants filtered down through the Middle Ages, some of it persisting until modern times. The solanaceous Belladonna, Henbane, and Mandrake, for example, were employed in the earliest folk medicine of the Continent for a wide range of medicinal purposes, because of their tropane alkaloid content. They likewise played important roles in witchcraft and sorcery in the Middle Ages; this is perhaps one of the reasons why such medicinally valuable plants as Belladonna and Henbane were not accepted in the London Pharmacopoeia until 1809.

One of the most widely prescribed cardiac drugs, Digitalis, was used in England and Wales as far back as the tenth century. The cardiotonic properties of Foxglove were introduced to modern medicine only in 1775, when Dr. Withering discovered its edema-reducing effects from treatments prescribed by country women in Shropshire. The plant had been official, however, for other uses as early as 1650 in the London Pharmacopoeia.

Perhaps the most astounding contribution made to modern medicine by folk pharmacy is Ergot. Used medicinally in Asia from ancient times, this fungal infection of rye and other cereals was valued during the Middle Ages in Europe by midwives in cases of difficult childbirth. Furthermore, when fruiting bodies of the fungus were accidentally milled into flour and baked into bread, whole towns were poisoned, many people died, some hallucinated, and some became permanently insane. Today, alkaloids from ergot are still used as relaxants of involuntary muscles to help induce childbirth and, as strong vasoconstrictors, to arrest postpartum hemorrhages and to treat migraine. There is evidence that ergot, because of its intoxicating properties, may have been involved in the Eleusinian mysteries of ancient Greece.

It was Pliny who was responsible for crystallizing an idea which originated probably with the Greeks, although it was found, in one form or another, in cultures around the world: (1) that nature serves man; (2) that plants were created to satisfy

St. Anthony's Fire is the medieval name for the violent reaction caused by the ingestion of Ergot *(Claviceps purpurea),* which was sometimes accidentally milled with flour. The "plague" took the form of mass poisoning, or sometimes hallucinations and permanent insanity. The seventeenth-century picture below shows St. Anthony withstanding satanic temptations and other ills.

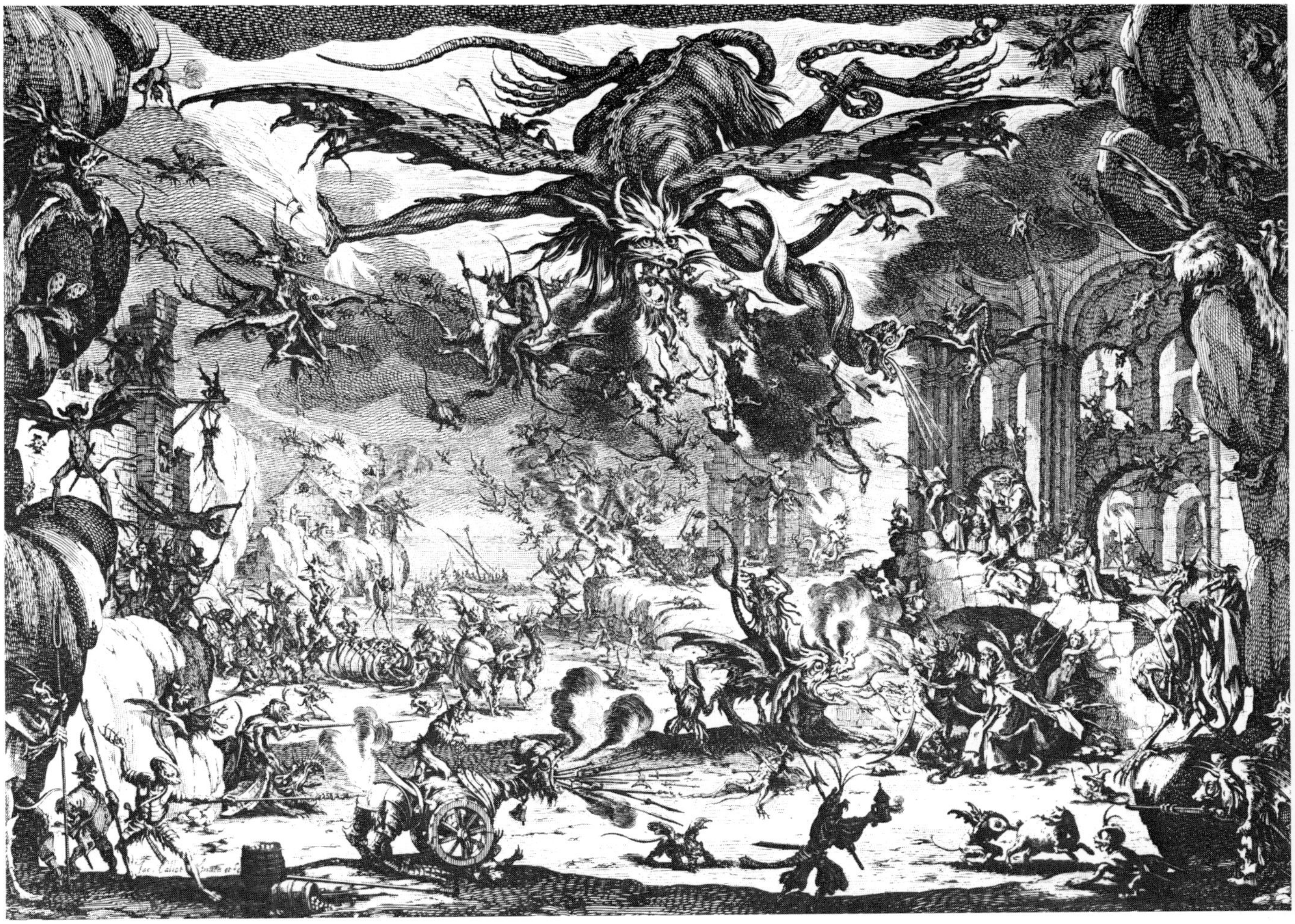

man's needs; and (3) that, therefore, all plants not obviously useful (as foods, fibers, lumber) might well possess medicinal properties.

This was the germ of an idea that in Medieval Europe developed into the famous Doctrine of Signatures. The idea was promulgated as a doctrine by Paracelsus, a Swiss physician who lived from 1443 to 1541.

Paracelsus postulated not only that herbs were put on earth for man's use, but that many were stamped by the Creator with a clear sign or signature of the purpose for which they were to be used. A heart-shaped leaf, for example, meant that the plant was a remedy for cardiac diseases. Many of the vernacular names of plants in Europe stem from belief in the Doctrine of Signatures: beard grass, crowfoot, foxtail grass, horsetail, goose foot, etc.

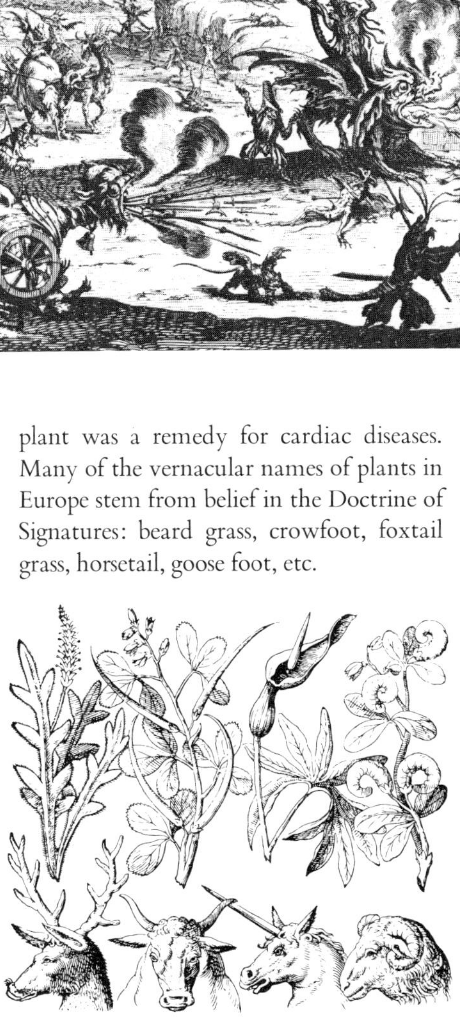

Illustrations for Giambattista della Porta's 1588 treatise on the Doctrine of Signatures draw analogies between plants and animals, suggesting that consumption of a particular plant could make a person either more energetic or calmer.

Foxglove *(Digitalis purpurea)*, source of the digitalis used in heart ailments: an herbal contribution to modern medicine.

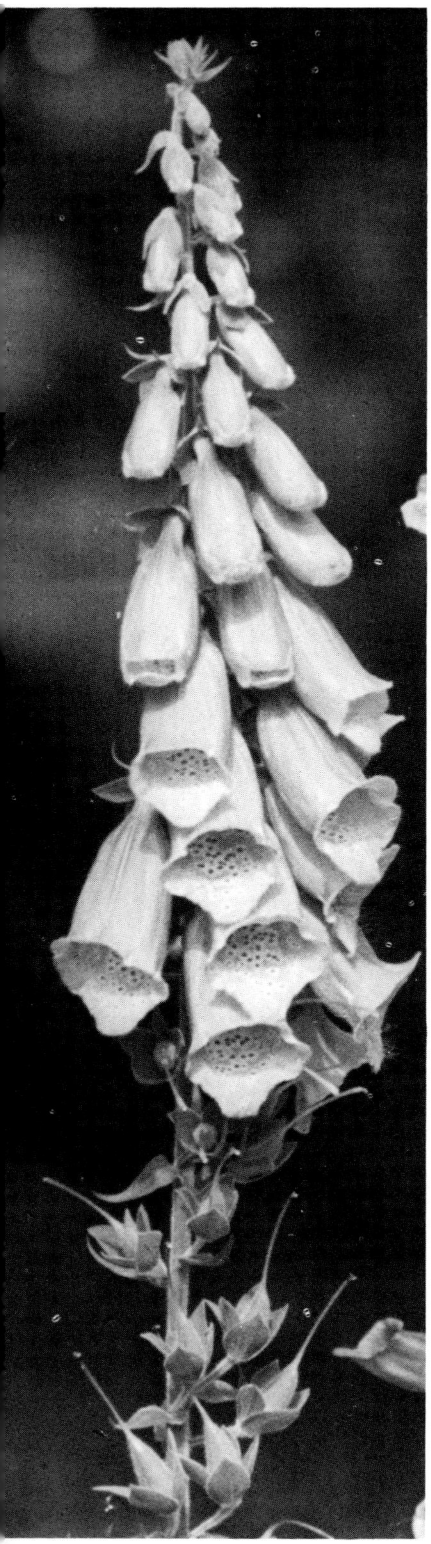

It was not until about 1470 that the hold that Dioscorides and other classical writers had on European botany and medicine began to weaken. At that time, the herbalists began to study plants themselves and to provide original descriptions and illustrations, and herbals—compendia of true and false information—began to appear. At first, they were but garbled versions of Dioscorides. It was not until about 1670 that botany began to divorce itself from medicine, to the mutual advantage of both sciences. It was not long before the Doctrine of Signatures was totally discredited. Yet the reputation that plants had acquired over such a long period was not easy to dispel and has often clung to them. But, through the ages, by trial and error, many plants that carried no special signatures gained fame as healing agents, and some of these have lingered on and, as in the case of Foxglove, have been supported by the impartial searchlight of modern chemical and pharmacological research.

PROTOHISTORICAL SOCIETIES OF THE PRESENT

A continent of rich and varied tropical floras—and apparently the home of man—Africa harbors millions of natives still living in primitive societies. Yet ethnobotanical studies are totally lacking for great areas of the continent. Recent publications on the toxic and medicinal plants of east, south, and west Africa suggest that investigations of some of the healing plants still used by the natives would lead to medically valuable discoveries.

Undoubtedly, one of the most important gifts of Africa to modern medicine has been physostigmine, an alkaloid isolated from the Calabar Bean of Nigeria. Exceedingly toxic, this bean, product of a forest liana, was administered as one of the many ordeal poisons of Africa and Madagascar to determine guilt or innocence. The beans have also had other uses in native healing practices. Physostigmine, the principal alkaloid, is now a major tool in modern ophthalmology, used to cause protracted dilatation of the pupil and as an aid in treating glaucoma.

Another African gift to modern medicine comes from several species of *Strophanthus* which, with a variety of medicinal uses as well, were employed by the natives in preparing arrow poisons and contain potent glycosides acting on heart muscle. One species is the source of ouabain, a cardiac stimulant now administered for acute heart failure and pulmonary edema. Another species yields glycosides valuable in the emergency treatment of acute cardiac asthma. It was the famous British explorer of Africa, Dr. David Livingstone (1813–1873), who first noted the toxicity and cardiac activity of *Kombe,* one of these species.

Four plants used in aboriginal civilizations.

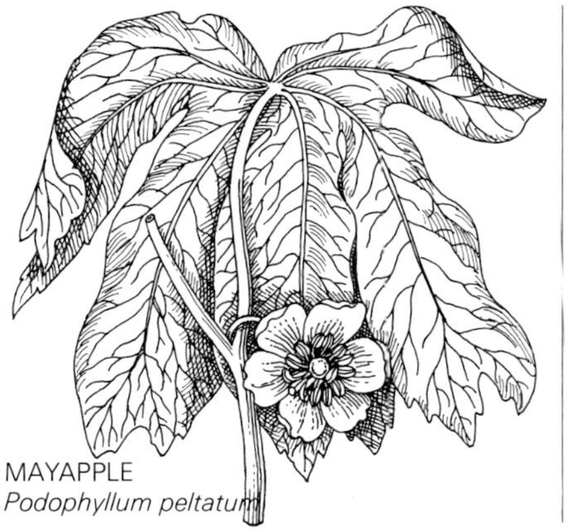

MAYAPPLE
Podophyllum peltatum

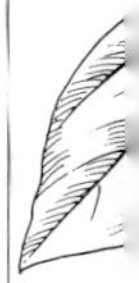

It was an African species of *Rauvolfia*—the so-called African Snake Wood—that, to a large extent, replaced the once supreme Indian Snake Root as a source of reserpine. This African species had a host of indigenous medicinal uses, including the treatment of snakebite, leprosy, jaundice, venereal diseases, rheumatism, and skin rashes, and it was valued as a vermifuge, purga-

The Tasaday tribe, 27 persons living a Stone Age existence in caves in the Philippine rain forests, were discovered by anthropologists in 1966. In their isolation, tribes such as this one preserve customs that had long disappeared from most parts of the earth; they thus offer a wealth of historical testimony about life in the Mesolithic and Neolithic cultures. In some cases, these anachronistic communities are a valuable source of information concerning herbal medicine, since plants are the only means of healing available to them.

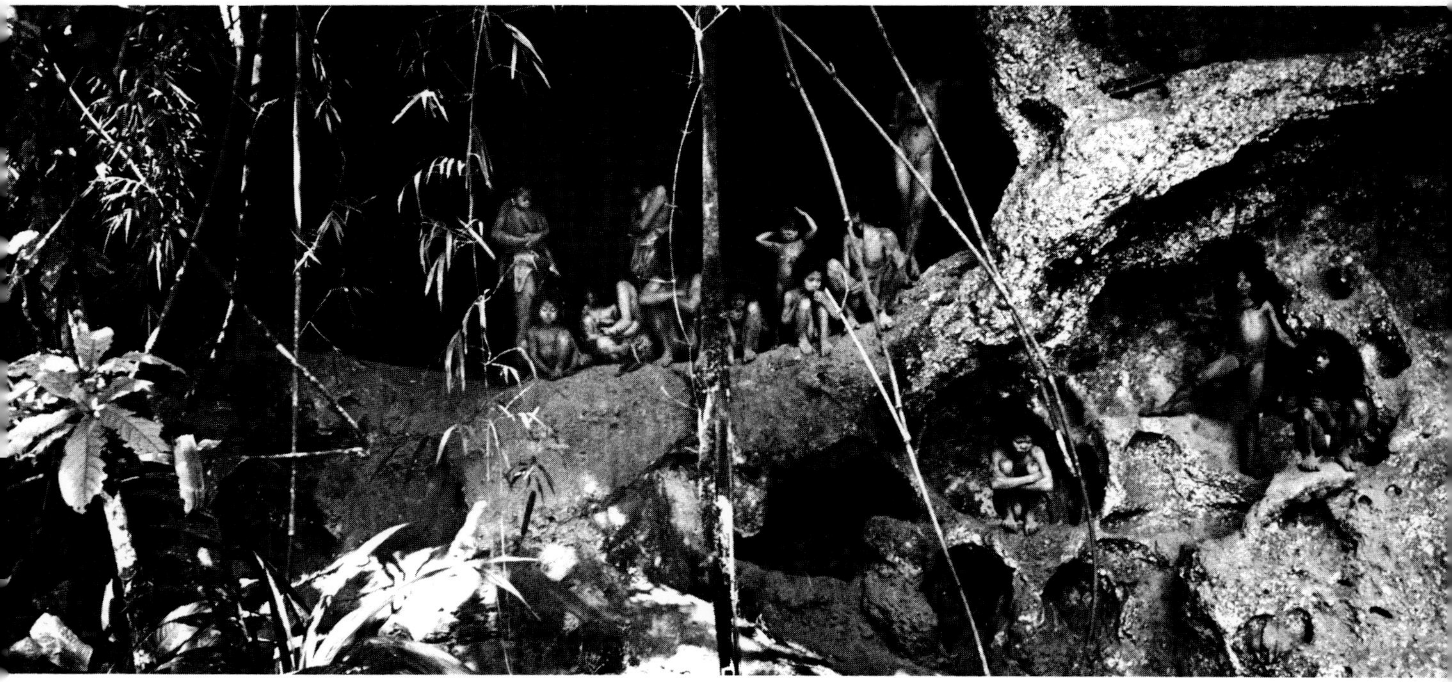

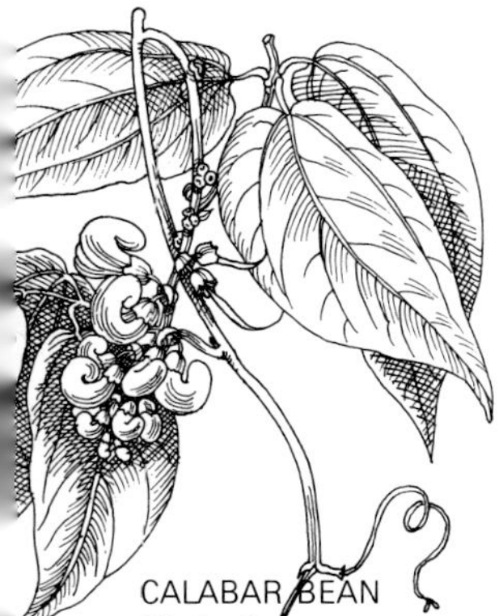

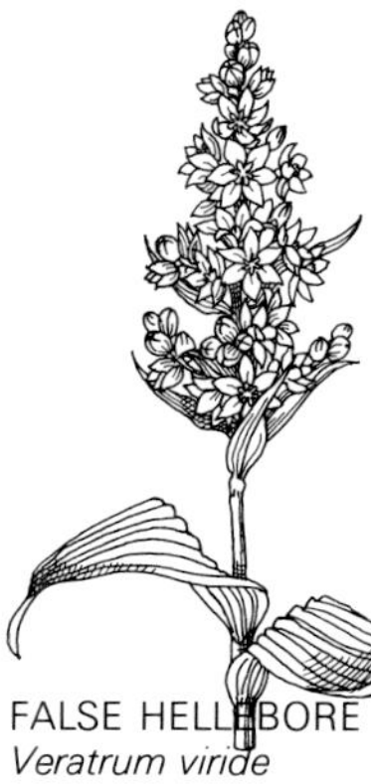

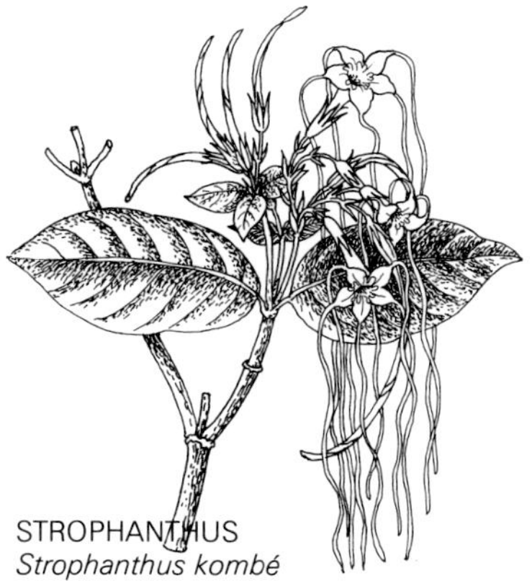

tive, emetic, and abortifacient and as an excellent inducer of sleep.

The flora of the Americas has been a prodigious provider of economic plants now used the world around. This has been true especially of healing plants.

Although its flora is rather limited, North America has given modern medicine a number of drug plants, most of them with histories of folk uses among the Indians.

Early Spanish missionaries along the Pacific coastal areas learned from the native inhabitants about the virtues of a bark employed as a mild cathartic. They called it *Cascara Sagrada* or "sacred bark." This medicinal plant has maintained its position as a major item in the United States Pharmacopoeia.

The North American Indians are responsible also for two healing plants that have only recently assumed importance in medicine: the False Hellebore and the May Apple.

Podophyllum—the May Apple or American Mandrake—had numerous uses in native

Indians smoking: one of the curiosities of the New World reported by a Frenchman named Thevet in his book *Singularités* (1558).

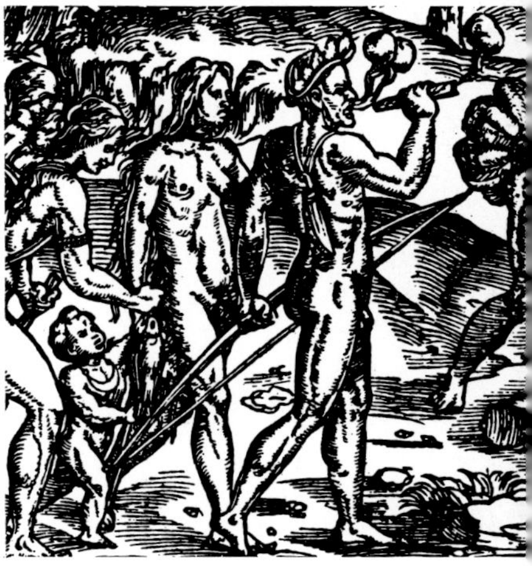

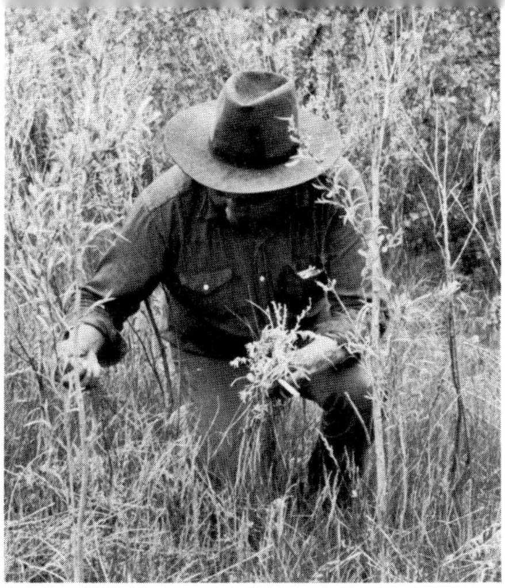

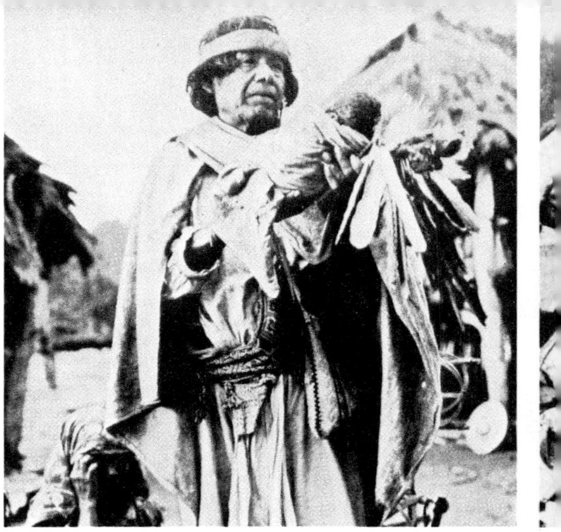

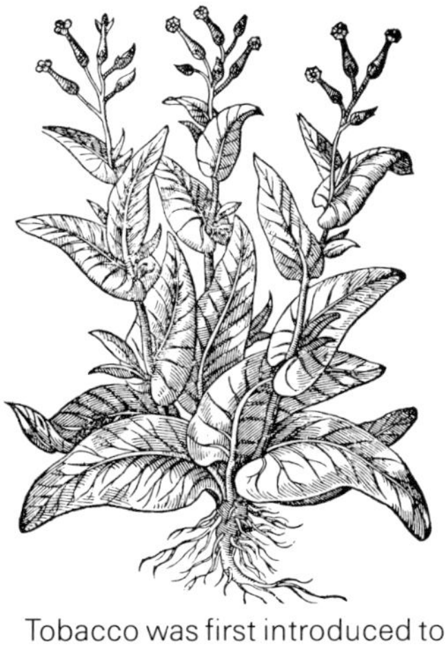

Tobacco was first introduced to Europe as a medicine. This is the first printed illustration of the plant to appear in England (1570).

medicine: the Cherokee employed the juice of the rhizome to relieve deafness; the Iroquois committed suicide by ingesting the raw rhizome. Despite its toxicity, it was valued likewise as an emetic, purgative, and anthelmintic (expelling intestinal worms). Adopted by the early white settlers for a host of purposes—including treatment of typhoid, dysentery, and hepatitis—the drug yields a resin now considered effective against venereal warts. Other species with similar chemical constituents have likewise long been employed in folk medicine in several parts of Asia.

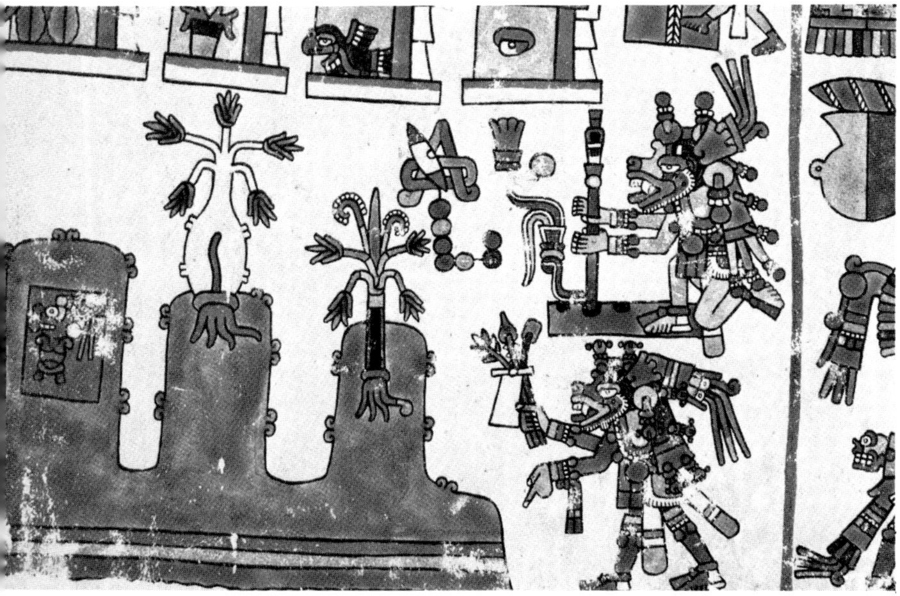

Pictures of healing plants in the Badianus Manuscript of 1552, the first herbal to appear in the New World. Written by a Mexican Indian, the work discussed nearly 200 species.

Another extremely toxic plant valued by the Iroquois Indians to treat nasal catarrh was False Hellebore. It was adopted by white settlers as a veritable cure-all. Recent research has isolated alkaloids now widely used—often with reserpine—to relieve hypertension.

The so-called Indian Tobacco, once smoked by North American natives and employed against pulmonary disorders, now yields alkaloidal constituents used in preparations to help break the cigarette smoking habit.

Some of the New World cultures, subdued and in great part destroyed by the Europeans, in many respects knew more than their conquerors about actual healing plants and their utilization. The first herbal of the New World, the *Badianus Manuscript* of 1552, recently discovered in the Vatican Library, illustrated in color, described the medicinal values of nearly 200 species: one interesting aspect of this early work is that its author was himself a Mexican Indian. In 1865 a Spanish physician, Monardes, wrote an extensive book on Mexican drug plants, based partly on personal experimentation with them on patients. The King of Spain sent his own physician, Dr. Francisco Hernández, to study Aztec drug plants: the result was an encyclopedic work on the natural history of "New Spain," in which some 1200 healing plants were discussed, usually in great detail, and many of them so carefully illustrated that their identification is rarely in doubt. The dried root and resin of Jalap, a Morning Glory, was, for example, the source of a powerful cathartic that is still employed. Sarsaparilla was esteemed highly in the treatment of bladder and kidney problems because of its strong diuretic properties. Tobacco powder served to relieve headache, stupor, dizziness, and nasal problems—and it should be noted that tobacco was first introduced to Europe as a medicine and was so used until the present century. The ecclesiastical writer Sahagún, whose *Historia de las Cosas de Nueva España* considered every aspect of Mexican life, devoted many pages to native medicine, including brief discussions of the

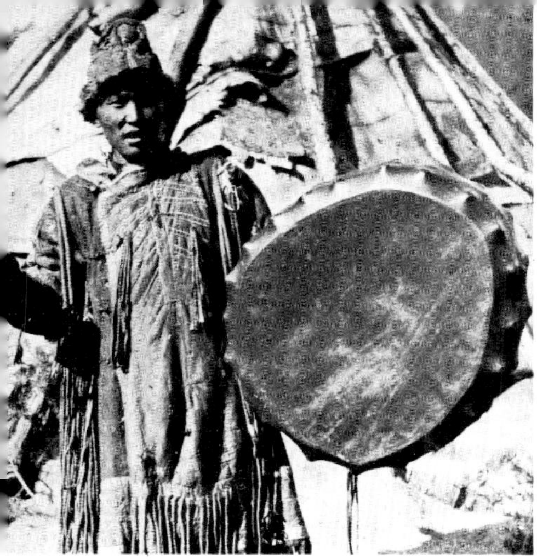

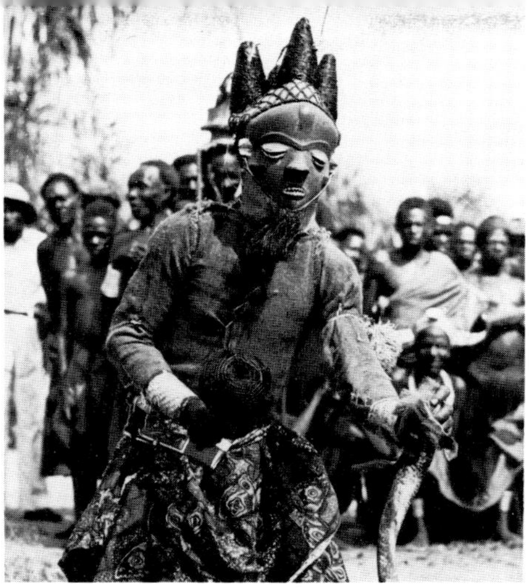

The shaman or medicine man was a dominant figure in many aboriginal civilizations in both hemispheres.

The four photographs at left depict *(from left to right)*:

A North American Sioux Chieftain gathering medicinal herbs.

A shaman of the Mexican Huichol community in the western Sierra Madres holding a newborn baby.

A Karagass shaman of Siberia, who beats the deerskin drum and consumes fly agaric mushrooms to induce a trance.

A masked witch doctor in Nioka-Kakese, former Belgian Congo, performing a ritual dance as he holds a basket filled with dried seeds and an antelope horn full of powder.

healing properties of local plants and plant products.

It was in Mexico that the use as "supermedicines" of psychoactive plants—the hallucinogens—was developed to an extraordinary degree in magico-religious and medical rituals. Of the many species of hallucinogenic plants so employed in Mexico, three groups are preeminent as "divine remedies": Peyote, Teonanacatl, and Ololiuqui. Employed ritualistically—even to the present time–and for healing purposes, they all have chemical constituents of value in modern medicine: mescaline from Peyote and psilocybine from the two dozen or so species of sacred mushrooms known to the ancient Aztecs as *teonanacatl* ("divine flesh") have found use in modern psychiatry; the ergoline alkaloids—chemically related to LSD—from the Morning Glory known to the Aztecs as *ololiuqui* are the same compounds occurring in Ergot, which has been employed by midwives in Europe from early times right up to the present day in the management of childbirth. These ergoline alkaloids constrict involuntary muscles and are vasoconstrictors—both properties being of extreme importance in modern gynecology. But their use as hallucinogenic "medicines" among the Mexicans was of the greatest importance to these people.

South America is the world's principal center for the use of arrow poisons or curare. Almost every tribe and sometimes almost every medicine man has a special formula. Although many plants enter into these formulas, the major active ingredient belongs usually to the genus *Strychnos* or to species of several menispermaceous genera. It is from extracts of the latter that alkaloids, especially tubocurarine, have become so important in modern medicine. Tubocurarine is a potent muscle relaxant. Supplies of the active constituents are still extracted from curare, a brownish paste prepared by Indians in the western Amazon. Although tubocurarine has been syn-

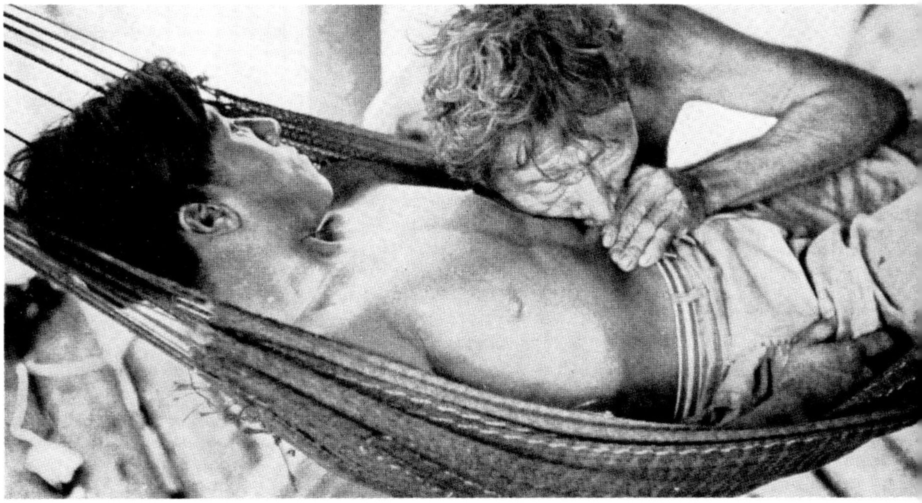

In Venezuela, a shaman treats an illness by sucking out the spirit or "sickness projectile" believed to have been sent by a mysterious power.

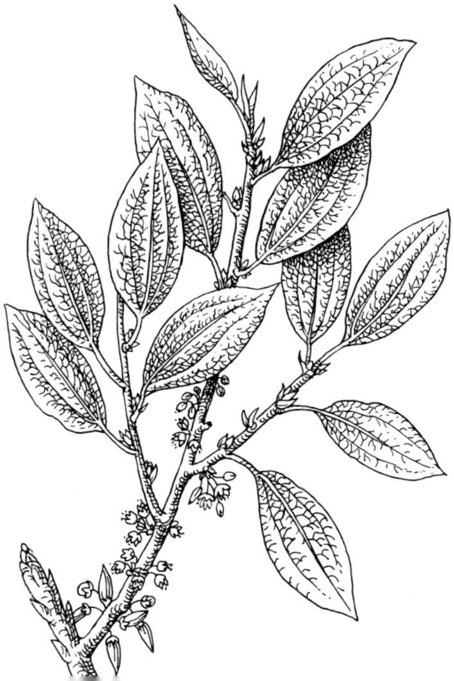

Left: The Cola plant, the most famous medicine in Peru. It was used as an analgesic, anorectic, and stimulant, and may even have been effective as an anesthetic. The plant's active principle, cocaine, is important in modern medicine.

thesized, the synthetic alkaloid is inferior to the natural alkaloid for medical use. Thus, here we have a major drug that is closely linked to folk medicine: the drug was discovered from native toxicology, and the Indian population is still its source.

Since the ancient Peruvians did not develop anything approaching written records, we know less about their pharmacopoeia.

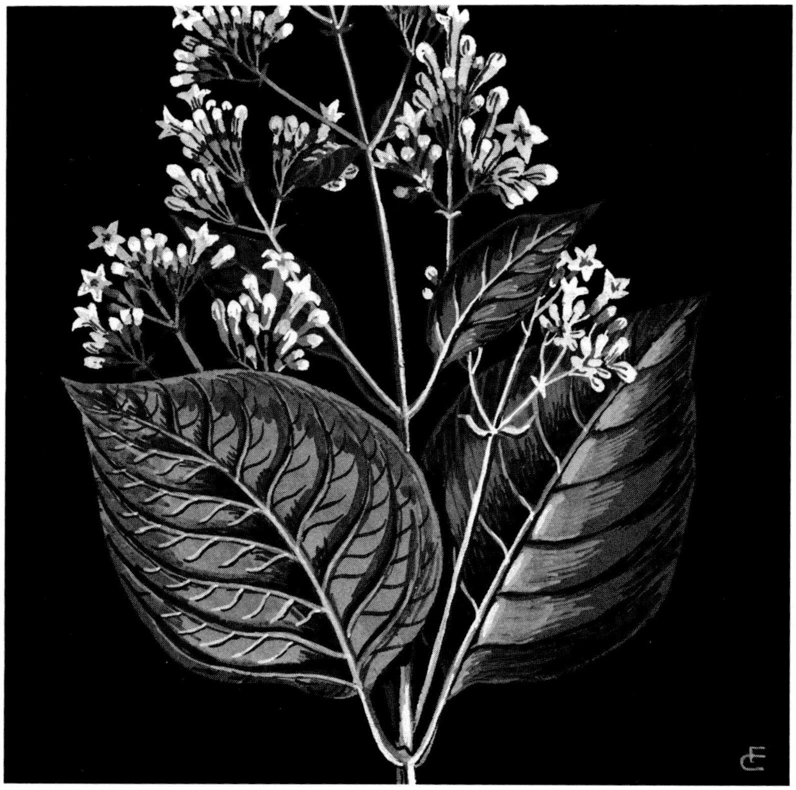

Quinine, western medicine's greatest debt to ancient Peru, is extracted from the bark of the Cinchona tree. Used by Ecuadorian Indians to relieve fever, the plant came to be called Jesuits' Bark in the seventeenth century and was later cultivated by the Dutch and British in Asia.

Their flora was replete with medicinally valuable plants, but unfortunately we know little about the extent of its use. The Incas had a bevy of "doctors": *hampicamayoc, oquetlupuc,* or *sircac* (possessors of medicine and surgery) and *colla-huaya* (traveling apothecaries who dispensed medicines).

Undoubtedly the most famous medicine in Peru was Coca, which was prescribed generally for its analgesic, anorectic, and stimulating properties. Once confined apparently to the priestly and noble castes, Coca was released for general use shortly before the Spanish conquest of Peru. There is even the suggestion—still unproven—that the Incas employed a poultice of masticated Coca leaves to relieve pain prior to the common Peruvian trepanning operation. The active principle of Coca, cocaine, has assumed an important role in modern medicine, especially in ophthalmology. Modern Indians living in the Andes still take a tea of Coca leaves to relieve many common ailments, especially digestive ills. The Peruvian pharmacopoeia had many healing plants, including tree Daturas and Ipecac. The Incas likewise had strong purgatives: *Huillcautari* fruits, and the root of Huachanca. Huachanca enjoyed fame also as an effective abortifacient. To relieve certain eye infections, the leaves of Mactellu were esteemed.

The most important medicine plant to have come to western medicine from ancient Peru, however, is Quinine, from the bark of several species of *Cinchona.* It was highly valued as a febrifuge by Ecuadorian Indians, from whom Jesuit missionaries learned of its properties in the early 1600s. Known from that time on as Jesuits' Bark, it was exploited for many years by this religious order. For two centuries, all bark was supplied by wild trees, until the Dutch successfully brought it under cultivation in their tropical Asiatic colonies. And today, despite very effective, synthetic antimalarial drugs, quinine maintains a place among our major drugs of plant origin. This Indian fever bark has saved probably more lives than any other drug.

These are but a few of the important healing plants that can trace their modern medical use to protohistorical societies of the present or very recent times. There are many more, and there are literally scores of modern drugs of lesser importance that have come to the healing arts from beliefs and customs of medicine men and from uncivilized man. Can there be any doubt that many more potential life-saving medicaments remain unnoticed by modern

MORNING GLORY *(Ipomoea violaceae)*, the pride of so many gardens in all parts of the world, is a native of South America. Known there as ololiuqui, it has a long history as a hallucinogenic agent.

science in the wealth of folklore lurking in the hinterlands of the world?

* * *

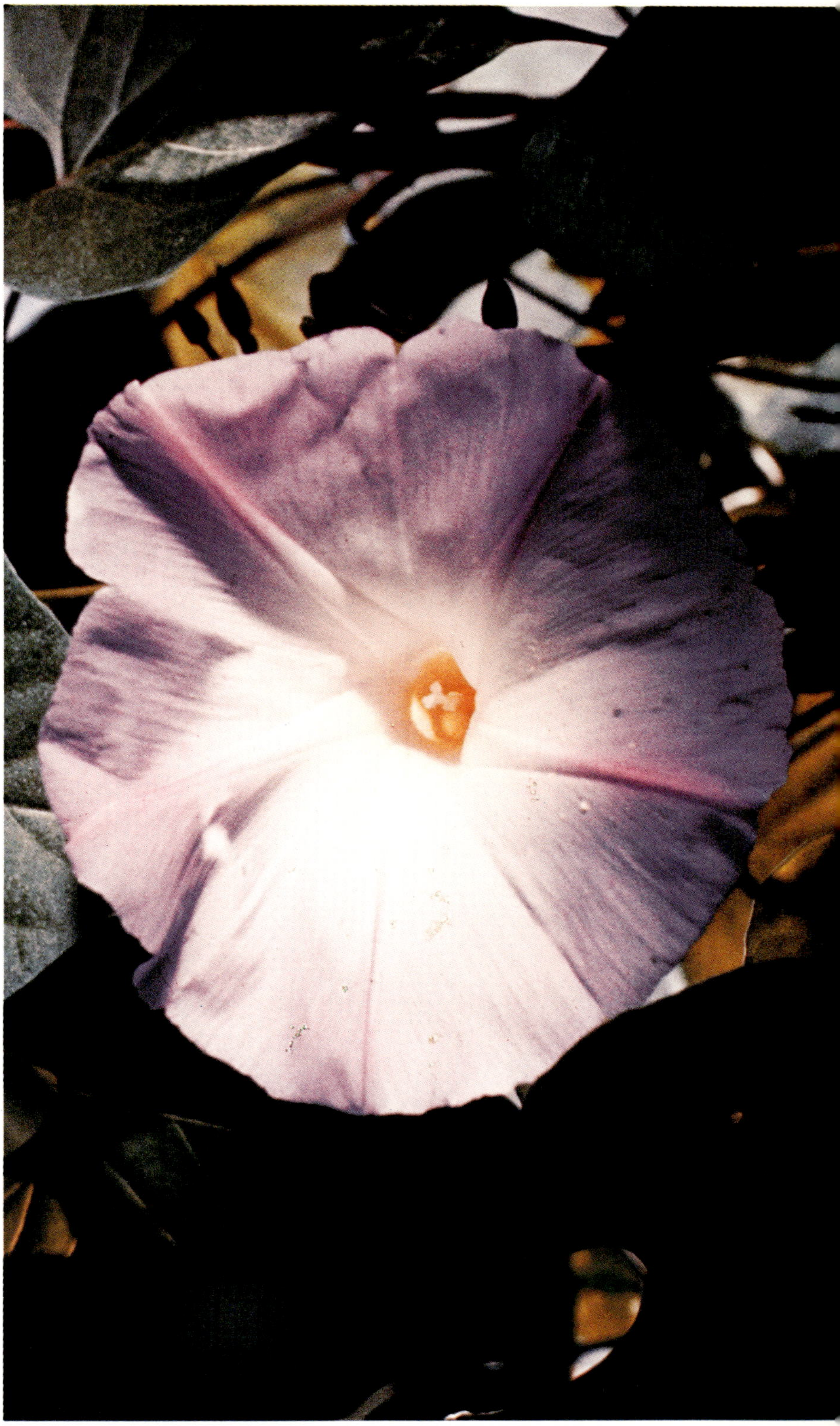

Serious and critical evaluation of native uses of plants still provides science with a remarkable and extensive reservoir of new ideas and potentialities when it is wisely interpreted. The extent is great: one investigator has noted more than 700 species of plants medically employed in the northwestern part of the Amazon alone—a region still very poorly explored.

The overwhelming number of our medicines coming from plants used in protohistorical societies should convince modern scientists of the value of ethnopharmacological investigation. There still lingers in many scientific circles, however, distrust of the value of a study of primitive medicine. Recent analytical evaluation of Aztec medicine has indicated that "although magic and religion were quite important in the Aztec treatment of disease, there was a strong empirical underpinning which has not received the attention it merits" (B. Ortiz de Montellano, *Science* 188 [1975] 215). Of 25 plants studied, 16 were found to produce the effects claimed in native medicine; 4 would possibly be active; 5 seem, from present knowledge of their chemistry, not to possess the effects claimed. This study thus implies that 80 percent might in reality be effective medicines. More research must obviously be done to assure that such a high percentage might be effective, but it is clear that, while magico-religious elements were important in Aztec medicine, a strong empirical basis existed for their use of healing plants—a basis not yet sufficiently recognized by science.

RICHARD EVANS SCHULTES

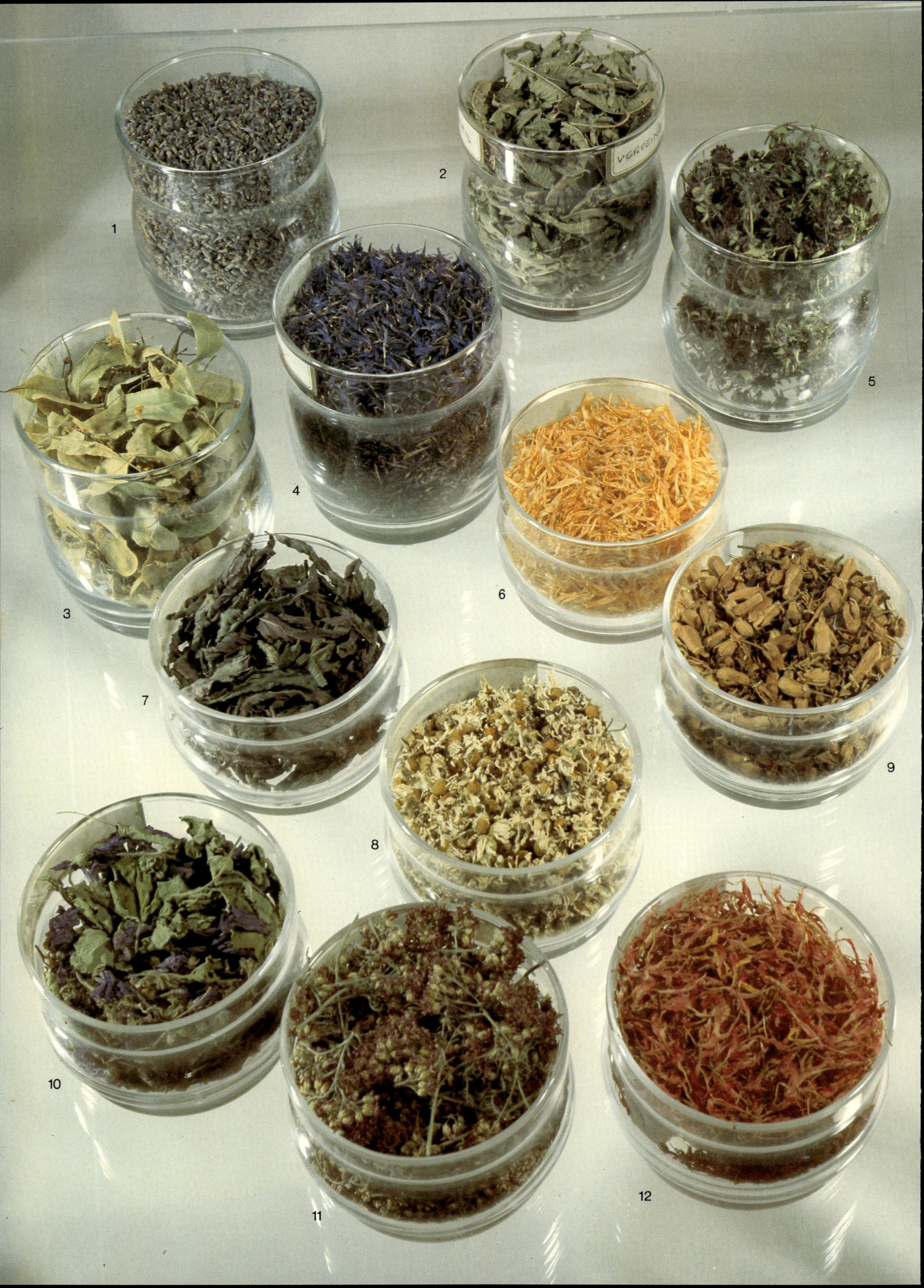
1
2
5
3
4
6
7
9
8
10
11
12

The Basic Techniques of Herbal Preparations

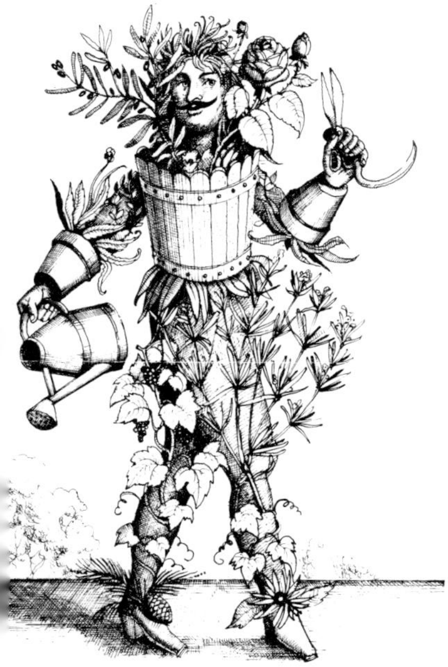

Left: Once herbs are dried, they can be loosely packed in glass jars or in cannisters. Each container should be labeled with the name of the plant and the date when it was picked. The illustration shows the following:

1 Lavender
2 Vervain
3 Bigleaf linden
4 Cornflower
5 Thyme
6 Marigold
7 Mint
8 German chamomile
9 Bitter orange
10 Pansy
11 Yarrow
12 Balm

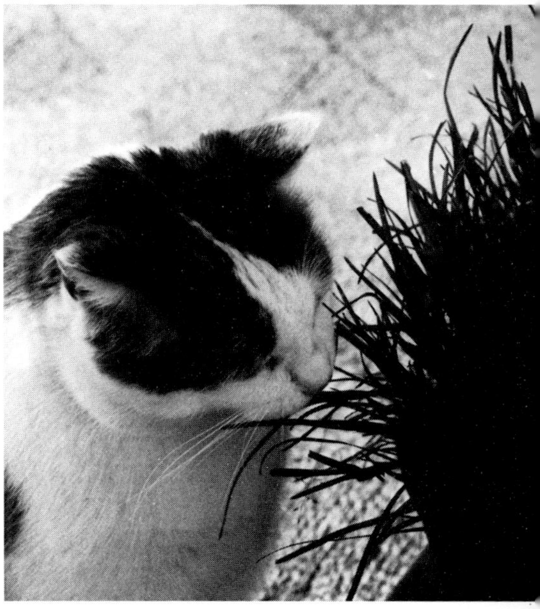

Above right:
Cats eat blades of grass in order to stimulate their digestion. Within a few minutes after swallowing grass, they regurgitate feathers, hairs, and other nondigestible matter.

Early man was very close to nature, living in daily contact with the plants and animals of the forest, hills, and valleys which were his home. Thus he was sensitive to the behavior of animals and the properties and powers of plants, and it is of more than passing interest that some traditional medicinal uses of plants originating in those early days have found confirmation in modern science. Our forefathers knew nothing of chemistry and pharmacology, but relied entirely on their natural powers of observation, on their intuition. This we have largely lost in modern civilization, in the age of technology, living as we do hurried and under pressure, ever remote from nature.

Valuable knowledge concerning the medicinal actions of plants was often acquired by careful observation of animal behavior.

Cats and dogs, for instance, cure their stomach upsets by eating sharp grasses, while sick sheep look for yarrow. A wild boar suffering from henbane poisoning uses the fresh roots of the carline thistle as a cure. Mice lay up stores of peppermint plants, to keep fit throughout the winter. In the first days of spring, starving bears look for flavorful "bear's garlic" or ramsons. Ants plant thyme all over their habitations. If chamois injure themselves, they roll in alpine plantains. Swallows take the juice of the common celandine (swallowwort) to open the eyes of their young, and jackdaws keep their nests free from fleas with tomato leaves. Cattle with rheumatic pains lie down in a patch of crowfoot, and lizards suffering from snakebite find a cure in chamomile.

This inherited, intuitive knowledge of which plant is the right remedy for a given ailment is one of the most fascinating aspects of nature, and it is not surprising that, by copying the animals, man soon learned how to use nature's healing powers for himself.

Later, becoming more sophisticated in his approach, man would look for special features in a plant, such as shapes or colors which bore a resemblance to human organs. Heart-shaped leaves, or red coloration, supposedly offered a clue to the specific medicinal use of the plant. Even while adhering literally to this Doctrine of Signatures, human beings by trial and error accumulated a vast store of medical knowledge based on their own observations and, above all, on their experience. Thus, from animals, from the appearance or aroma of plants, and finally from empirical evidence, man learned how plants could be of service to him not only for food, but also to keep him in good health.

At first, herbs were taken in their crude form—one simply swallowed a leaf, some bark, a flower, or a root, the dose being a matter of individual judgment.

The health of earlier human beings, however, was determined to a large extent by the variety in their natural diet. In spring, it was believed that bear's garlic, watercress, and dandelion provided not only nourishment but also vitality and resistance to disease. In June, people would eat fennel and buckbean; in July borage, marsh mallow, and also balm could be found; followed by marjoram, thyme, and

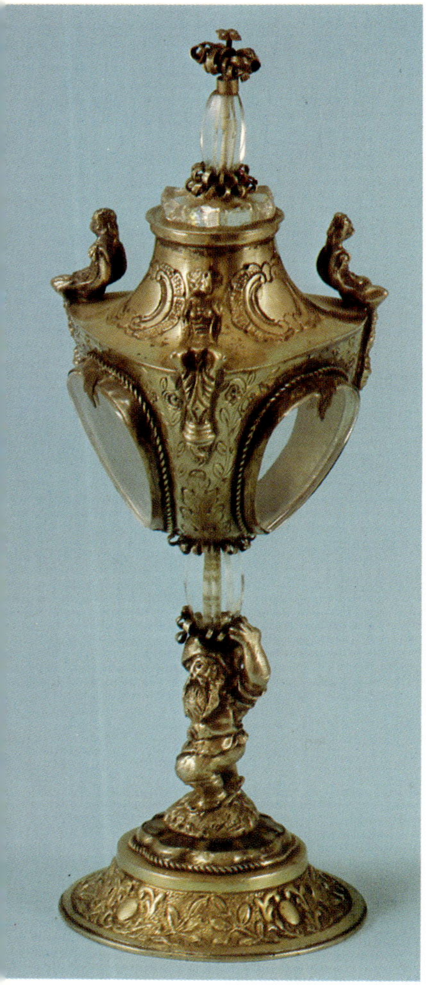

So-called radiation container. This rock crystal (21 cm high) mounted in silver emitted rays and thus was believed to prevent eye ailments. Swiss Pharmaceutical History Museum, Basel.

bedstraw in August. Autumn brought an abundance of berries—cranberries, blueberries, rose hips, elderberries, barberries, haws, and rowans. Thus, in the cycle of the seasons, the human organism was kept and refreshed in a natural way, being part of the cycle of nature, and only occasionally did the need for remedies arise.

As people moved farther away from nature, they appear to have become more prone to disease and their illnesses began to assume more ominous characteristics. The complex chain of cause and effect would be difficult to explain in the space allotted here. In any event, as human beings' health deteriorated, they began almost frantically to look to the plant world for a cure. For millennia, the natural gifts of plants were the only remedies known to man, and he learned to prepare them in different ways, for the benefit of his health.

Medicinal plants were at first taken raw: rightly so, for their natural form is undoubtedly the simplest and best. In fresh herbs, the natural content of enzymes, vitamins, and other active principles is most perfectly retained.

With some plants, raw consumption is still the custom. We eat dandelions, for example, in salads to improve the secretion of bile and to invigorate the system. Other herbal ingredients found in salads are nasturtium, in the belief that it is a natural equivalent of penicillin; nettles, a traditional remedy for anemia; watercress for glandular disorders; bear's garlic for high blood pressure; ground ivy to protect us against inflammation of the kidney and bladder. Such herb salads are prepared by adding a handful of chopped herbs to lettuce or chicory leaves, and then mixing this combination with a dressing of oil, vinegar, and seasonings.

Gradually, for a number of reasons, those simple original methods were replaced by others. No doubt the wish to preserve herbs and utilize them more fully played a role in this change. In the course of time, the processing of natural remedies also became a science. One of the prime movers in this process was Galen (A.D. 130–200), personal physician to the Roman emperor Marcus Aurelius and regarded as the father of pharmaceutics. Even nowadays the term "galenical" is still applied to tinctures, extracts, ointments, mixtures, pills, and other medicinal compounds based on plant ingredients.

Today we know that herbal remedies, those cures discovered by primitive man and developed through the ages, remain one of nature's greatest gifts. Elsewhere in this book the reader will find suggestions for remedies of minor ailments that he can prepare (see Reference Section II).

In the pages that follow, we offer background information, basic techniques, and pointers, as a supplement to the specific recipes of the Reference Section.

GATHERING MEDICINAL HERBS

Most medicinal herbs grow wild in our flora. It is astonishing that nearly every species is accorded its own place in Nature so that it can develop its active principles in the best circumstances. The fact that we have for centuries been cultivating sage, balm, rosemary, linden, and other plants in our gardens shows how eager people have been to have these helpful plants near them. People interested in gathering and harvesting healing plants themselves should heed the following rules.

Where should wild herbs be sought? Avoid fertilized terrain and areas that have been sprayed with insecticides. Do not pick plants along highways or hiking paths. Plants should be picked in isolated areas away from contamination by traffic and chemicals.

Because it is so difficult to know whether a field or a plant is free of chemical treatment and other types of pollution, great care must be exercised. One safeguard is to gather herbs out in the country on property

Dried plant parts. Even after the drying process, plants should retain as much as possible of their original color (as can be seen in the color picture at right).

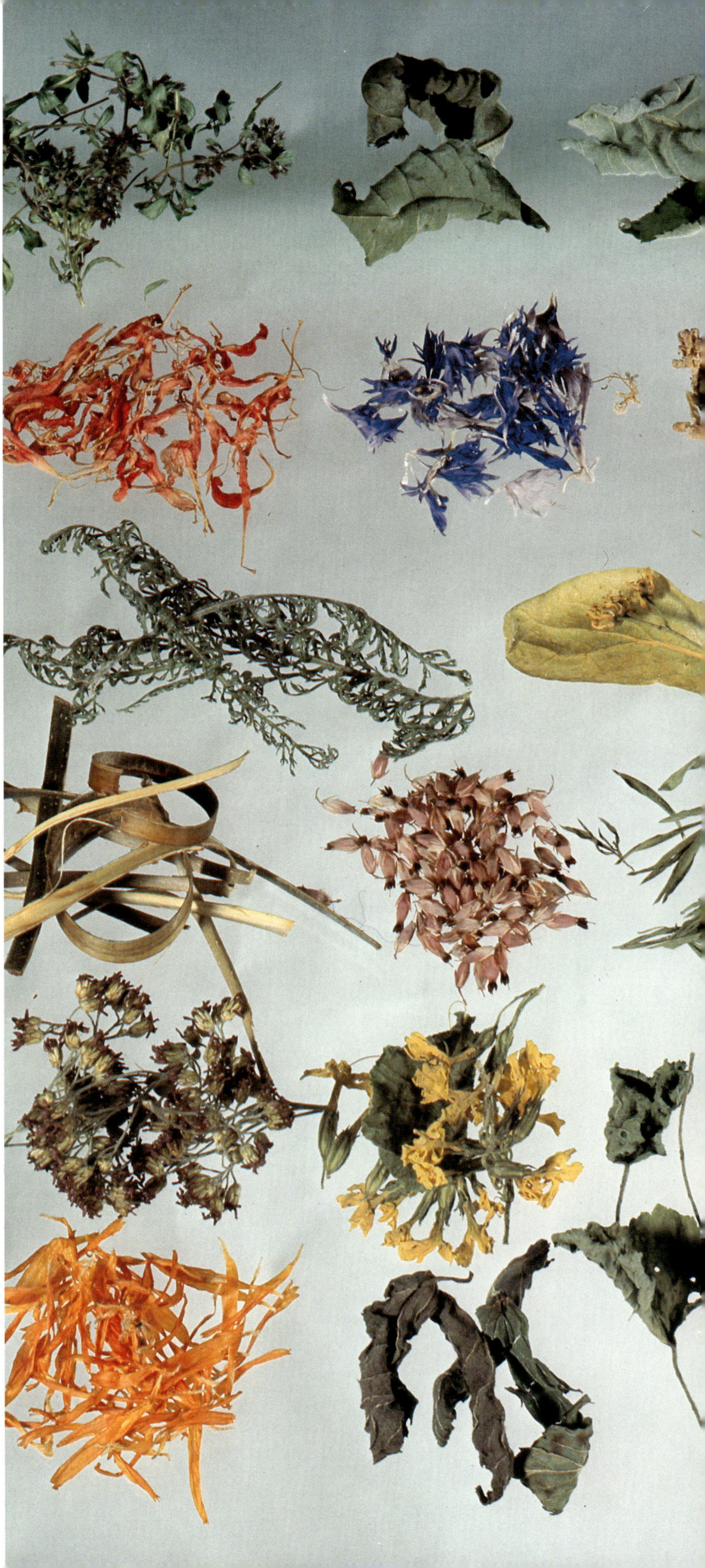

belonging to a friend or relative who can assure you of the safety of the surrounding flora. If you have a garden, you can cultivate many herbs yourself.

However, the surest way to obtain good-quality herbs or plant parts is to buy them from a reputable supplier, either an herbalist or a health-food dealer. Such professionals usually raise the herbs themselves under good conditions and are adept at drying and preserving them correctly. Pharmacies sometimes sell supplies of the more common medicinal herbs, such as chamomile and peppermint, for the preparation of teas. If you do plan to gather your own herbs from a safe, clean site, there are a few additional rules to keep in mind.

Plants must be approached and handled with the utmost care. Before picking a plant, be sure to check in a guidebook to be certain of its habitat, flowering season, color, shape, and dimensions, as well as any further identifying signs such as a special odor. Do not pick any plant unless you can be certain of its identity. It is all too easy, for instance, to confuse a plant such as yellow gentian with certain poisonous hellebore species.

The exact season for gathering plants is an extremely important consideration. In Reference Section III of this book, the reader will find precise recommendations for the gathering of each healing plant. In general, avoid picking plants that are extremely dry or wet (from dew or rain). Choose a clear, sunny day. Avoid early morning or the evening hours.

Take only healthy plants and plant parts. Beware of plants containing mildew, decay, parasites, or snails. Separate the plant from any surrounding blades of grass, leaves, earth, and stones, but do not wash them (except the roots).

HERB TEAS OR TISANES

By drying herbs, one can have a supply of herbal teas all through the year, since in dried form they can be preserved long past

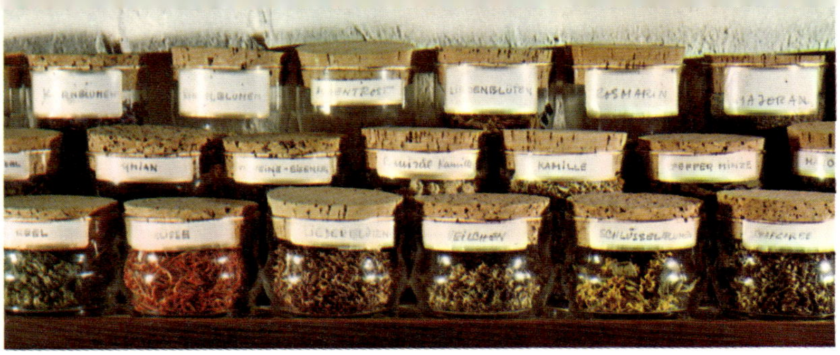

The stock of herbs should be preserved in a warm, dry place away from the light. Medicinal herbs should be replaced every year, since they lose their healing properties after lengthy storage.

their flowering season. Drying is a natural method of preservation by which fermentation is prevented, and fungi and bacteria are deprived of the conditions they need to flourish: bacteria need a moisture content of 40–50 percent to multiply, and fungi require at least 15–20 percent. Nevertheless, dried herbs should not be totally dry; if treated properly, they should retain a moisture content of 10 percent.

DRYING

The freshly gathered plants are spread in a thin layer on a linen sheet or on a nylon sieve in a wooden frame, or they may be tied in bunches and hung in the attic. Concrete floors are not suitable. Care must be taken to protect herbs from damp and from insects and vermin. The herbs should be very carefully picked over. After removal of any adhering earth, they are quickly washed, cut up lengthwise, and chopped into very small pieces (about 1 mm long). Very strong smelling plants, like lovage for instance, are dried separately from the others. Flowers (poppy, mullein, St. John's wort, arnica, and others) need to be dried very quickly and out of direct sunlight, and must be protected from daylight. Roots and barks may be dried in the sun. Herbs should not be handled during or after the drying process, and dried material should not be mixed with fresh.

COMBINED TEA

For relief from coughs

20 g (⅔ oz) coltsfoot blossoms
15 g (½ oz) English plantain leaves
15 g (½ oz) cowslip blossoms with calyx
15 g (½ oz) common (or high) mallow blossoms and leaves
10 g (⅓ oz) mullein blossoms
15 g (½ oz) licorice
10 g (⅓ oz) roselle

Pour 1 cup (¼ liter) cold water over 1 heaping teaspoon of the herb mixture. Let stand 8 hours at room temperature. Warm and strain. Drink sweetened with honey. Take 1 cup 2–3 times daily.

STORING

When dry, the herbs are put up in glass jars or other storage containers (do not pack them tightly), which are then closed and stored in a dry, warm, dust-free room. The containers should be labeled and dated, and herbs need to be replaced every year. Any residues may be used for baths. Herbs should always be stored in a dry place, and protected from light.

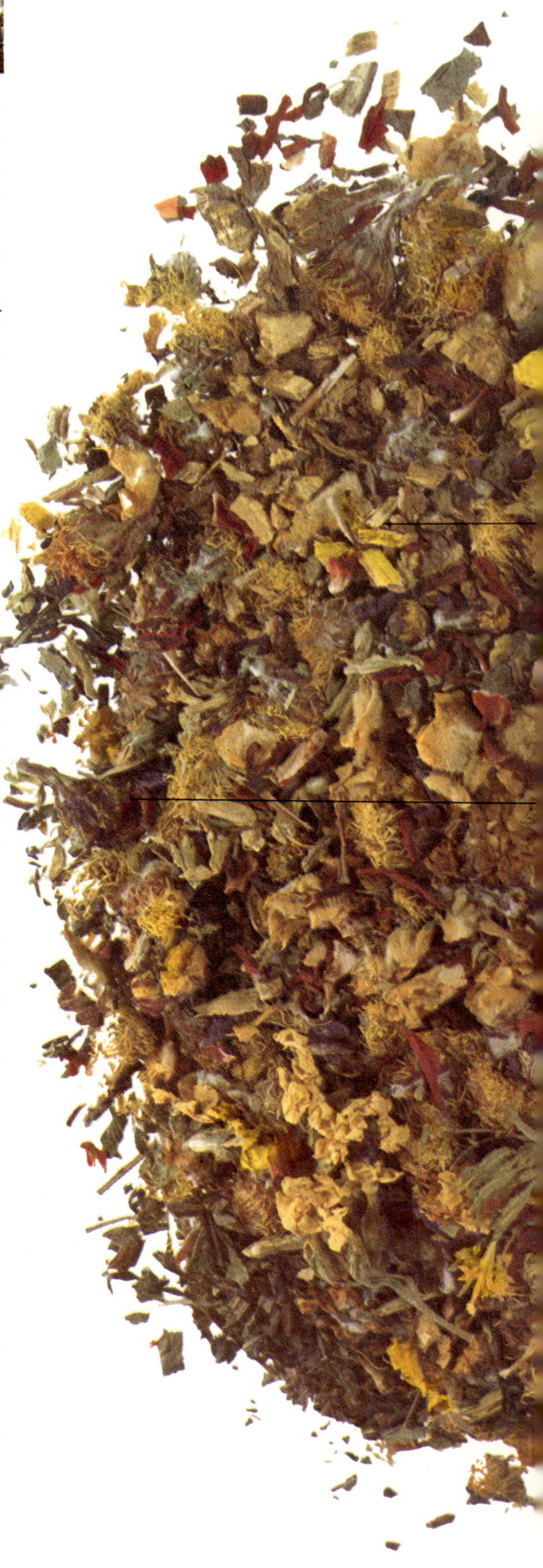

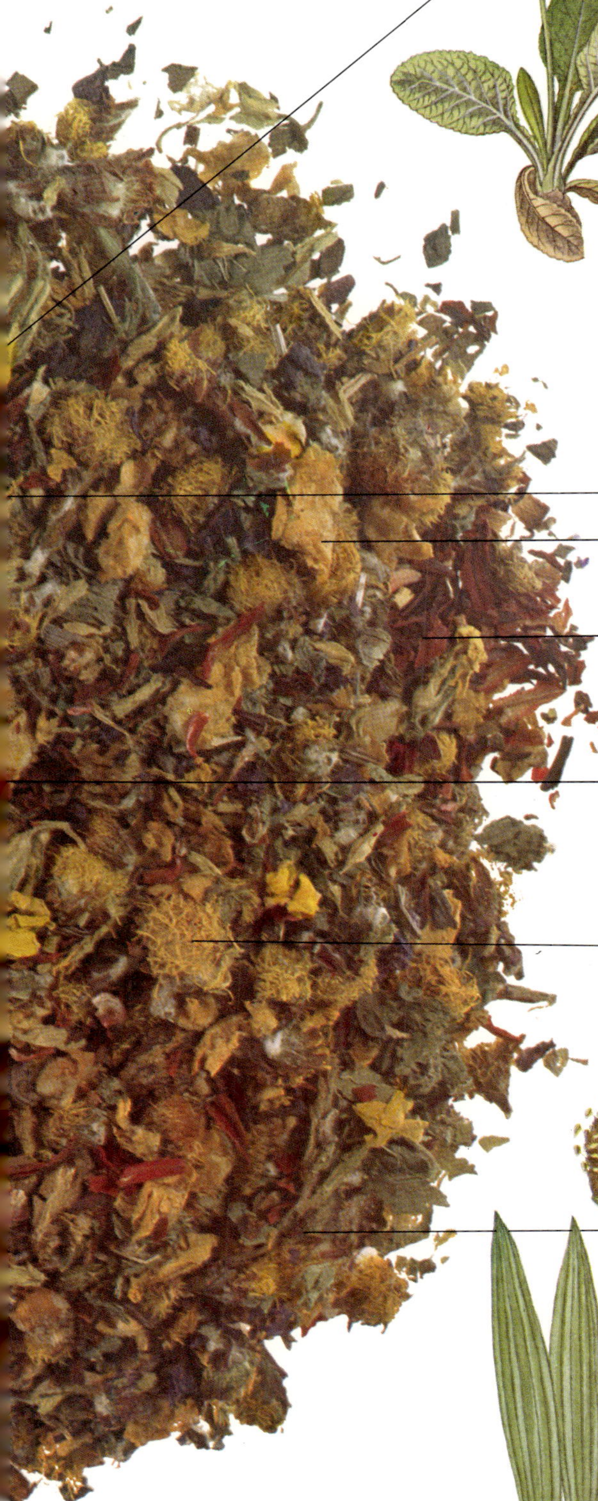

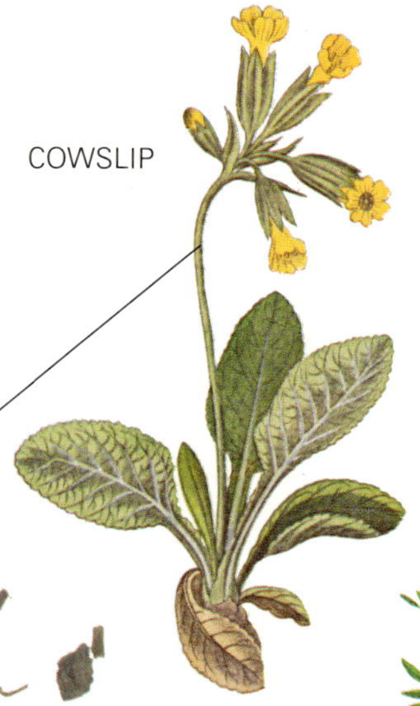

COWSLIP

COWSLIP *Primula veris*
A tisane of the golden-yellow, honey-scented cowslip is an old gipsy remedy for bronchial catarrh, easing the cough by its soothing action.

LICORICE *Glycyrrhiza glabra*
Licorice is a common constituent of mixed tisanes by virtue of its soothing action on the inflamed respiratory passages and its stimulating action in helping to get rid of phlegm.

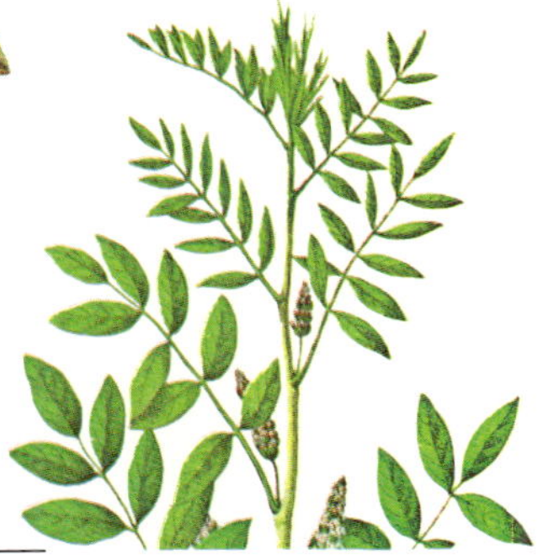

LICORICE

MULLEIN
Verbascum densiflorum
Mullein is a common constituent of mixed tisanes for coughs. Indeed it is used more often in this form than by itself. In addition to helping to soothe the cough, it has a useful mildly sedative action.

ROSELLE
Hibiscus sabdariffa
Widely cultivated throughout the tropics, roselle, or Jamaica sorrel as it is also know, is a constituent of jellies, sauces, and acid drinks to which it lends a much esteemed and prized flavor.

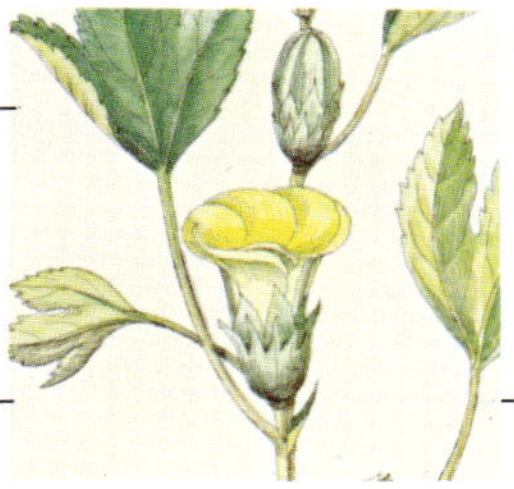

ROSELLE

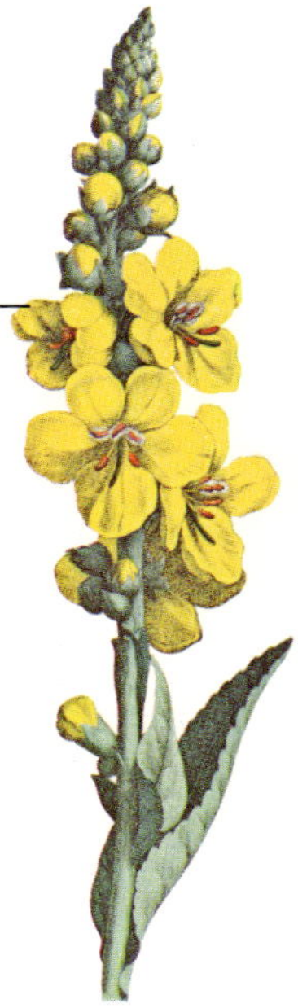

MULLEIN

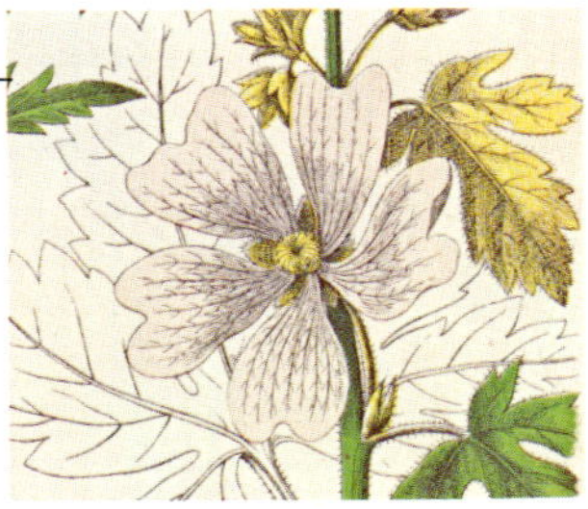

COMMON (HIGH) MALLOW

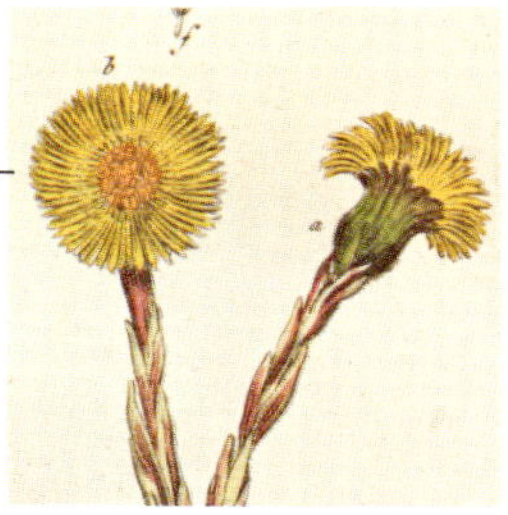

COLTSFOOT

COMMON MALLOW *Malva sylvestris*
Both the flowers and the leaves of the common mallow contain soothing mucilage which eases coughs.

COLTSFOOT *Tussilago farfara*
Coltsfoot, whose name *tussilago* indicates its cough-easing properties, is also known as coughwort. It is one of the most popular domestic cough remedies. As such it is as popular in China as in the occident. It owes its soothing action to the mucilage it contains.

ENGLISH PLANTAIN
Plantago lanceolata
Also known as ribgrass, this common weed of lawns is seldom used alone for coughs. As an ancillary, however, it has a mild soothing action.

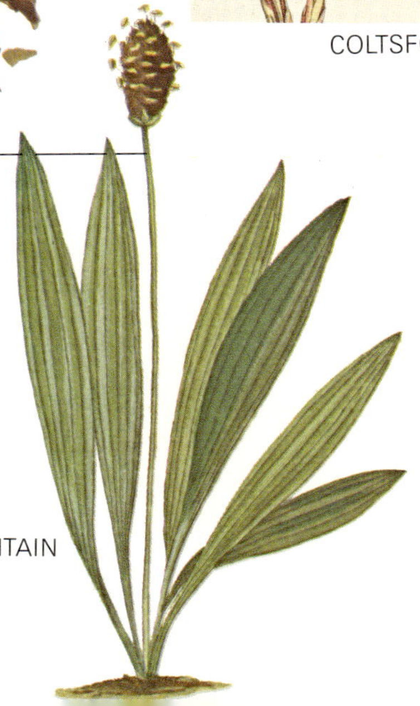

ENGLISH PLANTAIN

COMBINED TEA FOR STOMACH AILMENTS

SWEET FLAG

Basic ingredient: stimulates appetite and has a tonic effect on the stomach.

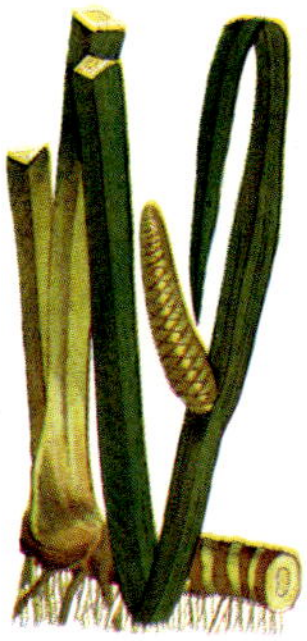

+

YARROW AND PEPPERMINT

Secondary ingredients: assist the effectiveness of sweet flag; stimulate the digestive capacity and gall secretion.

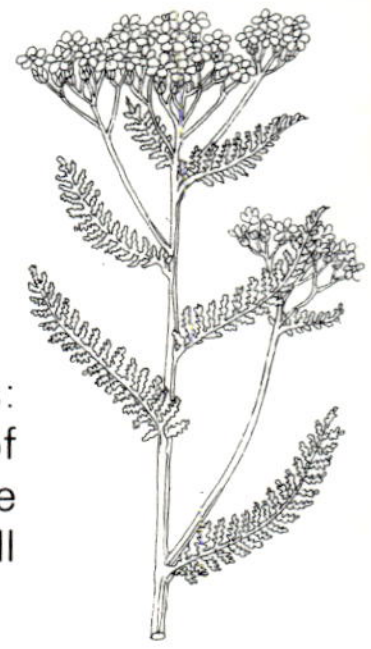

EXTERNAL APPLICATION OF HERBS TO SKIN

Discard the outermost leaves from a fresh head of winter cabbage. Take a few of the fresh inner leaves, wash well, and dry off lightly. Remove the large ribs from the leaves. Tap on the leaves to soften them, and place them on the skin. Hold them in place with a loose bandage. Leave in place for at least 1 hour. Repeat 2–3 times daily.
Application of winter cabbage relieves rheumatic and neuralgic pains and promotes the healing of inflamed wounds.

HERBAL BATH

With stimulating, strengthening effect on the circulation and nerves.

20 g (⅔ oz) rosemary leaves
20 g (⅔ oz) lavender blossoms
10 g (⅓ oz) chopped oregano herb

Pour 1 liter (1 quart) boiling water over this herbal mixture. Let stand, covered, ½ hour. Strain the liquid and add it to the hot bath water. Bath temperature should be 35°–37°C (95°–98.5° F). Rest ½ hour to 1 hour after bath. Because the bath has a stimulating effect, it should not be taken at night.

MACERATION, DECOCTION, INFUSION

Depending on the type of herb used, different methods are used to prepare herb teas or tisanes. Herbs containing a high proportion of volatile oils and mucilage are best steeped in cold water *(maceration)*. A teaspoonful of the dried herbs is placed in a cupful of cold water and left to stand for a full twelve hours at room temperature. The mixture is then gently warmed, strained, and the liquid sweetened with honey.
A *decoction* is made of plant materials which are not so easily extracted. A teaspoonful of the dried material is placed in an enamel saucepan (*not* a metal one) containing 1 cup of water and boiled for 2–3 minutes over a low fire. The strained-off liquid may be sweetened with honey. Decoctions should only be taken on medical advice.
The most familiar method of making a tea is by *infusion*. A teaspoonful of dried herbs is placed in a previously warmed cup, and boiling water is added. The infusion is covered and left to stand for 5–10 minutes, strained, and sweetened with honey.

GENERAL DIRECTIONS FOR THE USE OF HERB TEAS

Two or three times daily, always after meals, a teaspoonful of herbs is used to make about 1 cup of tea (halve these quantities for children). It is advisable not to drink this before meals, as it would dilute the gastric juice and interfere with digestion. If the patient has a fever, the tea should be taken lukewarm. Honey, a gentle remedy in its own right, is much more suitable as a sweetener than sugar. Treatment with herb teas should never be followed for a prolonged period; nor should it be stopped too early. As a rule, the tea is taken daily for 1–2 months, provided no additional symptoms develop.

THE MOST COMMON HERBS FOR HOME TEA PREPARATIONS

Below are some of the most frequently used herbal teas, with an idea of some of their uses.

Angelica root: flatulence.
Balm leaves: headache, insomnia.
Bearberry leaves: bladder problems.
Bigleaf linden blossoms: colds.
Birch leaves: bladder trouble.
Centaury herb: heartburn.
Coltsfoot blossoms: coughs, colds.
Cowslip blossoms: headache, insomnia.
Dog rose hips: colds, bladder trouble.
English plantain leaves: colds.
European elder blossoms: chills, fever.
Fennel fruits: flatulence, coughs.
Garden sage leaves: sore throat, coughs.
German chamomile blossoms: indigestion, colds.
Hawthorn blossoms: nervous stress.
Horsetail herb: circulation, bladder.
Lady's mantle herb: menstrual complaints.
Lavender blossoms: headache, nervousness.
Marigold blossoms: indigestion, gall bladder.
Mullein blossoms: coughs, inflammation.
Peppermint leaves: flatulence, nausea.
Rosemary leaves: circulation, nervous heart.
St. John's wort blossoms: digestive problems.
Silverweed herb: diarrhea, indigestion.
Snakeroot herb: bronchitis, sore throat.
Stinging nettle leaves: bladder troubles.
Thyme herb: colds, indigestion.
Valerian root: dyspepsia, tension headaches.
White deadnettle herb: bladder disorders.
Wormwood herb: indigestion.
Yarrow herb: flatulence, indigestion.
Yellow gentian root: indigestion, appetite loss.

COMBINED TEAS

There are definite rules for the combination of herbs in a tea mixture or composite. As with any medical prescription, expert

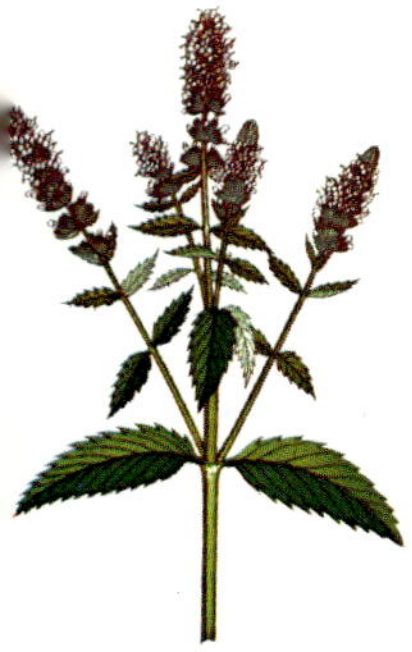

+ FENNEL
To enhance taste. Also has secondary effect as antiflatulent.

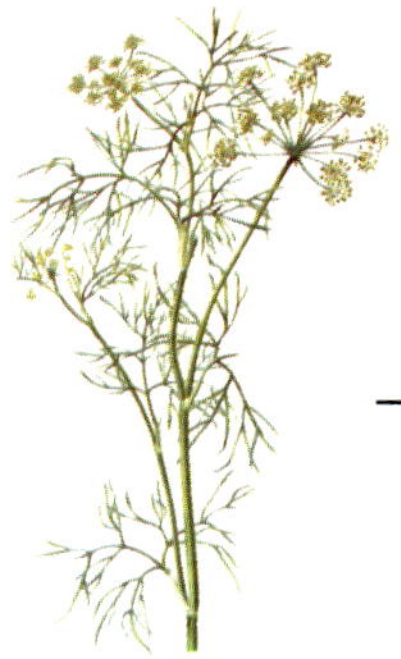

+ CHAMOMILE
To enhance appearance of the tea. Also has antispasmodic effect and relieves inflammation.

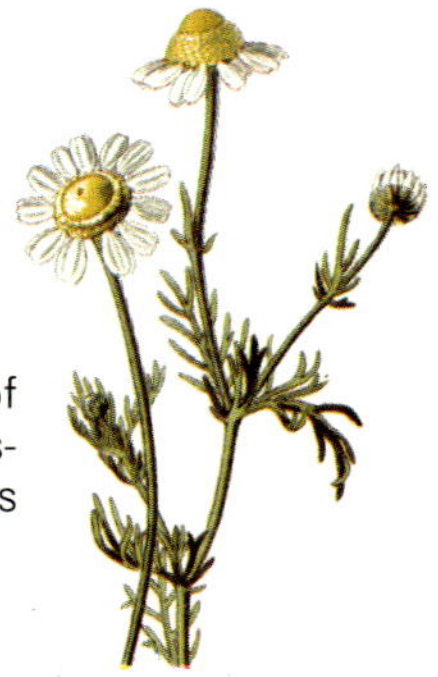

knowledge of the chemical and botanical compatibility of different plants is required if one is to use the right herbs together in the correct proportions.

Every formula includes the basic remedy plus an adjuvant to complement or enhance it. Often a corrigent is added (that is, a plant used to improve flavor and tolerance) as well as a plant to improve the appearance of the mixture. Herbs commonly used for their appearance include yellow mullein flowers *(Verbascum thapsiforma)*, blue cornflowers *(Centaurea cyanus)*, Oswego tea *(Monarda didyma)*, and orange-colored marigold flowers *(Calendula officinalis)*.

EXTERNAL APPLICATION

Herbs are sometimes applied directly to the skin or to wounds, so that their volatile oils may penetrate and stimulate the tissues. The fresh parts of the plant—usually the leaves or bruised roots—are cleaned, and then placed on the skin in a single layer. After about 20 minutes the herbs are removed and the application is repeated with fresh herbs. In some cases the herbs may be left in place overnight.

HERB BAGS

If fresh herbs are not available for external application, dried plants (leaves and roots) may be put in a small bag of gauze or cotton (about the size of a hand), immersed in hot water, and then placed on the area requiring treatment. The sack is covered with a piece of wool or flannel and left to act for 20–30 minutes.

HERBAL BATHS

The valuable natural substances contained in herbs, when added to the bath, cleanse and stimulate the skin. A handful of the prescribed herbs is briefly brought to the boil in a liter (1 quart) of water, filtered, and the liquid added to the bath water, together with a few pinches (2–3 g) of sea salt. Another method is to sew the herbs into a small bag and put this in the bath water. Herbal baths may be beneficial in a number of ways: rosemary is strengthening, lavender refreshing, valerian and lime blossom are sedative, chamomile cleanses, hawthorn stimulates the circulation, thyme is good for the nerves. Depending on the effect required (sedative, stimulating), herbal baths are taken either in the morning or evening.

HERBAL OINTMENTS

Applied in ointment form, the active principles of herbs are able to act on the skin for extended periods and thus accelerate healing, particularly in cases of injury, contusions, and effusions. In the old days, lard was used as the ointment base. This was later replaced with salt-free butter and finally with Vaseline or some other petroleum jelly. One or two heaped tablespoons of the herb or herbs are brought to the boil in about 200 grams (7 ounces) of Vaseline. The mixture is thoroughly stirred and strained. When cold the ointment is put into jars, ready for use as required.

COMPRESSES

Herbal compresses will achieve a similar effect, with the additional advantage of the therapeutic action of heat. One or two heaped tablespoons of the herb or herbs are brought to the boil in 1 cup (200–300 cc) of water. A cotton wool pad or some linen or gauze is dipped in the strained liquid, and after letting the excess liquid run off, is placed on the affected area while still warm. It is covered with a piece of woollen material. (The compress can be bandaged in place, if desired.) When cold, the

OIL FROM SAINT JOHN'S WORT

Crush 125 g (4 oz) fresh, just-opened blossoms in approximately 1 teaspoon olive oil. Pour ½ liter (1 pint) of olive oil over the whole and mix well. Place in a clear glass container and leave standing uncovered in a warm spot to ferment for 3–5 days. After fermentation seal the container well. Place in the sun for 3–6 weeks, until oil has become a bright red. Press through a cloth and pour off the watery layer. Keep well sealed in a dark-colored bottle. Taken internally, the oil can relieve stomach pains. Externally, the oil relieves pain and helps heal burns and wounds.

MARIGOLD SALVE

1 handful (2 oz) freshly picked marigold flowers
200 g (7 oz) Vaseline or other petroleum jelly

Melt Vasoline in a pot over low heat, add marigold flowers. Bring the mixture just to the boil. Stir well. Sift through a dish towel, pressing out the residue. Let cool.
Marigold salve is recommended for skin ailments, sores, and poorly healing wounds.

As a treatment for strained or inflamed eyes, a gauze compress can be moistened with chamomile or fennel tea, wrung out, and placed over the eyes.

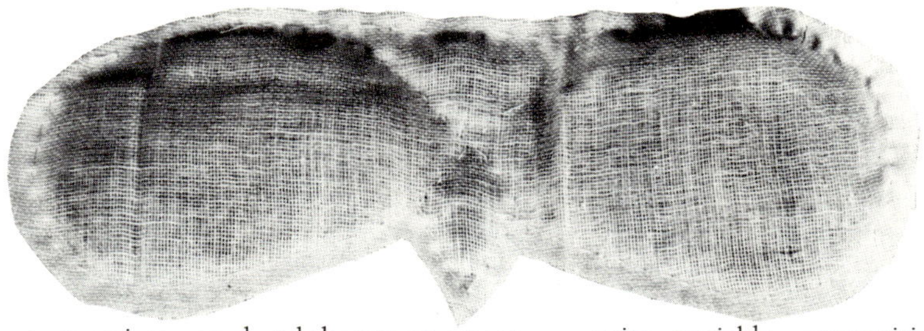

compress is removed and the process repeated if necessary. The cotton wool, linen, or gauze should be very clean (gauze can be bought sterile in special packages).

OILS

Herb oils are very useful where ointments or compresses may prove impracticable. St. John's wort red oil is widely known as a suntan oil. A handful of the fresh or dried herb is placed in olive oil and left to stand in the sun for 2–3 weeks. It is then filtered and any water collecting on the surface is removed. Herb oils need to be stored in containers of brown glass.

EXTRACTS

The making of extracts is a process for the pharmacist. There are three different types of extracts:

In *liquid extracts,* the volume of fluid extract equals the quantity of air-dried plant drug used.

Soft extracts are evaporated fluid extracts of ointment-like consistency.

Dry extracts have been completely evaporated and the residue dried and powdered.

In phytotherapy, extracts of different concentrations are mixed to make compound remedies such as elixirs, essences, and spirits. *Elixirs* were first prepared by the Greek alchemists. They used *xerion,* a mineral dusting powder, hoping to change baser metals into gold. The Islamic name for this was *al-iksir,* describing very finely powdered substances, mostly gray antimony, and toward the end of the Middle Ages the term came to be used for the "most sublime," the most highly refined substance. It was not until much later that the term "elixir" came to mean an essence capable of prolonging life and finally, more generally, to mean a clear, sweetened liquid, usually hydroalcoholic, used as the vehicle for certain medicinal principles.

The term *essence* is used for preparations of quite variable composition containing plant extracts. *Spirits* are solutions of volatile substances in alcohol.

TINCTURES

Tinctures are alcoholic solutions containing, in comparatively low concentrations, the active principles of crude drugs, such as herbs and plants. Their preparation, generally by maceration or percolation, is a technical procedure carried out in pharmacies or, more usually today, in the laboratories or factories of pharmaceutical companies. (Tinctures can sometimes be prepared on one's own, as can be seen in Reference Section II.)

Fifteen to 25 drops of the tincture are taken in a few tablespoons of water three times daily, about a half-hour before meals.

POWDERS

For internal use, dried plants or roots are reduced to a powder (in a mortar and pestle) and a small pinch—as much as one can pick up on the tip of a knife (i.e., about 1 gram)—is taken three times daily with a little water, before or after meals. For external use, the powdered herbs are mixed with oil, Vaseline or other petroleum jelly, or a little water and applied to the skin to treat wounds, inflammations, contusions, and the like.

SYRUPS

Syrup formulations of medicaments are intended chiefly for children and people with sensitive palates. Plant extracts tend to be bitter to the taste, and are therefore sweetened with sugar to make them go down more easily.

The general method is to place 100 grams (4 ounces) of dried or fresh herbs in 1 liter (1 quart) of water. Boil for 1 minute, and let the mixture stand for 2 or 3 days, then

ARNICA TINCTURE

Pour ½ liter (1 pint) 70 percent alcohol over 50 g (2 oz) dried or 25 g (1 oz) fresh arnica blossoms. Seal tight in a clear glass container and place in the sun. After 10–14 days, strain through a towel and press out the residue. After 1 day let it run through a coffee filter paper.

Arnica tincture is used as a gargle for inflammations of the mouth and throat. It is also helpful when used on a compress for bleeding, sprains, or slowly healing wounds.

COLD MARIGOLD COMPRESS

Pour ½ liter (1 pint) boiling water over 1–2 teaspoons of the marigold herb (leaves, stalks, blossoms). Let stand 15 minutes. Make cool compress by moistening gauze or linen in the liquid and gently wringing out.

Compresses can be applied for 1 hour several times daily. Compress must be re-moistened at intervals when it begins to dry out.

Marigold compresses are helpful in treating bruises, contusions, or slowly healing wounds.

press and filter. Cane sugar is then added, at a ratio of ½ kilogram (1 pound) sugar to the liter (quart).
Syrups are particularly useful in the treatment of coughs, mucous congestion, and bronchial catarrh.

HERBAL WINES

Fresh plants extracted in wine serve as a general tonic as well as specific remedies. Wine is altogether a good preservative for fresh plants. As a rule, a handful of fresh or dried herbs is steeped for a week in good-quality red or white dry wine, or sherry, Port, or Malaga. It is then strained and poured into bottles.
Directions for use: a small glass three times daily, half an hour after meals.

PRESSED JUICES

Fresh plant parts are pressed by hand or mechanically. This method is commonly used to produce juice from stinging nettle, bear's garlic, dandelion, (lemon) balm, juniper, and horsetail juice. Pressed juices are rich in vitamins and salts in the case of those plants containing vitamins and mineral salts, but have poor keeping qualities, so that they need to be freshly prepared.
Directions for use: a teaspoonful of the pressed juice diluted with a few tablespoons of water, to be taken three times daily, half an hour before meals.

FACIAL STEAM TREATMENTS

In conclusion, mention may be made of the cosmetic uses of medicinal plants. Certain herbs such as chamomile, yarrow, marigold, St. John's wort, horsetail, and rosemary are particularly beneficial to the skin. Depending on the plant used, the facial skin is cleansed, soothed, tightened, smoothed, or refreshed.
Directions for use: a handful of the appropriate herb is brought to the boil in some water in an enamel saucepan and then removed from the stove. The face is then held in the steam rising from the pan, so that the vapor plays over every part of the face. When no more steam is rising, the pan may be returned to the stove and brought to the boil for a second time. A towel is used to cover the head entirely during the treatment, to minimize the loss of steam. Afterward the face is washed in cold water. One steam treatment per week is sufficient.

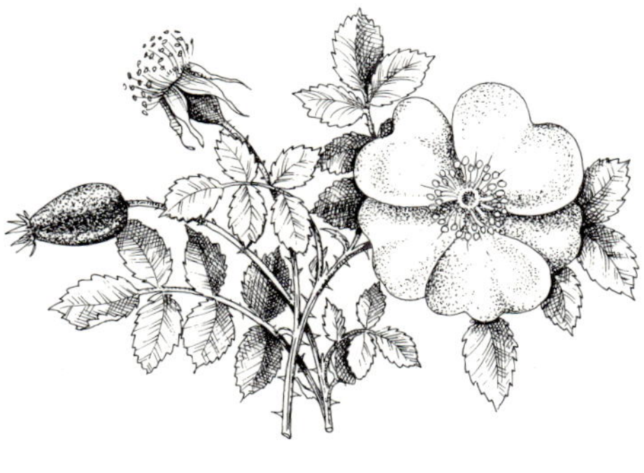

FACIAL HERBAL COMPRESSES

If facial steam treatment is not practicable, compresses may be used instead. One or two tablespoons of the appropriate herb are brought to the boil in 1 cup (200–300 cc) of water, which is then strained. A cotton wool pad or a piece of clean linen or gauze is dipped in the solution, and after letting the surplus run off, is placed on the skin while still warm. As soon as the compress has grown cold, the process is repeated. To complete the treatment, the face is washed in cold water.

BRUNO VONARBURG

* * *

This chapter, we should emphasize once again, is general in intention and scope. Little information is provided here on the type of herb to be used in each particular case, or on mixtures, dosages, and the duration of treatment. Such specific indications are found in Reference Section II, which is the complement to this chapter on basic techniques and products.

ROSE HIP WINE

Take 1 liter (1 quart) ripe rose hips, cut them in half, and remove pits. Crush the hips and mix with 500 g (1 pound) sugar. Add 3 liters (3 quarts) white wine. Let stand at least 1 week in tightly corked glass container. Filter the liquid and place it in bottles. Take 1 small wine glass daily to increase vitamin C supply or to help mild bladder ailments.

PEPPERMINT FACIAL STEAM BATH

Pour 1–2 liters (1–2 quarts) boiling water over 1 handful peppermint leaves in a basin. Hold the face directly over the steam. Cover the head and basin with a towel, so that as little of the steam as possible escapes. Inhale deeply for 5–10 minutes. As soon as the steam subsides, add more boiling water. After the steam bath, wash face with cool water.
Peppermint steam baths bring relief from colds and throat catarrh, and also can contract and invigorate greasy skin.

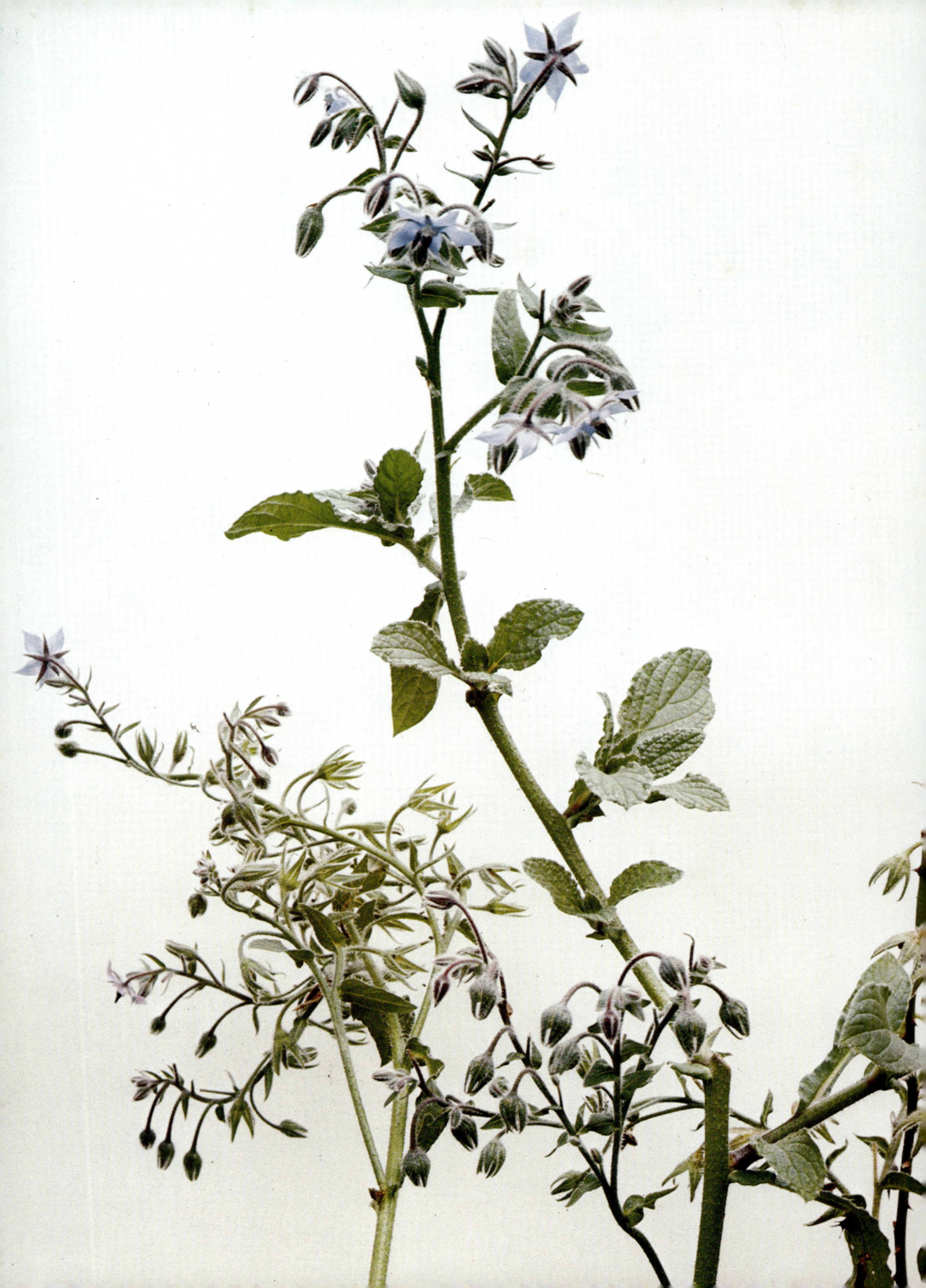

Healing Substances and Their Effectiveness

Reference Section III

A closer look at the healing plants. The following pages present a breakdown of the 247 plants: the specific parts that are used, with the contents (active principles) and healing effects of each plant part. The reader learns how and when to harvest, gather, and store the plants. The following abbreviations are used:

- sap
- fruit/berry
- leaf
- blossom
- whole plant with root
- wood
- bud
- herb (plant without root)
- moss
- nut
- fungus
- bark
- seeds
- rind
- stem
- straw
- rootstock and tuber
- roots
- bulb

Borage *(Borago officinalis)*, used by Arabian nursing mothers to aid lactation.

Right: Early medieval medicine was primarily an herbal art practiced by monastics.

For a long time, much was said by critics of herbal remedies concerning the "fuss," as they described it, that herbalists made about collecting herbs at a particular time of the day or year or in relation to the weather. This was held to be so much hocus-pocus. How wrong these critics proved to be. Research has shown that herbalists were absolutely right, and the amount of the active principle of the herb or plant varies considerably according to the time of day or the season, as does the part of the plant where it is to be found.

The yield of morphine from the poppy in the morning, for example, is often four times greater than that obtained in the evening. In the case of the periwinkle, the active principle is present throughout the plant after three weeks' growth, then disappears, to reappear around the eighth week. Flowering often coincides with an increase in the active principle; however, in some plants it decreases. This is why the harvest time of the plant is so important; and why one must know which part of the plant contains the active principle.

This information has slowly accumulated over the ages, and much of it is incorporated in country folklore. Until quite recent times, every country housewife knew what herb was effective for a certain illness, which part of the plant to use, when to harvest, and how to preserve it until it was needed. Fortunately, much of this folklore has not been allowed to die, and it is on this long experience that the knowledge of the modern herb farmer, pharmaceutical industry, and individual herbalist is based.

It is this information that is summarized in the accompanying Reference Section III. Obviously, all the details could not be given in the available space, but the essentials are here to guide those who wish to have the satisfaction, or fun, of gathering and processing their own herbs preparatory to using them as remedies for their own or their family's minor ailments.

Many persons will prefer to buy herbal remedies already prepared by local herbalist or pharmacist; others, however, will prefer to collect their own herbs or plants during country walks and make their own herbal remedies.

One need not be a "back to Nature" enthusiast (or fanatic) to realize that we are all part of Nature. If Nature produces herbs that heal, why should we not use them ourselves? Of course, mistakes will be made and failures occur, but it is by our mistakes that we learn and, as anyone who has chatted with old countryfolk soon learns, there is something intensely satisfying in having gathered from plants around us the cough remedy or cure for

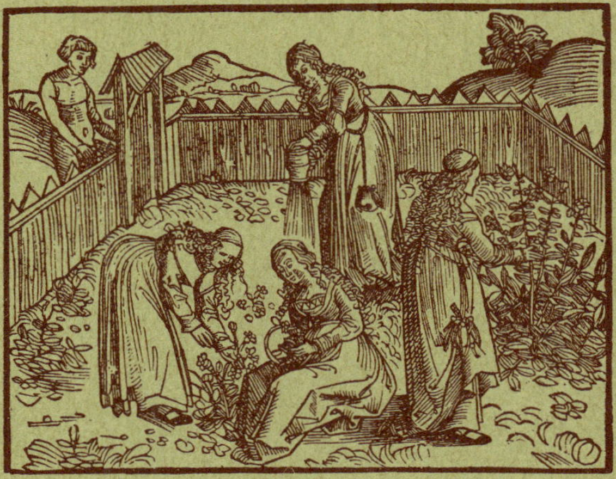

indigestion that never seems to fail. For those who have neither green thumbs nor an innate love of the countryside, the information provided here will allow them to appreciate some of the finer and more intriguing points about herbs that heal. When read in conjunction with other sections of this book, this outline provides an insight into the infinite variety of Nature's healing bounty.

What is required today is a symbiosis between man and Nature, whereby doctors and their associate research workers turn their attention to exploring the healing riches of Nature and harness them for the service of suffering humanity.

William A.R. Thomson, M.D.

Plant	Part used	Components and effects	Harvesting and further processing
AGAR AGAR 103		*Contains:* Up to 90 percent mucins. *Effect:* Swells in intestine, retains water; stimulates intestinal peristalsis; mild purgative.	Algae is gathered from the sea (May–September).
AGRIMONY 6		*Contains:* Tannins, glycosidal bitter principle, nicotinic acid amide, silicic acid, iron, vitamins B and K, some essential oil *Effect:* Promotes gastric secretion and secretion of bile, mild antispasmodic, astringent, constipating, anti-inflammatory.	Gather leaves or stalks with leaves in May and June, shortly before flowering. Dry in shade, not over 40°C.
		Contains: See leaf (above). *Effect:* See leaf.	Gather flowering stalks, June–mid-August. Dry in shade, not over 40°C.
ALDER BUCKTHORN 190		*Contains:* Anthraquinone compounds, tannin primers, ferments, traces of alkaloids, bitter principle. *Effect:* Mild purgative, mild stimulant for bile secretion. Fresh bark: emetic.	Gather bark from cut branches in late spring (April–May). Dry quickly in sun or by artificial heat. Store year before use.
		Contains: Anthraquinone glycoside, rhamnoxanthin, saponin, flavone and phenol glycosides, tannin, amygdalin. *Effect:* See bark (above).	Gather unripe green to red fruit in late summer (August–September). Dry in sun or shade.
ALPINE RAGWORT 213		*Contains:* Alkaloid fuchsisenecin, flavonol rutin, essential oil. *Effect:* Styptic.	Gather foliage at time of flowering (July–August). Dry in shade.
AMERICAN AND ASIATIC GINSENG 158		*Contains:* American ginseng: saponins, panaquilin, panacin, essential oil. Asiatic ginseng: saponins, panax acid and other acids, essential oil, glycosides, vitamin B, sugar, mucin, starch. *Effect:* Improves physical and psychic performance, regulates brain function and blood pressure, raises resistance.	Unearth roots of 6–8 year old plants in the autumn. Dry by artificial heat or in the sun. Asiatic "red" ginseng is produced by treatment with steam or hot water.
AMERICAN PENNYROYAL 116		*Contains:* Essential oil with menthone and pulegone, flavone, tannin, acids. *Effect:* Stimulates digestion and flow of bile, antirheumatic.	Gather at time of flowering (July–August). Dry in shade.
ANGELICA 16		*Contains:* Essential oil with phellandrene, angelica acid, coumarin compounds, bitter principle, tannin. *Effect:* Stimulates digestion, inhibits flatulence, expectorant.	Unearth in late autumn (September–October). Dry in shade or sun.
		Contains: Essential oil, fatty oil, coumarin compounds, bitter principle. *Effect:* Stimulates the stomach, diuretic, diaphoretic.	Gather the ripe seeds in summer (July).
ANISE 169		*Contains:* Essential oil with anethole, fatty oil, choline. *Effect:* Expectorant, carminative.	Gather ripe, dry fruit July–September.
ARNICA 27		*Contains:* Essential oil, flavone, nonglycosidic bitter principle, substances not yet known that act on the heart and arteries, acetylene compounds, tannin. *Effect:* Promotes healing, disperses bruises, vasodilator, stimulates respiration.	*Flower:* Gather at time of flowering (June–August). Dry quickly in shade, not over 35°C. *Rootstock:* Unearth in April–May or September–October. Dry in heat. *Leaf:* Collection possible throughout the summer. Dry quickly in shade.
ARTICHOKE 74		*Contains:* Cynarine, bitter principle, tannin, mucilage, enzyme. *Effect:* Stimulates liver function, promotes flow of bile, reduces blood fat level.	Gather leaves shortly before flowering or when the fruit is ripe. Dry in heat or in the sun. Do not use the edible green leaves of the flower top (ineffective).

Plant	Part used / Components and effects	Harvesting and further processing
ASH 95	*Contains:* Quercitrin, including flavonoids, mannite, tannin, essential oil, coumarin compounds, malic acid. *Effect:* Mild purgative, promotes elimination of urine and uric acid.	Gather in summer (June–August). Strip pinnate leaves from main stem. Dry in shade, not over 40°C.
	Contains: Coumarin compounds, glycosides (fraxin), mannite, tannin, essential oil. *Effect:* Reduces fever, diuretic.	Gather young branches and twigs in spring (April–May), pare bark. Dry in shade.
AUTUMN CROCUS 67	*Contains:* Alkaloid-like substance colchicin and its decomposition products, substances as yet undiscovered, fatty oil, phytosterol, sugar. *Effect:* Inhibits cell division, relieves pain and inhibits inflammation for acute attacks of gout.	Gather the brown, almost ripe seedpods from May–June, before the hay harvest. Dry spread out flat in shade or in the sun.
	Contains: Colchicin and its transformation products, chelidonic acid, phytosterin, various acids. *Effect:* Same as for seeds (above).	Unearth tubers in spring and early summer (April–June). Dry in sun or by artificial heat, not over 65°C.
AVENS 107	*Contains:* Essential oil with gein and eugenol, abundant tannins, bitter principles, flavone, resin, organic acids. *Effect:* Astringent, antiseptic, anti-inflammatory, slightly anesthetic, digestant.	Unearth rootstock with roots attached in spring (April–May) or during flowering (May–October). Dry in shade.
	Contains: Bitter principles, enzyme geasel, tannin, essential oil. *Effect:* Digestant, tonic.	Gather foliage at time of flowering (May–October). Dry in shade.
BALM 148	*Contains:* Essential oil with citral, citronellal, geraniol and linalool, bitter principle, acids, tannin (labiatic acid). *Effect:* Antispasmodic, sedative, carminative.	Gather leaves by cutting off young shoots. 2–3 harvests each year (June–September), as soon as shoots are approximately 30 cm high. Dry in shade, not over 35 °C.
	Contains: Same as leaf (above). *Effect:* Same as leaf.	Gather flowering tips of twigs, June–August. Dry in shade, not over 35 °C.
BALSAM POPLAR 179	*Contains:* Essential oil, flavones, phenolglycosides (populin and salicin, tannin). *Effect:* Diuretic, anti-inflammatory, stops itch.	Gather the young shoots in spring before sprouting (March–April). Dry in shade.
	Contains: Phenolglycosides, essential oil, yellow pigment, glycosides. *Effect:* Reduces fever, antirheumatic, diuretic.	Collect bark from young branches well into spring before sprouting (March–mid-April). Dry as quickly as possible in shade.
	Contains: See bark (above). *Effect:* See bark.	Gather leaves until early summer (May–mid-July). Dry in shade.
BARBERRY 35	*Contains:* Alkaloid berberine, etc., chelidonic acid, resin, tannin, wax. *Effect:* Digestant, promotes bile secretion.	Unearth roots in spring (March) or autumn (November). Pare off bark. Dry in shade.
	Contains: Fruit acids, vitamin C, pigment, pectin, rubber. *Effect:* Mild purgative.	Gather ripe berries. Dry in sun, in shade, or by artificial heat. Use fresh berries for juice.
BAY 135	*Contains:* Essential oil with cineol and pinene, fatty oil with lauric acid, oleic acid, palmitic acid, linoleic acid phytosterine, lauric alcohol. *Effect:* Aperitive, diuretic, external skin irritant.	Gather ripe fruit in summer (July–August). Dry in shade. Laurel oil is produced from fresh fruit by various processes (pressing or melting out).
	Contains: Essential oil, bitter principle. *Effect:* Aperitive.	Gather evergreen leaves in summer or all year long. Dry in shade.
BEAN 165	*Contains:* Glucokinin, amino acids, silicic acid, hemicellulose. *Effect:* Diuretic.	Gather ripe yellowish or white pods, not "green beans." Remove kernels from pods. Dry pods in shade or artificial heat.

Plant	Part used	Components and effects	Harvesting and further processing
BEARBERRY 23		*Contains:* Arbutin, partly methylarbutin, high tannin content. *Effect:* Urinary antiseptic.	Collection possible throughout the year, particularly favorable in the spring and summer. Dry in shade or sun.
BEARDED USNEA 236		*Contains:* Bitter fumaric acid. *Effect:* Increases resistance to infection, stimulates appetite.	Gathering possible throughout the year. Dry in a warm place.
BEAR'S GARLIC 10		*Contains:* Sulfurous essential oil, aldehyde, vitamin C. *Effect:* Beneficial effect on digestion, vermifuge, slight vasodilation.	*Entire herb:* Gather at time of flowering (April–June). Dry quickly in the shade, not over 40°C. *Leaves:* Gather in spring and summer, until leaves die. Dry in shade not over 40°C.
BEDSTRAW 101		*Contains:* Glycosides, flavone compounds, tannin, traces of essential oil, organic acids, abundant silicic acid. *Effect:* Slightly diuretic, stimulates metabolism, promotes milk curdling.	Gather stalks at time of flowering, May–September. Dry in shade or sun.
BELLADONNA 32		*Contains:* Tropeine alkaloids, flavone glycosides, coumarins scopoline and scopoletine, tannin, acids, phytosterol. *Effect:* Antispasmodic, relieves pain, inhibits secretion, mydriatic.	Gather leaves, flowering or fruit-bearing twig ends at time of flowering (July–August). Dry quickly in shade or artificial heat (60°C).
		Contains: Primary alkaloid hyoscyamine, secondary alkaloids atropine, scopolamine, belladonnine, cuskhygrine. *Effect:* See leaf (above).	Unearth roots in autumn after fall of leaves (October–November). Split thicker roots along length, clean all pieces, cut into pieces about 10 cm long. Dry in sun or shade.
BETELNUT PALM 24		*Contains:* Alkaloids, arecaidine, arecoline, fatty oil, tannin, Areca-red, essential oil. *Effect:* Stimulant, increases saliva, vermifuge.	Collect ripe berries, remove seeds, free from remainder of fruit wall.
BIGLEAF LINDEN 227		*Contains:* Essential oil with farnesol, mucin, flavonoids, hesperidine, etc., coumarin fraxoside, vanillin, carboxylic acids. *Effect:* Diaphoretic, mild sedative.	Gather flowers immediately after blooming in mid-summer (June–July), during dry weather. Dry carefully in shade, not over 35°C.
BILBERRY 237		*Contains:* Tannin, flavone, glucokinin, arbutin and hydroquinone (disputed). *Effect:* Reduces blood sugar slightly.	Gather leaves in June–July, before fruit ripens. Dry in shade, not over 55°C, or in the sun.
		Contains: Invert sugar, organic acids, myrtillin extractive, tannin, pectin, vitamins B and C. *Effect:* Astringent, diuretic, controls diarrhea.	Collect berries when ripe. Dry spread out flat in shade or in the sun. Process fresh berries for juice.
BIRCH 36		*Contains:* Saponins, tannin, traces of essential oil, bitter principle, glycosides. *Effect:* Slightly diuretic, weakly disinfectant.	Gather in spring and early summer, not later than 1–2 months after leafing (April–June). Dry in shade, below 40°C.
		Contains: Primarily high sugar content. *Effect:* Stimulates scalp and growth of hair base.	Tap the rising spring sap, early April, by cutting the branches or by tapping the trunk.
BITTER ALMOND 183		*Contains:* Hydrocyanic glycoside (amygdalin), fatty oil with oleic and linoleic acid, albumin, sugar, mucilage, enzymes. *Effect:* Slightly pain relieving, reduces irritation.	Gather ripe fruit in late summer (August–September). Commercially processed for medical purposes.
BITTER ORANGE 61		*Contains:* Essential oil, glycoside hesperidin, bitter principles. *Effect:* Mild sedative, stimulates secretion of gastric juices.	Gather the closed flower buds or open flowers. (Time of flowering not uniform; several blossoms per year.) Dry in shade.
		Contains: See flower (above). *Effect:* See flower.	Gather leaves in summer (May–July). Dry in shade.
		Contains: See flower, additionally carotenoids. *Effect:* See flower.	Pick fruit when ripe. Peel, free from white inner skin. Dry quickly in shade.

Plant	Part used / Components and effects	Harvesting and further processing
BLACK CARAWAY 170	*Contains:* Essential oil, coumarin derivates, tannins, saponin. *Effect:* Promotes bronchial secretion, soothes coughs.	Unearth in spring (March–April) or late autumn (September–October). Dry in shade or sun.
BLACK CHERRY 184	*Contains:* Hydrocyanic glycoside prunasine, enzyme emulsin, coumaric acid, tannin, scopoletine, traces of essential oil. *Effect:* Expectorant, soothes irritative cough.	Gather bark from young trunks in summer and autumn (July–October). Strip off outer bark. Dry inner bark carefully in shade.
BLACK COHOSH 58	*Contains:* Glycosides actaeine, etc., cimicifugin, bitter substance racemosin, estrogen substances, triterpenes, isoferulic acid, tannin. *Effect:* Stimulates menstruation.	Unearth rootstock with roots in autumn after fruit ripens. Cut lengthwise. Dry in sun or shade.
BLACK CURRANT 193	*Contains:* Tannin, traces of essential oil, enzyme emulsion. *Effect:* Diuretic.	Gather leaves after flowering and before berries ripen. Remove stems. Dry in shade.
	Contains: Vitamin C, dark pigment, fruit acids, potassium, flavone rutin, pectin, sugar, tannin. *Effect:* Supplies vitamin C, soothes coughs, quenches thirst.	Gather berries when ripe (July–August). Do not dry. Process while fresh.
BLACK HAW 241	*Contains:* Amentoflavone, coumarins scopoletine and aesculetine, arbutin, oleanolic and ursolic acid, sterol. *Effect:* Antispasmodic, soothing.	Branch bark obtained by stripping young and old branches in spring and summer. Dry in shade. Trunk and root bark obtained in autumn after fall of leaves. Dig out shrubs, strip trunk and clean root. Dry bark in shade.
BLACK HELLEBORE 119	*Contains:* Cardio-glycosides, hellebrin, saponin, aconitic acid, traces of essential oil. *Effect:* Regulates cardiac activity, similar to strophanthin and digitalis, hydragogue, irritates mucous membrane, induces diarrhea.	Unearth rootstock throughout the year. Dry in shade, in the sun, or by artificial heat.
BLACK MUSTARD 37	*Contains:* Glycoside-bonded allyl mustard oil, enzyme myrosinase, fatty oil, protein, phytinic acid, sinapine, mucin. *Effect:* Skin irritant, increases blood supply locally, stimulates circulation locally, rubefacient.	Gather the ripe, black pods in late summer (August–September). Tap seeds out of pods or thresh out if grown in fields. Leave to dry in a thin layer. Turn over frequently if large quantities.
BLACKTHORN 185	*Contains:* Traces of glycosides, possibly amygdaline, coumarin compounds. *Effect:* Mild purgative, diuretic, stimulates metabolism.	Gather flowers in spring (April–May). Dry in shade.
BLESSED THISTLE 63	*Contains:* Cnicin principle, flavonoids, tannin, traces of essential oil, copious mucilage. *Effect:* Increases gastric and bile secretion, tonic.	Gather leaves and flowering twigs when blooming (June–August). Dry in shade. Cut up after drying.
	Contains: Fatty oil with oleic and linoleic acid, albumin, cnicin bitter principle, arctin. *Effect:* Digestant.	Gather ripe fruit (seeds) in autumn (August–September).
BLOODROOT 205	*Contains:* Alkaloids chelidonine, sanguinarine, berberine, chelerythrine, etc. *Effect:* Expectorant, emetic, for external use against skin disorders.	Unearth rootstock with attached roots in early summer (May–June) or in autumn when the leaves have died (September–November). Dry carefully in sun or shade.
BLUE LUNGWORT 186	*Contains:* Mucins, silicic acid, tannin, saponin, allantoin, glycosides quercetin and Kampferol, vitamin C, mineral salts. *Effect:* Expectorant, mildly soothing, slightly diuretic, astringent, weakly binding.	Gather stalks at time of flowering (March–May). Dry in shade or in the sun.
	Contains: Same as flowering stalks (above). *Effect:* Same as flowering stalks.	Gather leaves during and after flowering (March–September). Dry in shade or sun.

Plant	Part used	Components and effects	Harvesting and further processing
BOLDO 164		*Contains:* Essential oil with ascaridol, alkaloids, flavanoids. *Effect:* Stimulates gastric and bile secretion, promotes uric acid elimination.	Gather evergreen leaves at any time. Dry carefully in shade, not over 40°C.
BROOM 76		*Contains:* Alkaloid (sparteine), secondary alkaloid (cytisine and others), tannin, bitter principle, traces of essential oil. *Effect:* Vasodilator, regulates cardiac activity.	Gathering possible from spring to autumn, preferably February–March or October. Dry in heat or sun.
		Contains: Sparteine, bitter principle, tannin, flavone glycoside, traces of essential oil. *Effect:* Diuretic.	Gather at time of flowering (May–June). Dry in heat or sun.
BUCHU 34		*Contains:* Essential oil with barosma camphor. *Effect:* Diuretic. Antiseptic in urinary canals.	Gather leaves (evergreen) throughout the year. Dry in shade, not over 40°C.
BUCKBEAN 150		*Contains:* Bitter principles, menyanthin, alkaloids, tannin, pectin, saponin, traces of essential oil, fatty oil, flavonoids. *Effect:* Stimulates digestive glands, choleretic.	Gather leaves May–June, while flowering. Dry as quickly as possible in shade.
BUGLEWEED 141		*Contains:* Tannin, traces of essential oil, lithospermic acid, phenolic substances. *Effect:* Sedative, astringent.	Gather foliage at time of flowering (July–September). Do not dry. Use while fresh or process to tincture and extract.
BUTTERBUR 161		*Contains:* Petasin and S-petasin, traces of essential oil, inulin, pectin, mucins, glycosidal bitter principle, resin. *Effect:* Antispasmodic, analgesic, dissolves mucus, diuretic and diaphoretic.	Unearth rootstock in late summer (August–September). Dry in shade or sun.
		Contains: Traces of essential oil, mucilage, tannin, albumin, resin, petasin. *Effect:* See rootstock (above).	Gather leaves in summer (June–July). Dry in shade.
BUTTERFLY WEED 31		*Contains:* Glycoside asclepiadine, bitter principle asclepione, cardenolides, traces of essential oil, resin, sterol. *Effect:* Diaphoretic, expectorant, influences heart and circulation.	Unearth rootstock in spring (March–April). Wash, split up. Dry in shade or sun.
CALABAR BEAN 166		*Contains:* Alkaloids, fatty oil, essential oil, stigmasterol, albumin, starch. *Effect:* Contracts pupils, reduces internal pressure of eye, stimulates peristalsis, slows heart.	Gather fruit when ripe. Free seeds from fruit husks.
CALIFORNIA POPPY 87		*Contains:* Alkaloids similar to opium poppy, protopine, allocryptopine, etc., flavone glycosides. *Effect:* Soporific, antispasmodic, analgesic.	Gather whole foliage at time of flowering (June–September). Dry in shade.
CAPE ALOE 11		*Contains:* Aloin, a bitter principle glycoside. *Effect:* Purgative, promotes bile secretion.	Cut off leaves in full sap. Sap is dried in the sun or by spray drying.
CARAWAY 46		*Contains:* Essential oil with carvene and limonene, fatty oil with oleic, linoleic, and petroselinic acids, nitrogenous substances, traces of tannin, coumarins, resin. *Effect:* Antispasmodic, effective against flatulence, promotes digestion, disinfectant, mild expectorant, milk-forming (folk medicine).	Gather fruit before fully ripe (July–August). Cut off umbels as soon as fruit turns brown. Allow to ripen fully in sun or shade. Comb down ripe fruit.
CARLINE THISTLE 45		*Contains:* Essential oil with carlina oxide, sesquiterpene carlenes, tannin, abundant inulin. *Effect:* Diuretic, diaphoretic, heals wounds.	Unearth roots in autumn (October) or spring (March–April). Dry in sun or shade.

Plant	Part used	Components and effects	Harvesting and further processing
CASCARA SAGRADA 191		*Contains:* Emodin glycosides and aloin-like glycosides, cascarosides, chrysaloin, chrysophanol, aloe-emodin, tannins, bitter principle, ferment, resin. *Effect:* Purgative, mild promoter of bile secretion. Fresh bark: emetic.	Gather bark from trunks and branches in spring and summer (mid-April–August). Dry in sun or shade with outside facing up. Store 1 year before use.
CASTOR BEAN 194		*Contains:* Toxalbumin ricin, enzyme lipase, alkaloid ricinine, fatty oil with purgative substance, ricinolic acid (as soap). *Effect:* Seeds: purgative.	Gather seeds at ripening time when 75 percent of a syncarp is ripe. Allow cut syncarps to ripen fully in sun, until seed capsules open. Seed kernels are processed by cold pressing to make castor oil.
CELANDINE 53		*Contains:* Alkaloids chelidonine, chelerythrine, coptisine, protopine, etc., chelidonic acid and other acids, traces of essential oil, saponin, carotenoid pigments, enzymes. *Effect:* Antispasmodic, relieves pain, promotes flow of bile, mild sedative, skin irritant.	Unearth roots in late summer and autumn (August–October). Dry in sun or shade.
		Contains: See root (above) but lower alkaloid content, no saponin. *Effect:* See root.	Gather foliage at time of flowering (May–June). Dry as quickly as possible in shade.
CENTAURY 50		*Contains:* Glycosidal bitter principles gentiopicrin and erythrocentaurine, nicotinic acid compounds, traces of essential oil, oleanolic acid and other acids, resin. *Effect:* Aperitive, digestant.	Gather foliage at time of flowering (July–September). Dry in sun or shade.
CHASTE TREE 245		*Contains:* Essential oil, fatty oil, flavonoid casticin, iridoglycoside agnuside and aucubin. *Effect:* Stimulates progesterone production.	Dark-brown to black berries picked at time of ripening (October–November). Dry in sun or shade.
CHAULMOOGRA 124		*Contains:* Fatty oil with chaulmoogra oil, hydnocarpic acid, protein, glycoside. *Effect:* Antileprosy drug, strongly irritant on gastrointestinal canal, vermifuge.	Gathe fruit at time of ripening, according to degree of ripeness. Free seeds from fruit pulp. Processed further to chaulmoogra oil (commercially).
CHICORY 57		*Contains:* Bitter principle, intybin, inulin.	Gather stalks and leaves at time of flowering (July–September). Dry in shade.
		Contains: Bitter principle, intybin, glycoside, cichorin. *Effect:* Mild stimulant for bile production, improves digestion.	Unearth roots in the spring (April) or autumn (October). Dry in heat or in sun.
CHINESE PAGODA TREE 219		*Contains:* Flavone glycoside rutin. *Effect:* Strengthens capillaries, styptic.	Gather flower buds in summer (July–August). Dry in shade.
CHIRATA 222		*Contains:* Bitter principles swertimarin, chiratin, tannin, resin. *Effect:* Stimulates gastric and bile secretion, tonic.	Gather the flowering or fruiting stalks at time of flowering (February–March). Dry in shade.
CINNAMON 60		*Contains:* Essential oil with cinnamaldehyde, cinnamic acid, eugenol, terpenes, tannin, starch, calcium oxalate, traces of mucilage. *Effect:* Stimulates secretion of gastrc juices.	Gather bark from trunks and branches of young shoots. Remove leaves, strip bark with copper or brass knife. Pare off outside bark. Dry inner bark in shade.
COCA 86		*Contains:* Alkaloid cocaine and subsidiary alkaloids, coca tannic acid, essential oil, nicotine, acids. *Effect:* Local anesthetic, reduces gland secretion, shrinks mucous membranes, reduces hunger and thirst, centrally stimulating, raises physical performance.	Gather young leaves throughout the year (4 harvests on average). Dry in shade.

Plant	Part used	Components and effects	Harvesting and further processing
COFFEE 65		*Contains:* Alkaloid caffeine, chlorogenic acid, trigonelline, fatty coffee oil, essential roast oil, tannin. *Effect:* Stimulates central nervous system, vasodilator (excluding abdominal vessels), promotes funtions of cerebrum, general stimulant, increases cardiac output, stimulates secretion of gastric juices and bile, diuretic, digestive.	Gather coffee cherries several times per year according to ripeness. Free seed kernels from pulp and shells by various technical processes ("wet" or "dry" process). Further processing for roasted coffee or coffee coal.
COLA 66		*Contains:* Caffeine, theobromine, catechin tannin, colarot, glycoside, essential oil, fatty oil, starch. *Effect:* Centrally stimulating, raises performance, raises spirits slightly (euphoric).	Gather nuts at time of ripening (varies according to region of origin). Remove seed kernels from fruit pulp, free from remains by washing. Dry in heat.
COLTSFOOT 232		*Contains:* Mucin, flavonoids rutin and hyperocarotene pigment taraxanthin, phytosterols arnidiol and faradiol, some tannin, essential oil. *Effect:* Expectorant, dissolves mucus, relieves irritation.	Gather flowers before fully blooming (end February–April). Dry carefully in shade.
		Contains: Mucin, abundant tannin, glycosidal bitter principle, inulin, sitosterol, saltpeter. *Effect:* Dissolves mucus, expectorant, astringent, anti-inflammatory.	Gather leaves in early summer (May–June). Dry in shade. Fresh leaves can be used until autumn.
COMFREY 223		*Contains:* Allantoin, tannins, mucilage, starch, inulin, traces of oil. *Effect:* Hastens wound healing, promotes formation of connective tissue, soothes irritation, inhibits inflammation.	Preferably unearth before budding in the spring (April) or after flowering in late autumn (September–October). Split root along length. Dry in heat (40°–60°C.) or in the sun.
COMMON NASTURTIUM 230		*Contains:* Benzyl mustard oil splitting glucotropaeoline, enzyme myrosin, unknown antibacterial substances. *Effect:* Antibacterial.	Gather foliage with flower and possibly seeds at time of flowering (July–October). Do not dry. Use while fresh or process.
		Contains: See stalk. *Effect:* See stalk.	Gather fruit at end of and after time of flowering. Use while fresh and process.
CORYDALIS 69		*Contains:* Alkaloids bulbocapnine, corydaline, etc. *Effect:* Antispasmodic.	Unearth tubers in spring before flowering. Dry in sun, shade, or artificial heat.
COTTON 110		*Contains:* Cellulose, water, wax. *Effect:* Highly absorbent.	Further processing degreasing, bleaching, etc.) done industrially.
		Contents: Resinous substance with phenolcarbonic acid, salicylic acid, betaine, sugar, traces of essential oil. *Effect:* Styptic.	Unearth after cotton harvest. Peel off crust thinly, about 1 cm wide, to strips 30 cm long. Dry quickly. Pluck the complete burst capsule or twist out the wool by hand.
COWSLIP 182		*Contains:* Saponin primulic acid A and auxiliary saponins, essential oil, sugar alcohol, volemite. *Effect:* Expectorant, diuretic.	Unearth roots before or during flowering (March–May) or in autumn (October). Wash well. Dry in shade or sun.
		Contains: Saponins, flavonoids, essential oil, carotenoids, pigments. *Effect:* As root, but weaker.	Gather fully blooming flowers with green calyx from March to May. Dry quickly in shade.
		Contains: Flavonoids, essential oil, carotenoids, pigments. *Effect:* Mild sedative.	Gather the flower corollae without calyx, March–May. Dry quickly in shade.
CURLED DOCK 199		*Contains:* Anthraquinone compounds (emodin), acids, tannin. *Effect:* Purgative.	Unearth in late summer and autumn (August–October). Dry at 50°–70°C. After slitting along length, also dry coarser parts in sun.
		Contains: Tannin. *Effect:* Controls diarrhea.	Gather the ripe, dry fruit (seeds), July–September.

Plant	Part used	Components and effects	Harvesting and further processing
DAMIANA 231		*Contains:* Essential oil with cineol, cymol, pinene; arbutin; hydrocyanic glycoside, bitter principle, tannin, resin. *Effect:* Nerve tonic, diuretic.	Gather leaves at time of flowering. Dry in shade.
DANDELION 224		*Contains:* Bitter principle taraxacin, ceryl alcohol, lactucerol, tannin, traces of essential oil, inulin, choline, waxy taraxacerin, sugar, resin, acids. *Effect:* Diuretic, stimulates secretion of bile, gastric juices, and pancreas, tonic.	Dig out tap roots in spring (March–April) or in early autumn (August–September). Dry in sun or shade.
		Contains: Taraxacin, ceryl alcohol, lactucerol, taraxacerin, inosite, choline, vitamins A and B, nicotinic acid, arnidiol and faradiol. *Effect:* See root (above).	Gather leaves from spring to late summer (April–August). Dry in shade. Gather young leaves for salad in spring (March–April) before flowering.
DILL 15		*Contains:* Essential oil, fatty oil, various acids.	Gather fruit when fully ripe, when turned brown. Spread out to dry, not in artificial heat.
		Contains: Essential oil. *Effect* (fruit and stalk): Stimulates secretion of gastric juices, combats flatulence, slightly antispasmodic.	Gather stalks preferably before blooming or after withering. Dry quickly, not in the sun, at about 40°C.
DOG ROSE 195		*Contains:* Abundant vitamin C, vitamins B and K, carotene, fruit acids, tannin, pectin, sugar, some essential oil with vanillin. *Effect:* Supplies vitamin C, mild astringent, weak purgative and diuretic.	Gather ripe, red hips while still hard during late summer and autumn (August–October). Halve, dry in shade, not over 50°C.
		Contains: Essential oil, fatty oil, lecithin, sugar, vitamin E. *Effect:* Weak diuretic.	Release kernels from the cut-open ripe fruit. Wash free from white cilium attached. Dry in shade, not over 60°C.
DWARF ELDER 203		*Contains:* Uninvestigated bitter principle, saponin. *Effect:* Diuretic, diaphoretic.	Unearth rootstock in spring (March) or autumn (October). Clean. Dry in sun or heat.
		Contains: Tannin, essential oil, traces of hydrocyanic glycoside, anthocyanin pigment. *Effect:* Laxative, diuretic, diaphoretic.	Gather the ripe, black berries August–September. Dry in shade.
EAGLE VINE 145		*Contains:* Bitter principle glycoside condurangin, essential oil, resin, organic acids, rubber-like substances, starch. *Effect:* Aperitive, digestive.	Bark of trunk and branches can be gathered throughout the year. Dry in sun or shade.
ELECAMPANE 130		*Contains:* Essential oil with bitter principles, resin, inulin. *Effect:* Relieves cough, expectorant, appetite stimulant, slightly diuretic.	Gather (unearth) in the autumn (September–October). Dry in the sun or at 50–70°C. Cut up large roots beforehand.
ENGLISH IVY 117		*Contains:* Hedera saponin and other saponins, hederin, helixin in the fresh leaf. *Effect:* Soothing, expectorant. Fresh leaf contains a blistering agent.	Gather young leaves in spring and early summer (April–July). Dry in shade. For external use: Collect leaves from shady woodland during late summer.
ENGLISH PLANTAIN 174		*Contains:* Glycoside aucubin, tannins, mucilage, chlorogenic and ursolic acid, potassium, silicic acid. *Effect:* Expectorant, soothes irritation, protects mucous membrane, astringent.	Gather leaves at time of flowering (May–September). Dry as quickly as possible in sun or shade at 30–50°C. The drug changes color and becomes ineffective if dried slowly.
		Contains: See leaf (above). *Effect:* See leaf.	Gather entire foliage at time of flowering. Dry, as for leaf.
ENGLISH VIOLET 242		*Contains:* Saponin, essential oil with methyl salicyalate. *Effect:* Dissolves mucus, expectorant.	Unearth rootstock during late summer (August–September). Dry in shade.
		Contains: Saponin, traces of essential oil with methyl salicyalate, mucin. *Effect:* As rootstock.	Gather leaves and flowers during spring (March–April). Dry in shade.

Plant	Part used	Components and effects	Harvesting and further processing
ENGLISH WALNUT 131		*Contains:* Tannins, juglone, flavones, essential oil. *Effect:* Astringent, anti-inflammatory.	Gather leaves in early summer (May–mid-June). Dry quickly in shade, not over 40°C. Leaves turn brownish-black if dried slowly.
EPHEDRA 83		*Contains:* Alkaloids ephedrine, pseudo-ephedrine, etc., tannins, saponin, flavone, essential oil. *Effect:* Vasodilator, raises blood pressure, stimulates circulation, anti-allergic.	Gather the fertile young branches of female plants in autumn, before the first frost, if possible after long dry spell. Dry in sun.
ERGOT 62	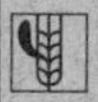	*Contains:* Alkaloids (some derivatives of glysergic acid), ergotamine, ergotoxine, ergotmetrine, etc. Tyramine, histamine, sterols, pigments. *Effects:* Stimulates uterine contractions, vasoconstrictor.	Gather ergots from ears of rye at beginning of ripening (end July–August) or after the harvest from the threshed rye. Dry at 35°–40°C.
EUCALYPTUS 88		*Contains:* Essential oil with cineole, tannin, ellagic and gallic acid, bitter principle, resin, wax, bacteriostatic substance. *Effect:* Expectorant, antiseptic, rubefacient.	The crescent-shaped new leaves of older branches can be gathered throughout the year. Do not take the heart-shaped primary leaves from younger trees. Dry in shade.
EUROPEAN BITTERSWEET 217	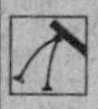	*Contains:* Solasodine, soladulcidine, glycosidic bitter principle, saponin, tannin. *Effect:* Stimulates central nervous system, slightly diuretic.	Gather before sprouting (March–April) or after leaves have fallen (October). Dry in heat.
EUROPEAN BLACKBERRY 198		*Contains:* Tannin, flavone, vitamin C. *Effect:* Slightly astringent, mildly binding.	Collect leaves June–August. Dry in shade or sun. Allow leaves to ferment for domestic tea. Leave in a pile for a few days until they turn greenish-brown.
EUROPEAN ELDER 204	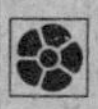	*Contains:* Flavone compounds rutin, isoquercitrine, Kampferol, etc., hydrocyanic glycoside sambunigrine, tannins, essential oil. *Effect:* Diaphoretic, increases resistance.	Gather the fully blooming umbels in June–July. Dry carefully in shade, not over 40°C. Pluck or comb off individual flowers.
		*Contains:* Invert sugar, fruit acids, tannin, vitamin C, anthocyanic pigments, traces of essential oil. *Effect:* Laxative, diuretic, diaphoretic.	Gather the well-ripened berries in autumn (September). Dry in shade or by artificial heat.
EUROPEAN HOLLY 128		*Contains:* Tannin, bitter principle, some theobromine, ursolic and ilexic acid, rutin, resin. *Effect:* Diaphoretic, weakly diuretic.	Gather the evergreen leaves throughout the year. Dry in sun or shade.
EUROPEAN MISTLETOE 244		*Contains:* Viscotoxin, basic proteins inhibiting tumors, choline. *Effect:* Lowers blood pressure, inhibits tumors.	Gather the leafy young branches in autumn and winter (October–December) or spring (March–April). Dry in shade, not over 45°C.
EUROPEAN POLYPODY 178	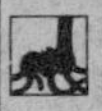	*Contains:* Glycosidal bitter principle, saponin, mucilage, traces of essential oil, sugar, resin. *Effect:* Soothes coughs, expectorant, expels intestinal worms, mild purgative, bile stimulant.	Unearth in autumn (September–November). Replant top of rootstock. Dry in shade or sun.
EUROPEAN SNAKEROOT 25	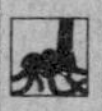	*Contains:* Aristolochid acid, essential oil, tannin, bitter principle, aristolochian yellow, resin, starch, sugar. *Effect:* Anti-inflammatory, kidney irritant.	Unearth rootstock in spring (March) or in autumn (September–October). Dry in shade.
		*Contains:* Aristolochic acid (less than root), essential oil, tannin bitter principle, allantoin, flavones, saponin, antibiotic substance. *Effect:* Same as rootstock (above).	Gather foliage before flowering (April–May) or during period of blossoming (May–July). Dry in shade.
EVERLASTING FLOWER 118	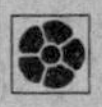	*Contains:* Flavonoids helichrysin, salipurposide, etc., coumarins, traces of essential oil, bitter principle, resin, phytosterin, hydrocarbons. *Effect:* Gastric, pancreas, and bile secretion.	Gather the flowers before fully blooming in summer (July–September). Dry in shade.

Plant	Part used / Components and effects	Harvesting and further processing
EYEBRIGHT 90	*Contains:* Aucubine-like compounds, tannin, essential oil. *Effect:* Inhibits inflammation of mucous membranes, particularly the eyes.	Gather at time of flowering (June–October). Dry in shade.
FALSE HELLEBORE 239	*Contains:* Steroid-alkaloid germidine, protoverine, jervine, veratramine, germidine, germitrine. *Effect:* Lowers blood pressure.	Unearth rootstock after leaves have died in autumn (October). Clean thoroughly, cut up along length. Dry in sun.
FENNEL 93	*Contains:* Essential oil with anethole and fenchone, fatty oil, albumin, sugar. *Effect:* Antispasmodic, inhibits flatulence, stimulates the stomach, expectorant.	Gather the ripe, split fruit in autumn (September–October). Cut off brown umbel. Comb fruit. Dry slightly in the shade.
	Contains: Essential oil with dillapiole and anethole, coumarins, sugar, starch. *Effect:* Inhibits flatulence, diuretic.	Unearth in spring (mid-March–April). Dry in shade, not over 35°C.
FENUGREEK 228	*Contains:* Mucins, alkaloid: trigonelline, albumin, fatty oil, bitter principle. *Effect:* Demulcent for chapped hands and lips, soothes disturbed digestion, stimulates lactation.	Gather stalks when ripe (about August–September). Thresh fruit.
FIG 91	*Contains:* Invert sugar, pectin, organic acids, fat, albumin, vitamins A and B. *Effect:* Mild purgative, soothing for coughs, slightly expectorant.	Gather the ripe fruit, preferably during the autumn harvest (September). Can be stored 6 months or more. Dry hanging up or spread out.
FIGWORT 210	*Contains:* Saponins, flavon-glycosides. *Effect:* Slightly purgative, useful in some chronic skin disease.	Stalks at time of flowering (June–August). Dry in shade or sun.
FLAX 139	*Contains:* Mucins, fatty oil with linoleic, linolenic, and oleic acids and saturated acids, protein, glycosides. *Effect:* Anti-inflammatory, mild purgative, analgesic, skin emollient.	Gather seed pods, mainly from threshings, when fully ripe (September).
FLEABANE 85	*Contains:* Essential oil with lime, tannin, flavone, gallic acid. *Effect:* Constricting effect on mucous membranes.	Gather at time of flowering (June–October). Dry as quickly as possible in the shade.
FOXGLOVE 78	*Contains:* Cardiac glycosides, saponins, flavones, tannin, organic acids, mucilage. *Effect:* Improves action of the heart, diuretic.	Gather leaves at time of flowering (June–September), if possible during a dry, sunny late afternoon. Dry as quickly as possible in shade or sun. Wear gloves when picking.
FRINGE TREE 54	*Contains:* Glycoside phyllirine, saponin. *Effect:* Stimulates secretion and flow of bile, mild purgative, heals wounds.	Unearth root in spring (March–April) or autumn (October). Wash thoroughly. Peel, dry bark in shade.
FUMITORY 97	*Contains:* Fumarine and other alkaloids, fumaric acid, resin, bitter principles, mucilage. *Effect:* Regulator of bile secretion, mildly diuretic, mildly purgative.	Gather at time of flowering (June–September). Dry in shade.
GARDEN CHAMOMILE 17	*Contains:* Essential oil, bitter principle, flavone glycosides, coumarin. *Effect:* Antispasmodic, diaphoretic, stimulates digestion, inhibits inflammation, promotes healing of wounds, similar to German chamomile.	Gather fully blooming flower tops in summer (June–August) in dry weather and, preferably, after a period of fine weather. Flowers picked when damp turn gray. Dry as quickly as possible in shade, not over 35°C.
GARDEN SAGE 202	*Contains:* Essential oil with thujone, linalool, camphor, borneol, triterpenic acids oleanolic and ursolic acid, labiatenic acid, bitter principles, flavonoids, resin, estrogenous substance. *Effect:* Astringent, anti-inflammatory, antiseptic, inhibits secretion of perspiration.	Gather leaves shortly before and at beginning of flowering in dry, sunny weather (May–July). Dry in shade, not over 35°C.

Plant	Part used	Components and effects	Harvesting and further processing
GARLIC 9		*Contains:* Essential oil containing sulfur with diallyldisulphide as odorant, allicin, alliin, vitamins A and C, nicotinic acid. *Effect:* Stimulates gall bladder and stomach secretion, promotes bile flow, inhibits fermentation and putrefaction in the stomach, vermifuge, antispasmodic, vasodilator, generally strengthening.	Unearth cloves when the leaves begin to wither (September). Store in a dry and cool place.
GERMAN CHAMOMILE 146	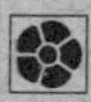	*Contains:* Essential oil with chamazulene and bisabol oil, coumarin, flavone glycosides, mucins, fatty acids, sugar. *Effect:* Antispasmodic, relieves flatulence, relieves pain, inhibits inflammation, promotes healing of wounds, antiseptic.	Gather flowers May–August, preferably in sunny weather. The maximum content of active agents is several days after blooming. Dry in shade, not over 35°C. Do not confuse with Roman or English chamomile *(Anthemis nobilis)* or false chamomile *(Boltonia)*
		*Contains:* Same as blossom (above). *Effect:* Generally same as blossom, but weaker.	
GERMANDER 225		*Contains:* Essential oil, bitter principle, tannin, nitrogen compounds, polyphenols. *Effect:* Stimulates secretion of gastric juices, slightly astringent, promotes healing of wounds.	Gather foliage at time of flowering (June–September). Dry in shade, not over 35°C.
GINGER 247	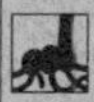	*Contains:* Essential oil with gingiberene and gingiberole, phellandrene, borneol, lineol, citral, resin mix gingerol, starch. *Effect:* Promotes secretion of gastric juice, carminative.	Unearth rootstock when leaves have died. Remove remains of stems and root fibers. Wash thoroughly, strip, leave in cold water overnight. Dry in sun. Root can also be used unstripped.
GINKGO 108		*Contains:* Flavonoid camphor oil, quercetin, luteolin, catechin tannins, resin, essential oil, fatty oil. *Effect:* Increases blood supply by dilating the blood vessels.	Gather the leaves in summer (June–August). Dry in shade or process fresh leaves to extracts.
GOAT'S RUE 98		*Contains:* Glukokinin galegine, flavone glycosides, saponins, tannin, bitter principle. *Effect:* Reduces sugar, milk forming.	Gather stalks at time of flowering (July–August). Dry in shade.
		*Contains:* Glukokinin galegine, flavone glycosides, saponin, fatty oil, sacharose. *Effect:* Stimulates renal secretion, hydragogue, controls inflammation, heals wounds.	Gather ripe seeds in August–September. Allow to dry out.
GOLDENROD 218		*Contains:* Saponins, essential oil, bitter principle, catechin tannin, flavonoids, acids. *Effect:* Stimulates renal secretion, hydragogue, controls inflammation, heals wounds.	Gather stalks at time of flowering (July–October), preferably from plants not yet blooming. Dry in shade, not over 40°C.
GOLDENSEAL 125	 	*Contains:* Alkaloids (hydrastine, berberine, etc.), traces of essential oil, resin, chologenic acid, fatty oil, sugar, albumin. *Effect:* Stimulates uterine muscles, vasoconstrictor, styptic.	Unearth rootstock with roots from 3-year-old plants in autumn after ripening of seeds. Clean carefully. Dry in the air spread out on cloth.
GRAPE 246		*Contains:* Tannin, inosite, organic acids, choline, mineral salts, borine compounds, flavone glykoside. *Effect:* Stimulates liver function, stimulates metabolism, astringent.	Unsprayed leaves can be gathered throughout the summer. Dry in shade.
		*Contains:* Tartaric and malic acid, mineral salts, dextrose and fructose, pectin, tannin, flavone glycosides, pigment, vitamins A, B, C. *Effect:* Laxative, diuretic, tonic.	Gather berries at ripening time (September–October). Use fresh or process to juice.
GRAPPLE PLANT 115	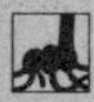	*Contains:* Glycoside harpagoside, harpagide, procumbine, sugar, stachyose. *Effect:* Anti-inflammatory, pain-relieving.	Unearth storage roots in autumn. Only use young side roots. Cut into pieces approximately 2 cm long before drying.

Plant	Part used	Components and effects	Harvesting and further processing
GREAT BURDOCK 22		*Contains:* Essential oil, abundant inulin, tannin, resin, mucilage, acids, antibiotic substance. *Effect:* Slightly diuretic and diaphoretic, promotes healing of wounds, stimulates hair growth (not proven).	Unearth root of 1-year-old plants still without stem in October–November or of 2-year-old plants (visible by stem) in April–mid-May. Clean carefully, split larger roots lengthwise. Dry, not over 70°C.
GREEN PEPPER 42		*Contains:* Capsaicin, carotenoids, flavonoids, vitamin C, traces of essential oil, sugar. *Effect:* Skin irritant, increases blood supply locally, promotes peristalsis.	Harvest fruit when fully ripe (end July–September). Dry in shade, with heat but not over 35°C. Whole fruit with calyx and stem is further processed to powder.
HARONGA TREE 114		*Contains:* Phenolic pigment, triterpene, betulin acid, anthraquinone compounds, tannin.	Gather bark and evergreen leaves throughout the year. Dry in shade.
		Contains: Phenolic pigment, hypericin, flavone, tannin. *Effect:* Increases secretion of pancreas, bile, gastric juices.	
HAWTHORN 70		*Contains:* Vitexine rhamnoside and other flavone bodies, triterpenic acids, ursolic and oleanolic acid, purine derivatives, choline and acetylcholine, organic acids, catechin, tannin. *Effect:* Vasodilator, lowers blood pressure, cardiac sedative.	Gather leaves in summer (May–July). Dry in shade.
		Contains: See leaf (above); additional essential oil, trimethylamine.	Gather flowers in early summer (May–June). Dry carefully in shade, not over 35°C.
		Contains: Flavonoids, triterpene acids, fruit acids, fatty oil, sugar, carotenoids, anthocyanic pigments, tannin, vitamins B and C.	Gather the fully ripe, red fruit in September–October. Predry in shade, dry fully in moderate artificial heat.
HEDGE HYSSOP 111		*Contains:* Glycoside gratioside, gratiogenin, gratiotoxin, essential oil, resin. *Effect:* Central and local stimulant, promotes bleeding, diuretic, strong purgative.	Gather stalks at time of flowering (June–August). Dry as quickly as possible in artificial heat (approximately 60°C).
HEMP AGRIMONY 89		*Contains:* Bitter principle, euparin, tannin, traces of essential oil, resin. *Effect:* Stimulates liver function, diuretic.	Gather at time of flowering (July–September). Dry in shade.
		Contains: Euparin, essential oil. *Effect:* Stimulates liver function.	Unearth in late autumn (October). Dry in shade.
HEMPNETTLE 99		*Contains:* Silicic acid, glycosidal bitter principle, tannin, saponin, acids, essential oils, resin, substance similar to pectin. *Effect:* Stimulates skin metabolism, astringent, dissolves mucus.	Gather stalks at time of flowering (July–September). Dry in shade.
HENBANE 126		*Contains:* Alkaloids (hyoscyamine and atropine), choline, tannin, traces of essential oil. *Effect:* Soothing, relieves pain.	1-year planting: gather at start of flowering (May). 2-year planting: in late summer of first year (July–August). Dry in shade or sun.
HERB ROBERT 106		*Contains:* Tannin, bitter principle geraniin, traces of essential oil, malic and citric acid. *Effect:* Astringent, inhibits diarrhea, styptic.	Gather foliage at time of flowering (May–October). Dry in shade.
		Contains: Same as stalk (above), but higher proportion of tannin, additional ellagic acid, resin, starch. *Effect:* Somewhat stronger than stalk.	Gather entire plant with roots at time of flowering (May–October). Dry in shade.
HIGH MALLOW 143		*Contains:* Mucins, pigment, malvine, tannin. *Effect:* Soothing, expectorant, astringent, anti-inflammatory.	Gather fully opened flowers, July–September. Dry carefully in shade, not too close together.
		Contains: Mucins (more than flower), tannin. *Effect:* See flower (above).	Gather leaves in summer, mid-June–mid-September. Dry in shade.

Plant	Part used	Components and effects	Harvesting and further processing
HOPS 123		*Contains:* Resin with picric acids, lupulon and humulon, essential oil, tannins, estrogenic substances, hopein. *Effect:* Mild sedative, soothes the stomach, external skin irritant.	Gather the female fruit pistils (hop cones) before full ripeness in late summer (August–September). Dry in shade. Lupulin extracted by knocking off and sieving the fresh fruit pistils.
HOREHOUND 144		*Contains:* Marrubiin bitter principle, tannin, essential oil. *Effect:* Expectorant, stimulates gall secretion, heals wounds.	Gather herb during blossom time (June–September). Dry in shade, not over 35°C.
HORSE CHESTNUT 5		*Contains:* Aesculus saponin with aescin, tannin, flavones, purine compounds, abundant starch, sugar, albumin, fatty oil. *Effect:* Haemostasis, increases venous tonicity.	Gather the fallen ripe chestnuts in autumn (September–October). Dry in sun or shade.
		Contains: Coumarin glycosides aesculin and fraxin, flavone quercitrin, saponin aescin, phytosterin, tannin, resin, pigment. *Effect:* Astringent.	Collect bark from young branches (not over 5 years old) in spring (March–April) or autumn (October–November). Dry in sun or shade.
HORSERADISH 26		*Contains:* Essential oil with mustard oil, glycosides, enzymes, vitamin B, antibiotic substances, asparagin, thiocyanogen compounds. *Effect:* Stimulates metabolism, promotes secretion, laxative, antiseptic, rubefacient.	Harvest roots in autumn and winter (September–February). Store in cellar in sand, or bury in earth outside.
HORSETAIL 84		*Contains:* Silicic acid, saponin, flavone glycoside, organic acids, nicotine, palustrine. *Effect:* Assists neutral healing processes, slightly diuretic.	Gather the green unfruitful summer fronds June–August. Take only plants without brown spots (fungus). Dry in shade (keep green color). Sort out discolored fronds.
HOUND'S TONGUE 75		*Contains:* Alkaloids, heliosupin, tannin, allantoin, essentixl oil, mucins. *Effect:* Astringent, controls diarrhea, soothing, relieves pain, encourages healing of wounds.	Gather stalks at time of flowering (May–June). Dry in shade.
		Contains: Alkaloids, cynoglossin, consolidin, bitter principle, cynoglossidin, tannin, mucin, allantoin. *Effect:* See flowering stalk (above).	Unearth root in spring (April) or autumn (September–October). Dry in shade.
ICELAND MOSS 52		*Contains:* Mucins, mainly lichenin, bitter fumaric acids (fumarprotocetraric acid, protolichesteric acid, and fumaric acid, partly usnine, some iodine. *Effect:* Reduces irritation of mucous membrane, stimulates appetite and digestion, weakly antiseptic, nutrient.	The lichen can be gathered throughout the year; preferably May–September in dry weather. Free from attached impurities such as foreign lichen and moss. Dry in shade or sun.
INDIAN HEMP 20		*Contains:* Cardio-glycoside cymarin and K-strophanthine, acetovanillin, androsterone, traces of saponin, tannin, resin. *Effect:* Slows heartbeat, regulates blood pressure, diuretic, irritates intestinal mucous membrane.	Unearth rootstock in autumn (September–October). Dry in shade or sun.
INDIAN SNAKEROOT 189		*Contains:* Complex alkaloid spectrum (reserpene, ajmaline, yohimbine, and many others). *Effect:* Lowers blood pressure, tranquilizer, antidepressant.	Unearth roots in December after leaves have fallen. Plants must be at least 18 months old. Clean thoroughly, dry in sun or shade, not in artificial heat.
INDIAN TOBACCO 140		*Contains:* Alkaloids lobeline, isolobeline, etc., lobelic and chelidonic acid. *Effect:* Respiratory stimulant, antispasmodic, anti-asthmatic.	Gather entire foliage with seed vessels and little flower at end of time of flowering (August–September). Dry in shade or artificial heat, not over 40°C.
IPECACUANHA 51		*Contains:* Alkaloids, saponins. *Effect:* Expectorant, promotes secretion of saliva, used in treatment of amoebic dysentery.	Root unearthed throughout the year, excluding wet period (3–4 year plant). Dry in the sun as quickly as possible.

Plant	Part used / Components and effects	Harvesting and further processing
IRISH MOSS 55	*Contains:* Mucins, proteins, amino acids; some iodine, bromine, and manganese salts. *Effect:* Soothes mucous membrane, laxative.	Gather algae washed up on shore or cut off during low tide. Free from impurities. Dry in sun, moistening frequently.
JABORANDI 168	*Contains:* Alkaloids (pilocarpine, pilosine, and secondary alkaloids), essential oil, traces of tannin. *Effect:* Stimulates salivary and sweat gland activity, stimulates parasympathetic nerve ends, miotic, reduces internal pressure of the eye.	Gather leaves throughout the year (four harvests on average). Strip off pinnate leaves. Dry in shade.
JAVA TEA 157	*Contains:* Saponin, sapophonin, essential oil, bitter principle glycoside, orthosiphonin, abundant potassium salts, urea, organic acids. *Effect:* Diuretic, slightly antispasmodic, promotes secretion and flow of bile, lowers blood pressure.	Gather leaves and tips of branches during flowering (July–August) from plants almost or just in bloom. Dry in shade.
JUNIPER 132	*Contains:* Essential oil with monoterpenes (alpha-pinene, etc.) and sesquiterpenes (alpha-cadenes, etc.) invert sugar, flavone glycoside, resin, tannin and bitter principle. *Effect:* Diuretic, antiseptic, digestant.	Gather the ripe, black, unshriveled berries in autumn (October). Dry in shade, not by artificial heat.
KAVA 172	*Contains:* Resin with lactones kawahin, yangonin, methysticin, etc., glycosides, starch. *Effect:* Makes insensitive to pain: soothing and relaxing, stimulates mental activity.	Unearth rootstock at any time of year. Free from roots, pare, split up. Dry in sun.
KHELLA 14	*Contains:* Furanochromone khellin, visnagin, khelloglycoside, fatty oil, protein. *Effect:* Antispasmodic, dilates bronchi, vasodilator, relaxes muscles (urinary tract).	Gather fruit in late summer (August–September) shortly before fully ripe. Dry in sun or shade.
KIDNEY VETCH 19	*Contains:* Saponins, tannin, xanthophyll. *Effect:* Externally promotes healing of wounds, mild digestant.	Gather flowers in early summer (May–July). Dry in shade.
	Contains: See flower (above). *Effect:* See flower.	Gather foliage at time of flowering (May–July). Dry in shade.
LADY'S MANTLE 8	*Contains:* Tannin, tannin glycoside, traces of salicylic acid, constituents still little known. *Effect:* Astringent, inhibits inflammation, slightly spasmolytic, sedative.	Gather flowering stalks or leaves only while flowering (May–September), preferably before mid-August. Dry in shade or sun.
LAVENDER 136	*Contains:* Essential oil with approximately 40 constituents, (including linalyl acetate and linalool), coumarin, tannin. *Effect:* Mildly soothing, carminative.	Gather flowers shortly before opening (June–September). Dry in shade, not over 35°C.
LEMON VERBENA 12	*Contains:* Essential oil with citral, limonene, dipentene, linalool, etc. *Effect:* Digestant, mild antispasmodic, soothing.	Gather leaves or flowering tips of branches at time of flowering in sunny weather (July–August). Dry in shade not over 35°C.
LICORICE 109	*Contains:* Saponin-like compounds glycyrrhizin with glycyrrhetic acid, flavonoids liquiritin, isoliquiritin, etc., coumarin, estrogenous substances, asparagin, starch, sugar. *Effect:* Promotes healing of gastric ulcers, expectorant, mild purgative, in larger doses raises blood pressure and causes edema.	Unearth roots and offshoots in late utumn (October–November). Wash. Dry in sun.
LIGNUM VITAE 112	*Contains:* Triterpensaponins, resin, rubber-like material, saponins, rubber, vanillin, traces of essential oil, guajacolum. *Effect:* Diuretic, diaphoretic, mild purgative.	Trees felled for technical use. Break up heartwood and sapwood produced during processing (without bark).

Plant	Part used	Components and effects	Harvesting and further processing
LILY-OF-THE-VALLEY 68		*Contains:* Cardiac glycosides convallatoxin, convallatoxole, convalloside, etc., saponins convallarin and convallaric acid, asparagin, chelidonic acid, other organic acids. *Effect:* Stimulates heart muscle, diuretic, strong irritant of stomach and intestine (in overdose).	Gather leaves at time of flowering (May–June). Dry in shade or artificial heat at approximately 60°C.
		Contains: Cardiac glycosides (see leaf, but higher proportion), essential oil with farnesol. *Effect:* See leaf (above).	Gather the fully open flowers in May and June. Dry in shade or by artificial heat (60°C).
		Contains: See leaf and flower. *Effect:* See leaf.	Gather foliage at time of flowering (May–June). Take fully blooming plants if possible. Dry in shade or artificial heat (60°C).
LOVAGE 139		*Contains:* Essential oil with phthalidene, terpineol, carvacrol, isovaleric acid, coumarin, angelica acid, benzoic acid, malic acid, resin, starch, sugar. *Effect:* Diuretic, stomachic, mildly carminative, mild expectorant.	Unearth roots of older, 2–3 year old plants in the autumn (September–October). Split the thicker roots along length. Dry in shade, not over 35°C.
MADDER 197		*Contains:* Anthraquinone derivatives such as alizarin (madder pigment) and purpurin carboxylic acid glucoside, organic acids, pectin, sugar, albumin, fatty oil. *Effect:* Antispasmodic in urinary passages.	Unearth root in autumn (September–October). Remove root fibres and outer skin. Dry in sun or shade.
MALE FERN 81		*Contains:* Filicin with phloroglucin derivatives aspidinol, albaspidin, flavaspidic acid, filixic acid, etc., tannins, fatty oil, traces of essential oil, resin, starch, sugar. *Effect:* Vermifuge (tapeworms).	Unearth rootstock in autumn (September–October). Free from subsidiary roots and dead pieces. Leave remains of stem standing. Dry in sun or by artificial heat (40°–50°C).
MARIGOLD 40		*Contains:* Bitter principles, little essential oil, saponin, carotenoids, pigments, xantophyll, flavone glycosides, triterpen-alcohol, acids, mucins. *Effect:* Heals wounds, anti-inflammatory, promotes bile secretion.	Gather whole flower tops or petals only, June–September. Dry carefully in shade, not over 35°C, not by artificial heat.
		Contains: See flower (above). *Effect:* See flower.	Gather foliage at time of flowering (June–September). Dry in shade, not over 35°C.
MARJORAM 156		*Contains:* Essential oil with thymol, carvacrol, acids, tannin, bitter principles. *Effect:* Astringent, expectorant, bile stimulant.	Gather at time of flowering (July–September), free from thicker stalks. Dry in shade, not over 35°C.
MARSH MALLOW 13		*Contains:* Mucins, traces of essential oil. *Effect:* Soothing for mucous membranes, emollient for inflammation.	Gather in summer (July–August), preferably after flowering.
		Contains: Mucins, starch, sugar, pectin, tannin, asparagin. *Effect:* Soothing, inhibits peristalsis, reduces inflammation, inhibits diarrhea.	Unearth in late autumn (October–November). Free from main root and root fibers, pare off cork layer and bark. Dry immediately at 50–60°C. Never dry before paring.
		Contains: Mucins, traces of essential oil, sugar, asparagin. *Effect:* Slightly soothing.	Gather at time of flowering (July–September). Dry in shade.
MASTERWORT 163		*Contains:* Essential oil with terpenes, palmitic acid and esters, coumarin compounds (bitter principles), tannin, resin, starch, fatty oil, hesperidin. *Effect:* Aperitive, digestant, expectorant, tonic.	Unearth rootstock in spring (March–April) or autumn (September–October). Split up larger roots. Dry in shade; in the autumn also in the sun. Do not confuse with roots of poisonous plants which look similar, such as White Hellebore *(Veratrum album)* and Monkshood *(Aconitum)*. Less danger of confusion in spring after sprouting.

Plant	Part used	Components and effects	Harvesting and further processing
MAYAPPLE 175		*Contains:* Resin (podophyllin) with podophyllotoxin and glycosides, fatty oil, wax, starch, calcium oxalate. *Effect:* Strong purgative, vermifuge, bile stimulant, inhibits cell division (inhibits some cancers).	Unearth the long rootstock following ripening of the fruit in the autumn (October–November). Wash and cut into pieces approximately 10 cm long. Dry in heat.
MILK THISTLE 215		*Contains:* Flavone bodies silybin (= silymarin), silydianin, and silychristin, essential oil, tyramine and histamine, bitter principle, fumaric acid, mucilage, fatty oil, albumin. *Effect:* Promotes secretion and flow of bile.	Gather the syncarps shortly before fully ripe (August–September). Allow to ripen fully in shade. Tap out seeds.
MONKSHOOD 2		*Contains:* Alkaloids (aconitine, mesaconitine, etc.), alkamines, organic acids, sugar, resin, fat, starch. *Effect:* Analgesic, reduces fever.	Unearth in autumn (September–October). Dry as quickly as possible in shade at 40°C.
		Contains: Same active components as tuber. *Effect:* Analgesic, reduces fever.	Gather at beginning of flowering (June–July). Dry in shade.
MOSSY STONECROP 211		*Contains:* Flavonol rutin, tannin, alkaloids, organic acids, mucilage, rubber. *Effect:* Astringent, heals wounds.	Gather flowering foliage throughout summer (May–August). Dry in sun or artificial heat.
MOTHERWORT 137		*Contains:* Bitter principle, leonurin, bitter principle glycosides, alkaloids, tannin, traces of essential oil, resin, organic acids (generally not yet studied). *Effect:* Mild sedative, inhibits flatulence, controls diarrhea, uterine stimulant.	Gather stalks at time of flowering (June–September). Dry in shade.
MUGWORT 29		*Contains:* Essential oil: cineole, thujone, bitter principle *Effect:* Aperitive.	Gather leaves and flowering stalk ends shortly after blossoming (July–September). Dry in shade with natural or artificial heat.
MULLEIN 240		*Contains:* Mucilage, saponins, flavonoids hesperidin and verbascoside, aucubin, yellow pigments, traces of essential oil. *Effect:* Protects mucous membrane, relieves irritation, expectorant.	Gather flowers without calyx, July–September during dry weather. Pluck out carefully. Dry in shade or by artificial heat (35°–40°C). The flowers turn brown in the presence of moisture and become ineffective.
NEW JERSEY TEA 49		*Contains:* Alkaloids ceanothyn, etc., tannin, phlobaphene, quercitrin, resin. *Effect:* Astringent, promotes blood clotting.	Unearth roots in spring (April–May). Wash, remove subsidiary roots, pare bark. Dry bark in shade or sun.
		Contains: Tannin, resin, bitter principle, some essential oil. *Effect:* Astringent.	Gather leaves in summer. Dry in shade.
NIGHT-BLOOMING CEREUS 212		*Contains:* Cardiac glycosides, pigment, flavonol and isorhamnetin glycosides. *Effect:* Stimulates heart muscle, regulates heart rhythm, diuretic.	Gather flowers or flowers and young juicy stems in summer (July). Dry in shade. More usual to process fresh for tincture.
NUX-VOMICA 221		*Contains:* Indole-alkaloids (strychnine, brucine). *Effect:* Stimulates gastric secretion, tonic.	Gather fruit according to ripeness (depending on geographic area).
OAK 188		*Contains:* Tannins (phlobatannin and phlobaphene in older barks). *Effect:* Astringent, inhibits inflammation, styptic, inhibits diarrhea, antiseptic.	Pare young bark in spring (April–May) from trunk growths or branches no more than 10 cm thick. The bark must be smooth and free from blemishes. Dry in sun, shade, or artificial heat.
		Contains: Acorn sugar (quercite), tannin, sugar, starch, fatty oil, albumin. *Effect:* Astringent, invigorating (acorn coffee).	Gather the ripe, fallen fruit (acorns) in autumn (September–October), then peel and roast.

Plant	Part used	Components and effects	Harvesting and further processing
OATS 33		*Contains:* Approximately 50 percent starch, albumin, saponins, vitamin B, calcium, trigonelline, flavone, fat, sugar. *Effect:* Nourishing, controls diarrhea, soothing.	Gather fruit and straw at harvest time (in August about 4 weeks after rye harvest), cut ripe stalks and bind together. Leave to dry upright. Thresh out fruit free from spelts.
		Contains: Much silicic acid, saponin, mucins, vitamin A, calcium. *Effect:* Stimulates skin metabolism, strengthens connective tissue.	Crush dry stalks (straw).
OLEANDER 153		*Contains:* Cardiac glycosides (oleandrin, oleandrigenin, neriin, flavones, rutin), tannin, resin. *Effect:* Helps heart and circulation, diuretic.	Gather leaves April–June before flowering starts. Dry as quickly as possible in sun or shade.
OLIVE 154		*Contains:* Fatty oil with oleic acid, linoleic acid, palmitic acid, stearic acid, and arachidic acid, some free fatty acids, phytosterin, traces of lecithin, enzymes, bitter principle, pigment. *Effect:* Soothing, anti-inflammatory, laxative, stimulates bile secretion, nutrient.	Gather the ripe, black olives in late autumn and winter (November–January). Olive oil extracted by pressing. Several pressings with different pressures and temperatures.
		Contains: Glycoside oleosid, bitter principle, oleuropein, etc., choline, flavonoids, organic acids, chinaalkaloids, tannin, carotenoids, traces of essential oil. *Effect:* Lowers blood pressure, antispasmodic, vasodilator, astringent.	Leaves can be collected throughout the year, preferably during warm weather (May–October). Dry in shade or sun.
OPIUM POPPY 159		*Contains:* Approximately 40 opium alkaloids, morphine, codeine, papaverine, narcotine thebaine, etc., albumin, rubber, resins, sugar, fat, mucins, wax. *Effect:* Strong pain-killer, anesthetic, antispasmodic, inhibits diarrhea, addictive.	Raw opium extracted by slitting the outer layer of the unripe poppy capsule. The milky juice escapes from the slit, hardens in the air, and is scraped off next day.
		Contains: Opium alkaloids in smaller quantities. *Effect:* Mild sedative, promotes sleep.	Gather foliage at time of flowering (June–August). Dry in shade.
OSWEGO TEA 151		*Contains:* Essential oil with phenolene, tannin, bitter principle, anthocyan monardeine. *Effect:* Mild aperitive, inhibits flatulence, weak menstrual regulator, diuretic.	Gather flowers and stalks at time of flowering (July–September). Dry in shade, not over 35°C.
PANSY 243		*Contains:* Saponins, flavonoids, salicylic compounds, tannin, mucilage. *Effect:* Diuretic, reduces fever, expectorant.	Gather at time of flowering (June–August). Dry as quickly as possible in the shade.
PAPAYA 44		*Contains:* Pectins, albumin-dissolving ferments, organic acids, resins, vitamins A, B, C, essential oil. In milky juice: numerous ferments (notably papain), fatty phospholipids, peptides, and free amino acids. *Effect:* Promotes digestion of fat, protein, and carbohydrates, vermifuge.	Milky juice is extracted by careful slitting of the green, unripe fruit. The juice dripping out is collected in cloths stretched out below. The coagulated latex is finally dried in the sun or quickly by artificial heat. Processed further to make powder.
PARAGUAY TEA 129		*Contains:* Caffeine, theobromine, tannins, chlorogenic acid, traces of vanillin, some essential and fatty oil, resinous substances. *Effect:* Mild stimulant, mild laxative, diuretic.	Gather branch tips at harvest time. Draw branches through open, smokeless fire to prevent fermentation ("Zapekier process"). Final drying by various desiccating processes.
PARSLEY 162		*Contains:* Essential oil with apiol, myristicene, similarly pinene and other terpenes, flavone glycoside apiin, furanocumarin bergapten, fatty oil with petroselinic acid. *Effect:* Digestant, carminative, diuretic, stimulates uterus.	Gather fruit from August to September. Cut off umbels just before fully ripe, since ripe fruit falls off easily. Spread out flat and leave to ripen in the shade.
		Contains: Essential oil, apiin, bergapten, isoimperatorin, mucilage, sugar. *Effect:* See fruit (above), but weaker.	Unearth root in autumn (October–November) or spring (April). Dry in shade, not over 40°C.

Plant	Part used	Components and effects	Harvesting and further processing
PASQUE FLOWER 187		*Contains:* Essential oil ranunculin or its transformation products protoanemonin or anemonin, glycosides, tannins, resin, little saponin. *Effect:* Strongly irritant on skin and mucous membrane, destroys red blood corpuscles.	Gather stalks at time of flowering (March–April). Dry in shade. Active agents are extremely volatile, it is recommended to process to tincture or extract.
PEPPERMINT 149		*Contains:* Essential oil with menthol menthone, jasmone, tannin (labiatic acid), bitter principle. *Effect:* Carminative, promotes secretion and flow of bile, antispasmodic.	Gather leaves at time of flowering (June–August) during dry, sunny weather. Dry in shade, not over 35°C.
PERUVIAN KRAMERIA 133		*Contains:* Catechin tannins, phlobaphene, methyltyrosine ratanhin, starch, mucilage, sugar, rubber, wax. *Effect:* Astringent, inhibits diarrhea, styptic, anti-inflammatory.	Unearth roots in autumn. Free from subsidiary roots. Dry in sun.
POKE 167		*Contains:* Saponin, formic acid, tannin, phytolaccin (not studied sufficiently), fatty oil, resin, sugar. *Effect:* Stimulates the metabolism, strong purgative, anesthetic, emetic, irritates skin.	Unearth root in late autumn (October–November). Clean carefully, cut into slices lengthwise or crosswise. Dry in sun or shade.
PRICKLY RESTHAAROW 155		*Contains:* Essential oil, ononin, flavone, triterpene, ononide, tannin, saponin (disputed). *Effect:* Hydragogue.	Unearth root in autumn (October), also possible in spring (April). Split thicker roots lengthwise. Dry in sun or shade.
		Contains: Essential oil, ononin, ononide, tannin. *Effect:* Diuretic.	Gather stalks at time of flowering (June–September). Dry in shade.
PSYLLIUM 173		*Contains:* Mucins, aucubine, enzymes, protein, fat. *Effect:* Purgative, soothes skin inflammation.	Gather the ripe seeds (August–September).
PUMPKIN 71		*Contains:* Unknown main constituent, fatty oil with linolein and oleic acid, amino acid cucurbitin, albumin, lecithin, resin, phytosterin. *Effect:* Vermifuge, slightly diuretic.	Harvest the ripe pumpkins in late summer (August–September). Remove kernels from fruit pulp. Dry in sun or shade; spread out flat.
PURPLE CONEFLOWER 82		*Contains:* Glycoside echinacoside, essential oil, echinaceine, resin, inulin, betaine, phenolic acid. *Effect:* Tonic, heals wounds.	Unearth roots in autumn. Process to extracts in fresh state. Dried root is practically ineffective.
PURPLE LOOSESTRIFE 142		*Contains:* Tannins, glycoside, salicarin, mucins, traces of essential oil, resin. *Effect:* Astringent, heals wounds.	Gather tips of twigs at time of flowering (June–August). Dry in shade.
PURPLE TRILLIUM 229		*Contains:* Glycosides trillin and trillarin, tannin, resin, traces of essential oil, fatty oil, saponin, starch. *Effect:* Astringent, styptic.	Unearth rootstock during late summer (August) or after leaves have fallen (October). Dry in sun or shade.
QUACK GRASS 7		*Contains:* Polysaccharide triticin, traces of essential oil, antibiotic substance, mucilage, silicic acid, potassium, inosite, mannite, glycosides. *Effect:* Diuretic, antiseptic, relieves irritation.	Unearth rootstock in spring (March–April) or early autumn (August–September). Wash carefully. Dry in sun or shade.
QUEEN-OF-THE-MEADOW 92		*Contains:* Essential oil with salicylic acid compounds spiraeine and gaultherin, spiraeoside, odorants, salicylic acid, citric acid, tannin. *Effect:* Diuretic, reduces fever, slightly analgesic, astringent, mildly binding.	Gather flowers in summer (June–August). Only take fully opened umbels. Strip or comb off individual flowers with the hand. Dry in shade, not over 40°C.
		Contains: Flavone glycosides; otherwise see flower (above). *Effect:* Same as flower.	Gather stalks at time of flowering (June–August). Strip flower off umbel, pluck off leaves. Dry in shade, not over 40°C.
QUINCE 73		*Contains:* Mucins, amygdalin, enzyme emulsion, fatty oil, tannin, protein. *Effect:* Anti-inflammatory, mild purgative, astringent.	Harvest fruit when ripe (end September–October). Free stones from fruit pulp. (Pulp processed to sauce or juice.) Dry at 40°–50°C.

Plant	Part used	Components and effects	Harvesting and further processing
RED BRYONY 39		*Contains:* Resin bryoresin, alkaloid bryonicin, glycosides, trimethyl-amine, essential oil. *Effect:* Strong purgative, antirheumatic, anti-inflammatory, rubefacient.	Unearth pumpkin like root in autumn (September–October). Wash and cut into slices about 1 cm thick. Dry in sun or shade.
RHUBARB 192		*Contains:* Anthraquinone compounds (rhein, rheum, and aloe emodin), chrysophanol, physcion, sennidine, rheidine, palmidine, tannins, glucogallin, tetrarin, catechin, gallic acid, flavone rutin, starch, pectin, phytosterol. *Effect:* Purgative; smaller doses astringent, aperitive.	Unearth rootstock from plants at least 4 years old during flowering (July–August) or in autumn (September–October). Remove parts of plant above ground. Split rootstock along length. Dry in sun or by artificial heat (open fire).
ROCKWEED 96		*Contains:* Iodine, mucilage, sugar, bromine. *Effect:* Stimulates thyroid activity.	Gathering possible throughout the year, depending on shore deposits. Dry carefully.
ROSELLE 121		*Contains:* Hibiscus acid and other fruit acids, red pigment. *Effect:* Mild purgative, quenches thirst.	Gather faded, pulpy, and reddened fruit calyces (August–September). Dry in shade.
ROSEMARY 196		*Contains:* Essential oil with borneol, camphor, cineol, borneol ester, etc., tannin, triterpenic and carboxylic acids, bitter principle, resin. *Effect:* Tonic, carminative, antiseptic.	Gather branches after flowering all through the summer (June–September). Dry in shade, not over 35°C. Tap leaflets off branches after drying.
RUE 200		*Contains:* Essential oil with methyl ketones, flavone glycoside rutin, furocumarins bergapten, rutarellin, xanthotoxin, etc., alkaloids. *Effect:* Antispasmodic, mild sedative, strengthens capillaries, promotes menstruation.	Gather foliage before flowering (June–August). Dry in shade.
RUPTURE-WORT 120		*Contains:* Saponins (including herniarin), essential oil. *Effect:* Astringent and diuretic properties.	Collect at time of flowering (June–August). Dry in shade.
ST. JOHN'S WORT 127		*Contains:* Essential oil, flavonoids, hyperine, rutin, red pigment hypericin, tannin, pectin, choline. *Effect:* Heals wounds, inhibits inflammation, astringent, antidepressant.	Gather entire blossoming stalks os only tips of twigs or flowers in summer (June–August). Flowers can be open or half-closed. Dry as quickly as possible in shade.
		Contains: See stalk (above). *Effect:* See stalk.	Use fresh to prepare St. John's wort oil.
SARSAPARILLA 216		*Contains:* Saponins parillin and sarsaponin, glycosides, sitosterol, stigmasterin, traces of essential oil, resin, sugar, fat. *Effect:* Diuretic, diaphoretic.	Unearth rootstock with roots throughout the year. Remove rootstock, clean roots. Dry in sun or shade.
SASSAFRAS 208		*Contains:* Essential oil with safrol, tannin, resin. *Effect:* Diuretic, diaphoretic, stimulates skin metabolism.	Fell trees in spring before sprouting or in autumn after leaves have fallen. Dig out roots. Cut in pieces. Dry in shade.
		Contains: See rootstock (above). *Effect:* See rootstock.	Strip roots. Remove outer cork bark. Dry inner bark in shade or by moderate artificial heat.
SAW PALMETTO 214		*Contains:* Essential oil, fatty oil with capric, caprylic, and lauric acids, fatty acids, carotene, tannin, sitosterol, invert sugar, estrogenic substance. *Effect:* Soothing, diuretic.	Gather the deep browny-red fruit at ripening time. Dry in shade.
SCOPOLIA 209		*Contains:* Tropane alkaloid hysoscyamine, atropine, scopolamine, coumarin compounds Scopoline and Scopoletine; choline, betain. *Effect:* Antispasmodic, narcotic, dilates pupils.	Harvest the roots by digging up the shrubs in autumn after leaves have fallen (October–November). Thicker roots can be split lengthwise. Cut in pieces 10 cm long. Dry.
SCOTCH PINE 171		*Contains:* Essential oil with terpenes, bitter principle pinipicrin, tannin, resin, vitamin C (in fresh state). *Effect:* Inhibits secretion of bronchial tubes, disinfectant, mildly diuretic, tonic.	Gather the young shoots in the spring (April–May), immediately after sprouting. Dry in shade.

Plant	Part used	Components and effects	Harvesting and further processing
		Contains: Same as shoots (above). *Effect:* Same as shoots (above).	Gather needles in the spring or throughout the year. Dry in shade.
		Contains: Resinic acids, essential oil. *Effect:* Limits secretion of bronchial tubes, antiseptic, irritates the kidneys, externally epispastic, and promotes blood supply.	Balsam is extracted by artificially tapping the trees (removing the bark or tapping the trunk). Further processing for turpentine and colophonium.
SCURVY GRASS 64		*Contains:* Mustard oil glycoside and transformation product butyl mustard oil, essential oil, bitter principle, tannin, vitamin C, mineral salts. *Effect:* Stimulates the metabolism, promotes gastric secretion, slightly diuretic, skin irritant.	Gather flowering stalks or only leaves, May–June. Dry in shade, not over 35°C. After blossoming, fresh leaves can be gathered for salad or to make juice.
SEA BUCKTHORN 122		*Contains:* Abundant vitamins B, C, E, carotenes, fatty oil with unsaturated fatty acids, fruit acids, flavones. *Effect:* Tonic.	Gather the ripe berries in autumn (September–October). Process fresh to juice. Preserve with honey or sugar.
SEA ONION 234		*Contains:* Cardiac glycosides scillaren A, glucoscillaren A, proscillaridin A, mucin, tannin, some essential oil, fatty oil. *Effect:* Diuretic, stimulates heart muscle, regulates cardiac rhythm.	Unearth tubers of white kind after blossoming and before leaves fall (September). Remove brown outer layer and glutinous inner parts. Cut central pulpy shell into strips. Dry in sun.
SEDGES 43		*Contains:* Silicic acid, saponin, tannin, little essential oil, glycoside, resin, mucilage, starch. *Effect:* Stimulates metabolism, diaphoretic.	Unearth rootstock in spring (March–May). Dry in sun or shade.
SENECA SNAKEROOT 176		*Contains:* Saponins, free salicylic acid, methylsalicylate, fatty oil, mucilage, resin. *Effect:* Expectorant.	Unearth roots in autumn (September–October). Remove leaves and stems. Clean. Dry in sun or shade.
SENNA 47		*Contains:* Anthraquinone compounds, flavones, tartaric acid, salts, mucin, essential oil, resin, traces of tannin. *Effect:* Purgative, inhibits resorption in intestine.	Gather leaves from June–December shortly before fruit ripens. Strip pinnate leaves from leaf stem. Dry in sun.
		Contains: See leaf (above). *Effect:* Purgative (milder than leaf).	Gather pods according to degree of ripeness. Dry off in sun.
SHEPHERD'S PURSE 41		*Contains:* Tyramine, choline acetylcholine, tannin, essential oil, resin, saponins, flavonoids, diosmine, acids, potassium, sodium salts. *Effect:* Stimulates the uterus, promotes blood clotting. (Constituents and effect still disputed.)	Gather stalks with flower and fruit, March–November; possible practically throughout the year in temperate regions. Dry as quickly as possible in shade at 35°–40°C.
SILVERWEED 180		*Contains:* Ellagic tannin, flavone, organic acids, stearins, choline, bitter principle, unknown substances with spasmolytic action. *Effect:* Astringent, controls inflammation.	Gather at time of flowering (May–August), preferably before August. Dry in shade.
SMARTWEED 177		*Contains:* Essential oil with tadeonal and terpenes, flavone compounds rutin and rhamnazine, tannin. *Effect:* Styptic, diuretic.	Gather foliage at time of flowering (July–September). Dry in shade, not over 45°C.
SMOOTH-LEAF ELM 233		*Contains:* Mucin, tannin, and bitter principle. *Effect:* Relieves irritation, astringent, anti-inflammatory.	Gather bark from young branches in spring before sprouting. Remove outer cracked bark. Dry inner bark in sun or by artificial heat.
SNAKEROOT 206		*Contains:* Saponins, some essential oil, tannin, bitter principle, allantoin. *Effect:* Anti-inflammatory, heals wounds, expectorant.	Gather the flowering foliage, May–July. Dry in shade.
		Contains: See stalk (above). *Effect:* See stalk.	Gather leaves at time of flowering (May–July). Dry in shade.

Plant	Part used	Components and effects	Harvesting and further processing
SOAPWORT 207		*Contains:* Saponins. *Effect:* Expectorant, mild diuretic, laxative, stimulates skin metabolism.	Unearth rootstock with roots in spring (April) or autumn (September–October). Dry in sun or artificial heat (50°C).
		Contains: Saponins. *Effect:* See rootstock (above), but weaker effect.	Gather foliage at time of flowering (July–September). Dry in sun or shade.
SPANISH CHESTNUT 48		*Contains:* Tannin, quercetin, fat, resin, sugar, pectin. *Effect:* Expectorant, antirheumatic.	Gather in autumn (September–October). Dry in shade.
		Contains: Tannin. *Effect:* Controls diarrhea.	Gather the ripe fallen fruit in autumn (October). Allow to dry.
SPIKENARD 21		*Contains:* Essential oil, tannins, spogenins, diterpene acids. *Effect:* Expectorant, diuretic, carminative.	Unearth in summer and autumn (July–October). Cut into pieces, slit thicker roots along length. Dry in heat or in sun.
SPRING ADONIS 4		*Contains:* Glycosides similar to digitalis. *Effect:* Aids the failing heart.	Gather at time of flowering. Dry quickly, by heating for ½ hour at 55°–60°C.
STINGING NETTLE 235		*Contains:* Nettle toxin, histamine, formic acid, chlorophyll, glucoquinine, iron, vitamin C. *Effect:* Promotes elimination of uric acid, slightly hydragogue, stimulates the metabolism, externally epispastic and antirheumatic.	Gather leaves of young plants (30–50 cm) during late spring and early summer. Dry as quickly as possible in shade, not over 50°C. Collect young tender leaves for vegetables in spring (March–April).
		Contains: Tannin, mineral salts. *Effect:* Astringent.	Unearth root with rootstock in autumn (September–October). Dry in sun or artificial heat.
		Contains: See leaves (above). *Effect:* See leaves.	Gather stalks at time of flowering. Dry in shade, not over 50°C.
STRAWBERRY 94		*Contains:* Tannin, vitamin C, essential oil, silicic acid, flavone. *Effect:* Astringent, diuretic.	Gather young leaves (May–June). Dry in the shade.
		Contains: Sugar, pectin, vitamin C, acids, iron compounds, aromatics. *Effect:* General tonic.	Gather the ripe fruit depending on climate (June–September).
STROPHANTHUS 220		*Contains:* Glycoside mixture k-strophanthin (primary glycoside k-strophanthoside, also k-strophanthin-beta, coumarin, etc.), alkaloid trigonelline, choline, fatty oil, enzyme, saponin, resin, mucilage. *Effect:* Stimulates heart, diuretic.	Gather the unopened dehiscent fruit at time of ripening. Peel off fruit skin, dry until capsules burst open. Remove seeds, free from needles.
SUNDEW 80		*Contains:* Naphthoquinone derivatives, plumbagin and hydroplumbagin, enzymes, flavonoids, traces of essential oil, organic acids. *Effect:* Soothes irritative cough, antispasmodic.	Gather foliage at time of flowering (July–August). Dry in shade.
SWEET FLAG 3		*Contains:* Essential oil with asarone, bitter principles, tannin, mucin, starch. *Effect:* Aperitive, increases secretion of gastric juices, tonic.	Harvest rootstock in autumn (September–October). Pull out with a hook from muddy ground. Free from leaves and roots. Clean thoroughly. Halve along length. Dry in shade.
SWEET VERNAL GRASS 18		*Contains:* Coumarin, silicic acid. *Effect:* Skin irritant, increases blood supply locally, reduces pain.	Gather the small plant parts which fall out during hay storage. Sieve out larger pieces.
SWEET WOODRUFF 100		*Contains:* Coumarin glycoside splitting coumarin, aperuloside, tannin, bitter principle, traces of nicotinic acid. *Effect:* Sedative, antispasmodic.	Gather foliage before flowering (April–early May) or while flowering (May–June). Dry in shade.
TANSY 56		*Contains:* Essential oil (often with thujone), bitter principles tanacetin I and II, glycosides, acid, resin, fat, sugar, carotenoids. *Effect:* Aperitive, promotes digestion, vermifuge.	Gather flowers June–September. Dry in shade, not over 35°C.

Plant	Part used / Components and effects	Harvesting and further processing
	Contains: See flower (above). *Effect:* See flower (above), but weaker.	Gather foliage at time of flowering (June–September). Dry in shade, not over 35°C.
THORNAPPLE 77	*Contains:* Alkaloids hyoscyamine, scopolamine, little atropine, tannin, traces of essential oil, acids. *Effect:* Antispasmodic, soothing, anesthetic, inhibits secretion.	Gather leaves at time of flowering (July–September), preferably early in morning. Dry in sun or by artificial heat (up to 60°C).
	Contains: Alkaloids, as leaf (above), additional fatty oil. *Effect:* See leaf (above).	Gather the ripe, black seeds during early autumn, as soon as the capsules burst.
THYME 226	*Contains:* Essential oil with thymol and carvacrol, cymol, linalool, borneol, tannin, bitter principle, flavonoids, triterpenic acids. *Effect:* Antispasmodic, relieves irritative coughs, disinfectant, digestant.	Gather flowering branches June–August in dry, sunny weather. Dry in shade, not over 35°C.
	Contains: See stalk (above). *Effect:* See stalk.	Gather whole branches before flowering (May). Dry in shade, not over 35°C. Strip off leaflets after drying.
TORMENTIL 181	*Contains:* Very high tannin content (tormentil tannin acid), tormentil-red, little essential oil. *Effect:* Constricts mucous membranes.	Gather in summer and early autumn (June–September), in morning if possible. Dry as quickly as possible in sun.
TURMERIC 72	*Contains:* Essential oil, curcuma pigments curcumin, etc., bitter principles, fatty oil, acids, resin, starch. *Effect:* Stimulates secretion of gastric juices, irritates mucous membrane, promotes bile flow.	Unearth rootstock when the leaves begin to die (December–January). Free main and subsidiary tubers from roots and leaves; wash. Scald with hot water or boil for 1 hour. Dry in sun.
VALERIAN 238	*Contains:* Essential oil, valepotriates (special valerian compounds), alkaloids. *Effect:* Relieves stress, relaxes muscle spasms.	Unearth in autumn (September–October). Wash roots thoroughly; comb with coarse comb. Dry in shade.
WATERCRESS 152	*Contains:* Mustard oil glycoside, sulfurous essential oil, vitamin C, iodine.	Collect stalks at time of flowering. Dry quickly in shade, not over 40°C.
	Contains: Mustard oil glycoside, essential oil, iodine, bitter principle. *Effect:* Stimulates metabolism, promotes bile secretion.	Gather leaves for use as salad or juice, preferably before flowering (end March–early May), but also during flowering. Use as quickly as possible.
WHITE DEADNETTLE 134	*Contains:* Catechin tannin, histamine, tyramine, methylamine, choline, flavones, acids, traces of essential oil, mucilage. *Effects:* Astringent, protects mucous membrane.	Gather the flower corollae in dry, sunny weather, May–September. Dry carefully in shade, not over 35°C.
	Contains: As for flower (above), but higher proportion of tannin, also xantophyll, possibly saponin. *Effect:* Astringent, protects mucous membrane, weak expectorant, diuretic.	Gather the flowering foliage, May–September. Dry quickly in shade, not over 35°.
WHITE WILLOW 201	*Contains:* Salicin and other phenoglycosides, enzyme, tannin, resin, oxalate. *Effect:* Reduces fever, antirheumatic and antineuralgic, antiseptic, astringent.	Gather bark from young branches (2–5 years) in spring when sprouting (April–May). Dry quickly in sun or shade.
WILD GINGER 30	*Contains:* Essential oil with asarone, acids, tannin, resin, flavonoids. *Effect:* Stimulates secretion of respiratory tract mucous glands, purgative, diuretic, emetic.	Gather entire plant at time of flowering (April–May). Dry in shade, not over 35°C.
	Contains: See whole plant (above). *Effect:* See whole plant.	Unearth rootstock in late summer, free from parts above soil. Dry in shade, below 35°C.

Plant	Part used	Components and effects	Harvesting and further processing
WILD PASSION FLOWER 160		*Contains:* Alkaloids harmine, harman, harmol, etc., sterol mixture, flavone glycosides. *Effect:* Mildly soothing, antispasmodic.	Gather foliage at time of flowering (May–July) or foliage with fruit at end of and after flowering (July–September). Dry in shade.
WINTER CABBAGE 38		*Contains:* Mustard oil glycoside glucobrassin, enzyme myrosinase, so-called anti-ulcer factor, vitamins A, B, C, mineral substances. *Effect:* Healing of gastric ulcers, relieves pain, heals wounds, anti-inflammatory.	Harvest cabbage heads in autumn or winter depending on climate. Store in a cool, dry place. Use only while fresh.
WINTERGREEN 102		*Contains:* Glycoside gaultherin (splitting essential oil with 99 percent methyl salicylate), enzyme gaultherase, aldehyde, 1 alcohol, 1 ester, tannin, mucilage, wax. *Effect:* Relieves pain, antirheumatic, antiseptic, diuretic, rubefacient.	The evergreen leaves can be gathered throughout the year, preferably in summer. Dry in shade. To extract the essential oil, soak leaves in warm water for 12–24 hours and then distill with steam.
WITCH HAZEL 113		*Contains:* Hamamelitannin and other tannins, traces of essential oil, flavonoids, choline, 1 saponin. *Effect:* Astringent, anti-inflammatory, styptic.	Gather leaves throughout the summer (June–August). Dry as quickly as possible in shade, not by artificial heat. Leaves change color if dried slowly.
		Contains: See leaf (above), but less tannin. *Effect:* See leaf.	Gather branch bark in spring after sprouting. Dry in sun or shade.
WORMWOOD 28		*Contains:* Essential oil with thujone, thujol alcohol, phellandrene, cadenes, proazulene artabsin, bitter principles absinthin and anabsinthin, flavone compounds, acids, lactone. *Effect:* Promotes secretion of gastric juice and bile, carminative.	Gather leaves and flowering twig ends at time of flowering (July–September). Dry in shade.
YAM 79		*Contains:* Dioscorine, saponins, copious starch. *Effect:* Expectorant, diuretic, antirheumatic.	Unearth rootstock in autumn (September). Dry in shade or sun.
YARROW 1		*Contains:* Essential oil with cineole and chamazulene, bitter principle achillein, tannin. *Effect:* Antiseptic, antispasmodic, expectorant, stimulates secretion of gastric and intestinal glands, choleretic, regulates kidney function, astringent, inhibits inflammation.	Gather whole stalk or blossom when blooming (June–September), free from thick pieces of stem. Dry in shade, not over 40°C.
YELLOWBARK CINCHONA 59		*Contains:* Alkaloids (quinine, quindidine, and numerous secondary alkaloids), tannins, bitter principles, quinic acid. *Effect:* Stimulates secretion of gastric juices, generally tonic. Quinine: Reduces fever and soothes pain. Quinidine: Effect on heart.	Bark obtained by various processes: felling and stripping of 6–8 year old trees or stripping during growth or unearthing the thickly set plants after 6–7 years. Bark dried in sun or by artificial heat (70°–80°C).
YELLOW GENTIAN 105		*Contains:* Bitter principles (gentiopicrin, amarogentin), fermentable sugar, pectin, mucilage, traces of tannin. *Effect:* Promotes saliva and gastric juice secretion, stimulates appetite, accelerates emptying of stomach, generally fortifying.	Unearth in autumn (August–October). Dry as quickly as possible. Root should not ferment or change color.
YELLOW JESSAMINE 104		*Contains:* Alkaloids, gelsemine, gelsemicine, sempervirine, essential oil, fatty oil, tannin. *Effect:* Vasodilator, reduces blood pressure, heart sedative, dilates bronchi, relieves pain.	Unearth rootstock in autumn (October). Dry in shade or sun.
YELLOW SWEETCLOVER 147		*Contains:* Melilotin and other coumarin glycosides, melilotic acid, flavones, mucilage, tannin, traces of essential oil. *Effect:* Anti-inflammatory, emollient.	Gather leaves and flowering tips of twigs at time of flowering (July–August). Dry slowly in shade, not over 40°C. Coumarin only forms during drying.

Epilogue: The Future

People ascribe
the greatest healing power
to drugs that come
from farthest away, drugs
that cost the most.
In my long experience
I have come to believe
that people go
to the ends of the earth
to look for something
they could find
right on their doorstep.
If only we could learn
to trust Nature . . .

Maurice Mességué

"The apparently instinctive practice of taking drugs is believed to exist among the lower animals. It is a fascinating subject for the speculative mind to ponder how this instinct arose and how, as primitive man struggled upwards, a belief in the power of drugs to remedy disease originated. . . . It is clear that faith in drugs, especially vegetable drugs, has been deep-seated and widespread amongst all peoples from the earliest times. It is as strong in modern civilization as it was amongst primitive man."

So wrote Sir David Campbell in his inaugural lecture as Professor of Materia Medica in the University of Aberdeen in 1930. Nigh on half a century later, in the *Pharmaceutical Journal,* the official publication of the Pharmaceutical Society of Great Britain, E. J. Shellard, Professor of Pharmacognosy in the University of London, wrote in reviewing a new book on healing plants: "There is undoubtedly a resurgence of interest in herbal medicine."

Nature's herbs and molds yield effective remedies to many human diseases and complaints. Six examples are shown below.

INDIAN SNAKEROOT
Rauvolfia serpentina
TRANQUILIZER

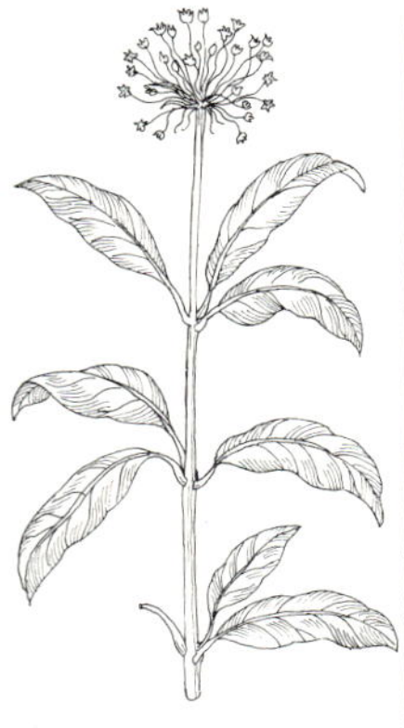

PENICILLIN
Penicillium potatum
ANTIBIOTIC

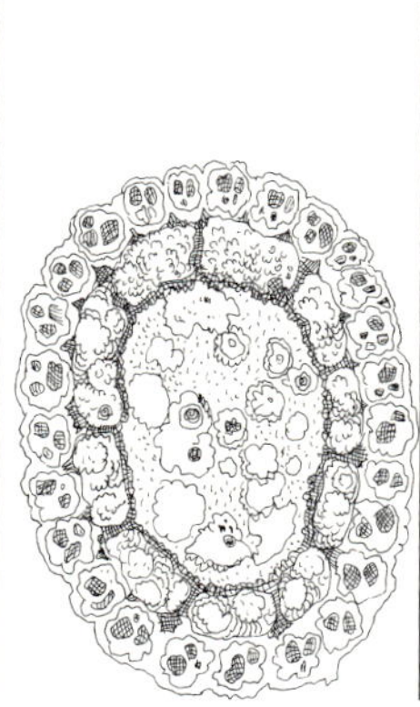

EUROPEAN MISTLETOE
Viscum album
HYPOTENSIVE DRUG

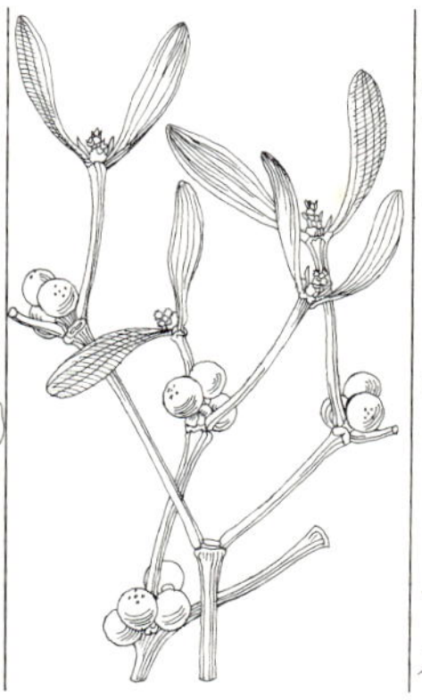

MA-HUANG
Ephedra
ANTI-ALLERGIC

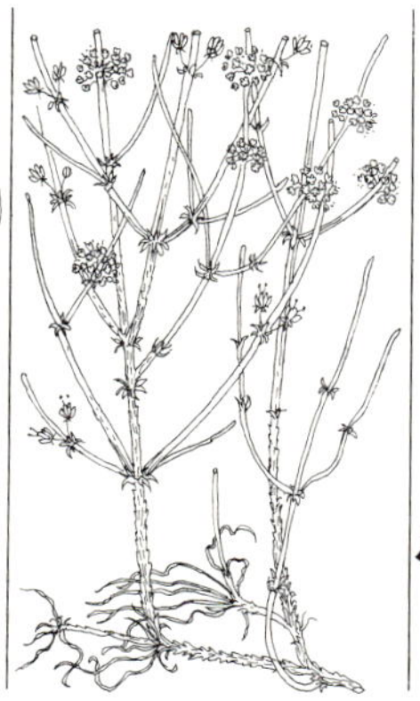

CURARE
Chondodendron tomentosum
ANESTHESIA

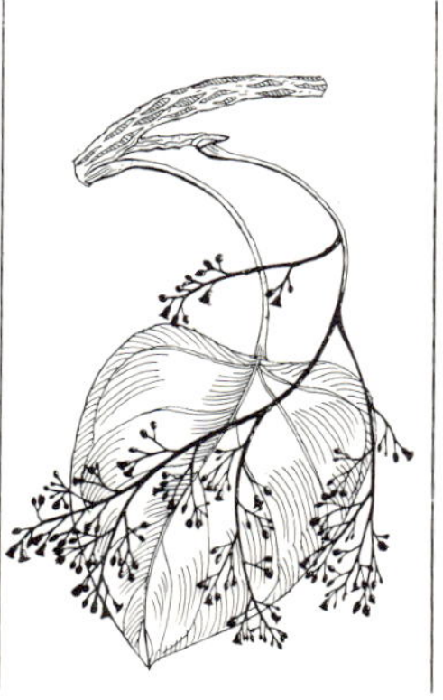

PERIWINKLE
Vinca rosa
ANTICANCER

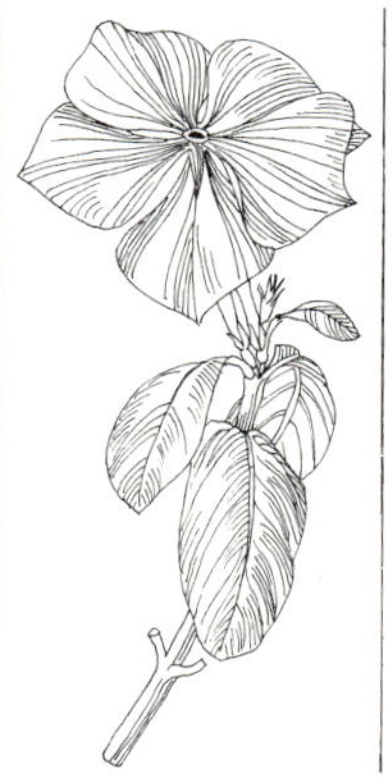

And this in spite of the fact that the era intervening between these comments by two of the doyens of the healing art had witnessed the most dramatic and outstanding outpouring of synthetic drugs in the history of the human race. The sulfonamides, admittedly backed up by the antibiotics, had brought infection largely under control. The tranquilizers had wrought something like a revolution in the treatment of disorders of the mind, and there was an almost infinite variety of man-made drugs to lower the blood pressure, bring comfort, if not necessarily a cure, to those afflicted with ischemic heart disease, and relieve the discomfort of allergic conditions such as hay fever. Anesthesia had been brought to an almost incredibly high level of efficiency, safety, and comfort so that surgeons were able to perform the most intricate operations, and a steady stream of anticancer drugs had come into the arena of practical therapeutics.

Why are neither the public (patients and prospective patients) nor the medical profession satisfied with this galaxy of man-made drugs? Why is there this resurgence of interest in herbs that heal? Inevitably the answer is complex, but certain salient points can be picked out from the morass of arguments which befog the issue. One is the increasing number of toxic effects resulting from the potent new synthetic drugs pouring forth (some would say gushing forth was a more appropriate phrase) from the research laboratories of the pharmaceutical companies of the world. Another is that we owed to Nature the greatest of all these therapeutic advances—the antibiotics.

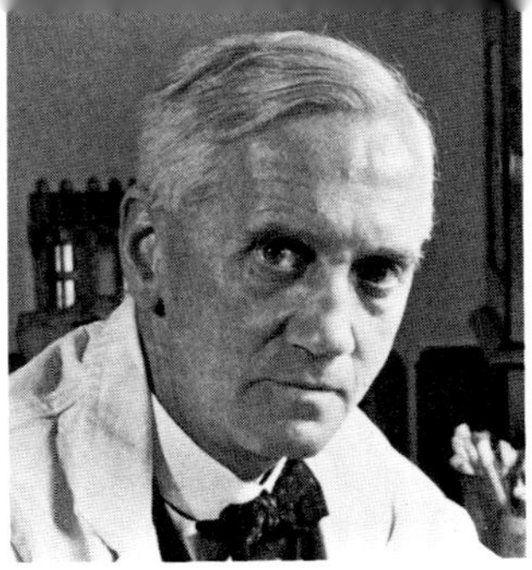

Sir Alexander Fleming (1881–1955), the shrewd, canny Scottish bacteriologist, whose refusal to discard a contaminated culture plate in his laboratory in St. Mary's Hospital Medical School, London, led to the discovery of penicillin, one of the greatest advances in medical history.

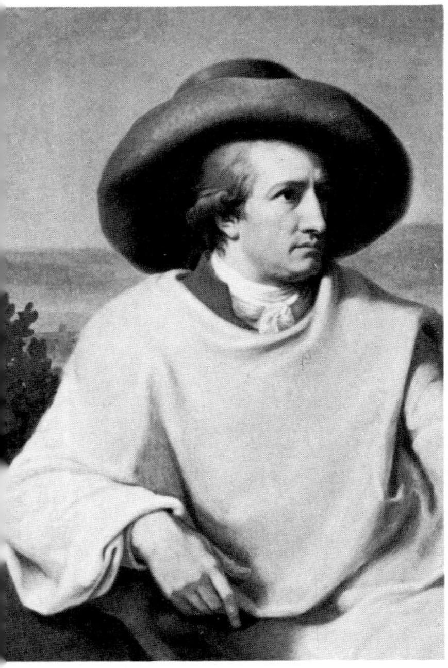

Goethe (1749–1832), a pioneer of the "back-to-Nature" school, whose philosophy was overtaken by the Darwinian era and the irruption of the synthetic school of pharmacology. Today, the traditional wheel is coming full circle, and thinking men and women are coming to realize how much truth there is in his comment:
"Nothing happens in living Nature that is not in relation to the whole."

The discovery of penicillin was not the result of high-pressured scientific research in a chromium-plated research institute. It was the result of the acute observation of a shrewd, cautious Scotsman. An utterly unplanned intervention of Nature in a laboratory procedure produced a result that technically was catastrophic, and 90 percent—nay, 99 percent—of bacteriologists would have discarded the contaminated culture plate without further thought. Sir Alexander Fleming, however, was of the old school who had been brought up to use the natural gifts with which Nature had endowed him: his sight, his hearing, his sense of touch. Further, his innate curiosity had not been destroyed, as it so often is, by unthinking obeisance to the man-made approach of the modern laboratory. The result was the retention of the "contaminated" bacteriological culture—and what we now know as penicillin.

Over a decade was to elapse before the synthesists in our midst were able to emulate Nature and produce penicillin on a commercial scale. And even then, all that *homo sapiens* could do was to produce a clumsy, expensive Heath-Robinson imitation of the delicate, efficient manner in which Nature produces it. To synthesize on a commercial scale is still impossible, and the best that leading research brains in the world have been able to produce in emulation of Nature is what is described as a semisynthetic method.

It was the means whereby pencillin was revealed to us that was largely responsible for a third factor in encouraging and stimulating this renewal of interest in herbs that heal. This was an increasing appreciation that we live in a natural world that provides the process of healing, a world that contains, among other things, herbs that are beneficial to man. In other words, we must realize that much more attention must be given to investigating the wealth of therapeutic possibilities that lie hidden in the secret fastnesses of Nature.

According to Goethe, "Nothing happens in living Nature that is not in relation to the whole." This may overstate the case, but there can be little doubt that the integration of man with Nature as a whole is more intimate than many have suspected in the post-Darwinian era. Neither does one need to be a "back-to-Nature" enthusiast to admit that to ignore Nature is asking for trouble. Again and again, as in the case of the use of ergot in midwifery and of digitalis in heart disease, the scientists (or synthesists) have gone astray and, instead of improving upon Nature, have held up progress toward the better understanding of the working of valuable drugs. What is required is close collaboration between the synthesists and the naturalists. As has been repeatedly shown, such collaboration can improve upon Nature, always provided the scientist is not too clever and does not carry purification too far. What is too often forgotten—or never realized—is that there is an art in the scientific study of drugs.

This neglect of Nature, of course, is no new phenomenon. As Wordsworth reminded us:

The world is too much with us; late and soon,
Getting and spending, we lay waste our powers:
Little we see in Nature that is ours.

"Yet," as I have pointed out elsewhere, "in Nature is to be found many a secret, the revealing of which has brought to light a healing drug, a soothing balm, or a solace to the distressed mind. Quinine, till well within living memory the only remedy for malaria; morphia, the pain-reliever *in excelsis* which the ingenuity of scientific man has failed to improve upon; emetine, still the most specific controller of amoebic dysentery; *Rauvolfia,* which introduced the much abused concept of tranquilizers; curare, one of the most valuable handmaidens of modern anesthesia, not to mention penicillin: all these we owe to Nature."

Yet, with certain notable exceptions, all that the so-called scientific doctors and research workers did was was to scoff at our forebears for their "childish" faith in herbs, ridicule them for the fuss they made about collecting their herbs at a certain time of day, a certain season, or a certain period of the moon (as so delightfully described by Maurice Mességué in his fascinating reminiscences, *Of Men and Plants),* and ended up by castigating it all as an unholy combination of magic, astrology, and superstition. How wrong time has proved these critics to be. Over the years research has shown that, like good gardeners, these old herbalists were right.

Thus the yield of morphine from the poppy at nine o'clock in the morning is often four times the yield obtained twelve hours later. The same diurnal variation has been shown with various other plants, including atropine. In other cases the active principle varies with the stage of germination. In the case of the periwinkle (the producer of one of our most valuable anti-cancer drugs), for example, there is virtually no active principle in the seeds. It appears during germination and by the end of three weeks is present throughout the whole plant—only to disappear and then reappear at around eight weeks. Flowering often coincides with an increase in the active principle, but in some plants there is a decrease. In other words, the old herbalists knew what they were doing. Equally important is the variation in the constituents of the same plant or species in different parts of the world.

While these may be the sins of omission of the blinkered modern scientist, two of his sins of commission are worthy of note. One is what Professor Shellard has described as his "quite unscientific belief that all plants must contain a well-defined 'active constituent.'" "It is true, of course," he adds, that there may often be readily isolated constituents having a pronounced pharmacological activity which can be exploited." "On the other hand, however," he notes, "a plant may yield two or more constituents having quite different pharmacological activities. The fact is that the therapeutic effects of any plant or plant preparation depend upon the sum total of the pharmacological actions of all the constituents present, some of which we may know nothing about."

There is also some evidence that in attempting to purify the active principle of a herb, one of two things may happen. One is that it loses some or all of its potency. The other is that it becomes almost dangerously potent: it is as if there was some braking, or balancing, mechanism in the plant itself which prevents the active principle from becoming too powerful.

This is a point that is admirably exemplified by digitalis, our great stand-by in the treatment of the failing heart. Digitalis comes from the leaf of the foxglove. We owe its introduction to modern medicine to Dr. William Withering. In 1775, Dr. Withering, a Birmingham physician, was asked to see an old woman waterlogged with dropsy. This he did and decided that she was not long for this world. A few weeks later, on inquiring how she was, he learned, much to his surprise, that she had made a most satisfying recovery. This she attributed to taking a herbal tea concocted by an old woman in Shropshire. When he analyzed this tea, Dr. Withering found, in his own words, that "it was composed of twenty or more different herbs." "But," he added, "it was not very difficult for one conversant in these matters to perceive that the active herb could be no other than the foxglove." Ten years later, in what is now one of the medical classics, *An Account of the Foxglove,* a detailed report of 163 cases, he demonstrated the value of the foxglove *(Digitalis purpurea)* in the treatment of heart failure.

The passage of time has only served to confirm the correctness of his views, but the scientists have not been prepared to leave well enough alone. To be fair to them, there were certain snags about the

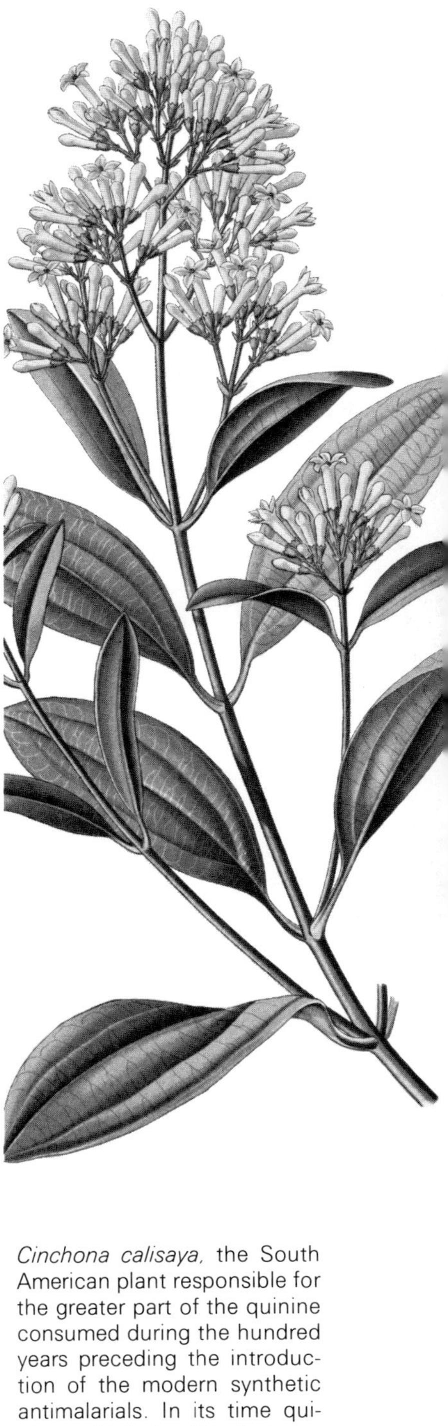

Cinchona calisaya, the South American plant responsible for the greater part of the quinine consumed during the hundred years preceding the introduction of the modern synthetic antimalarials. In its time quinine, which is still playing a useful part in the control of malaria, has saved a well-nigh uncountable number of lives.

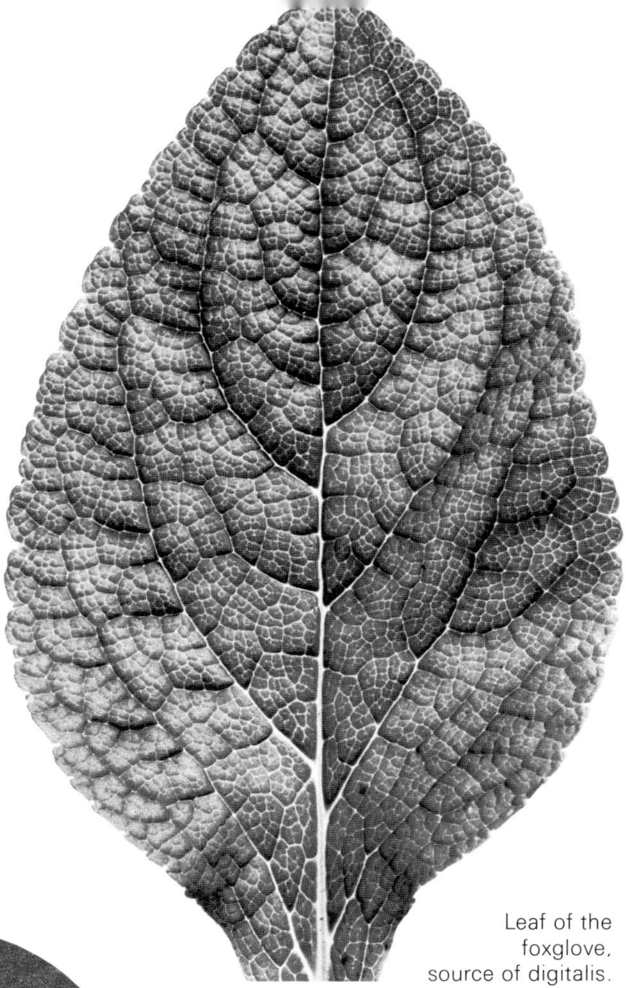

Leaf of the foxglove, source of digitalis.

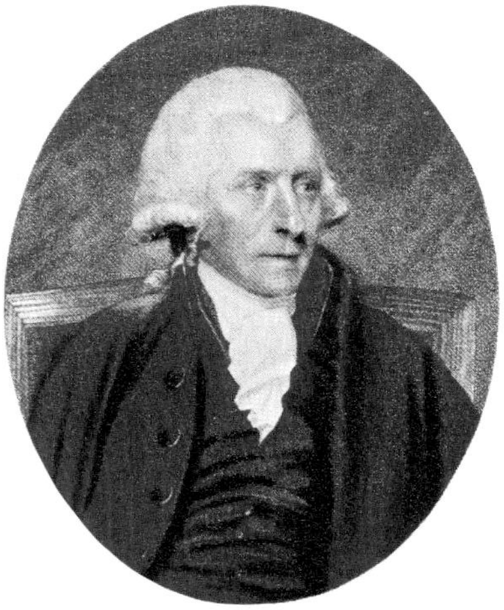

Dr. William Withering (1741–1799), the English physician, whose astute powers of observation of an old country folk remedy, led to the discovery of the healing powers of the foxglove *(Digitalis purpurea)* in heart disease. Today, just over two hundred years since Dr. Withering first reported his observations, digitalis, as the active principle derived from the leaf of the foxglove is known, still stands supreme as the drug for the failing heart.

preparation of digitalis. In the first place, it was difficult to produce a standardized preparation of the leaves of the foxglove that would always have the same effect in a given dose. Equally worrying was the fact that certain preparations, such as the tincture, tended to go off rather quickly, even if kept in reasonable conditions. Third, the margin between an effective dose and a toxic dose was relatively small, as Dr. Withering himself had pointed out.

In an attempt to overcome these drawbacks, research workers began isolating the active principles. This they succeeded in doing, and immediately the pharmaceutical industry cashed in and started producing a series of glycosides, as these active principles of digitalis are known, which they sold to doctors as the very last word in therapy. Undoubtedly some of these glycosides are useful and do not deteriorate over a period of time, but they are as potentially dangerous as the preparation made from the whole leaf. Not the least of their disadvantages is their very efficiency, and the fact that they can be given by injection into the bloodstream, thus ensuring a quick action.

This, however, is often not required. To push digitalis to the maximum dose in order to get a quick response is asking for trouble. Slow and sure is the golden rule, working up to a dose that produces the desired effect. This can be achieved as effectively, if not more so, by the use of the British Pharmacopoeia preparation known as digitalis leaf. There is no convincing evidence that any of the individual glycosides in use today have any advantage over digitalis leaf, whether from the viewpoint of efficacy, toxicity, or keeping properties. And it is not irrelevant to note a recent report showing that one in four patients with heart conditions treated by the most widely used of these digitalis glycosides was found to be suffering from an overdose of the drug, and of these patients one in sixteen died of digitalis poisoning. Equally significant is the comment of a member of the house staff of the Peter Bent Brigham Hospital, Boston, that "nowadays lanatoside (a glycoside obtained from *Digitalis lanata)* is replacing homicide as a leading cause of death."

As already noted, we owe some of our most valuable drugs to Nature's *largesse.* That this lesson is gradually penetrating the fastnesses of the pharmaceutical industry is illustrated by a recent working party organized by the United Nations. This was convened to cope with the current world shortage of opiates, and particularly one aspect which was looming in an acute form. This was a shortage of codeine, one of the most valuable constituents of opium. Chemists had to admit they could not synthesize it. This left only one solution: the larger production of another of the constituents of the poppy, thebaine, which can be readily converted in the laboratory into codeine. Although present in the poppy known as *Papaver somniferum,* the major source of medicinal opium, thebaine is present in much larger amounts in another member of the poppy family, *Papaver bracteatum.* The purpose of the working party, which was held in the

Ergot is the resting stage of the fungus *Claviceps purpurea,* a parasite which grows on rye. Ergot has proven effective in labor, migraine, and for many other uses.

United States and attended by representatives from seventeen countries and twelve pharmaceutical companies, was to study the problem of how best to isolate the maximum amount of thebaine from *P. bracteatum.* In other words, reversing what had almost become the routine procedure, the first approach here was by seeking the help of Nature—not the inmates of the research laboratory.

Another example of the stupidity of science in dealing with herbs that heal is the story of ergot, which is derived from a fungus, *Claviceps purpurea,* that parasitizes rye. Toward the end of the sixteenth century a German physician referred to the fact that ergot was being used by midwives for quickening labor. What might be termed the modern era of ergot dates back to 1808, when Dr. John Stearn, of New York, published a report entitled *An Account of Pulvis Parturiens,* in which he recommended this powder, the active ingredient of which was ergot, for the quickening of labor, not the least of its advantages being that it reduced the incidence of one of the dreaded complications—hemorrhage after the birth of the child, or postpartum hemorrhage as it is technically known. In due course, in the form of the liquid extract, the administration of ergot became almost a routine ritual at the end of labor.

As in the case of digitalis, however, the pharmaceutical industry decided that it could improve on Nature and at the same time supplement its income. The research workers were therefore alerted and told to isolate the active principle. This they did with great éclat, being utterly unaware of the chemical complexity of ergot and what a Pandora's Box it was going to prove to be. In retrospect the sequel is an admirable example of what C. E. Montague described as "rough justice."

In 1906 a British pharmaceutical company claimed to have isolated the active alkaloid, which they named ergotoxine. Twelve years later a Swiss pharmaceutical company made the same claim, naming their alkaloid ergotamine. In due course the two turned out to have identical properties, but the two companies differed violently, and in public, on their relative clinical merits. Be all that as it may, British obstetricians and midwives refused to have anything to do with either, and stuck to their British Pharmacopoeia preparation, the traditional liquid extract of ergot on which they had been born and bred professionally, and which had proved such a valuable adjunct to the successful culmination of parturition.

Finally the Medical Research Council stepped in to try and clarify the issue. The upshot was a brilliant justification of British obstetricians. In short, it was shown that, while ergotoxine and ergotamine were powerful stimulants of the uterus, causing it to contract, they were relatively inert when given by mouth, which was the method of giving the liquid extract. Conversely, when the liquid extract was given by mouth it had a potent action in stimulating the uterus to contract after labor is completed. To cap all, the final comment of those undertaking the investigation was: "We believed that the clinician was fully vindicated in his dogged belief in the efficiency of the old-fashioned preparation. . . . We are now able to prove the correctness of our conclusions by reporting the isolation of the substance to which ergot rightly owes its long-established reputation as the 'pulvis parturiens.' We propose to name it 'ergometrine.'"

In other words, both the British and the Swiss pharmaceutical companies were wrong. The alkaloid they had isolated had nothing to do with the value of ergot in midwifery. This action was due to the alkaloid isolated by the Medical Research Council investigators, one of whom was an obstetrician. This alkaloid was present in the liquid extract of ergot which the British and Swiss companies had slanged, but which British doctors and midwives had refused to give up—fortunately for all their parturient ladies.

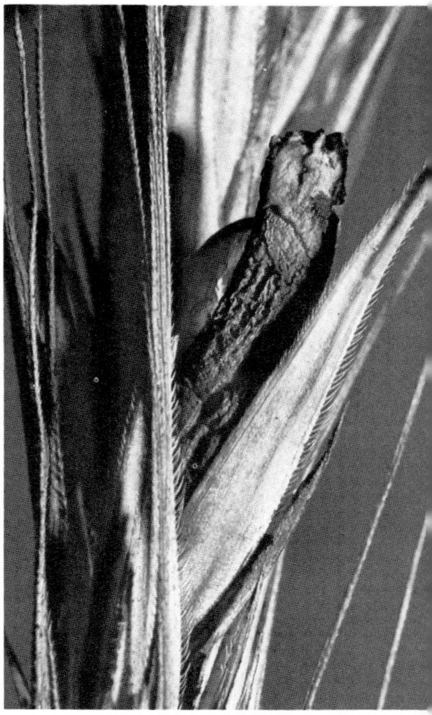

While morphia is the main constituent of *Papaver somniferum,* also known as the opium or white poppy, this invaluable herb contains many other pain-relieving drugs.

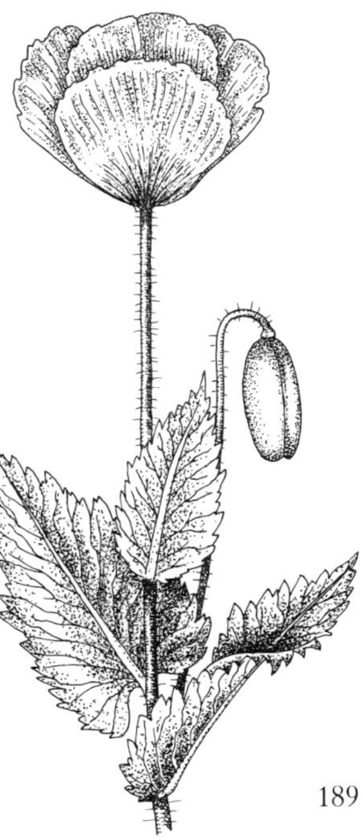

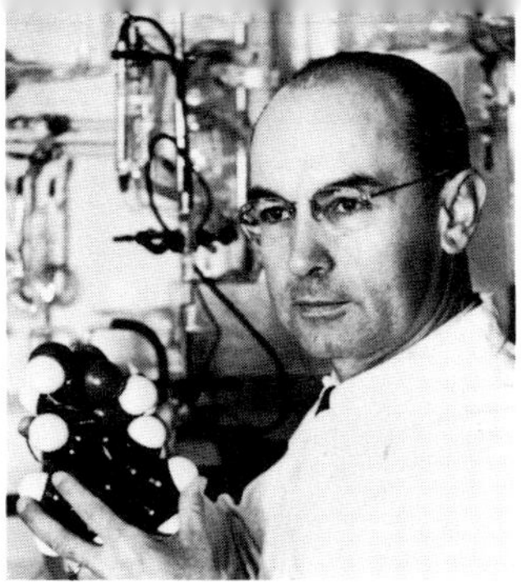

Dr. Albert Hofmann, the distinguished Swiss pharmacologist who discovered, in 1943, the hallucinogenic properties of lysergic acid diethylamide. LSD, as it is popularily known, is yet another of the drugs, or active principles, of ergot.

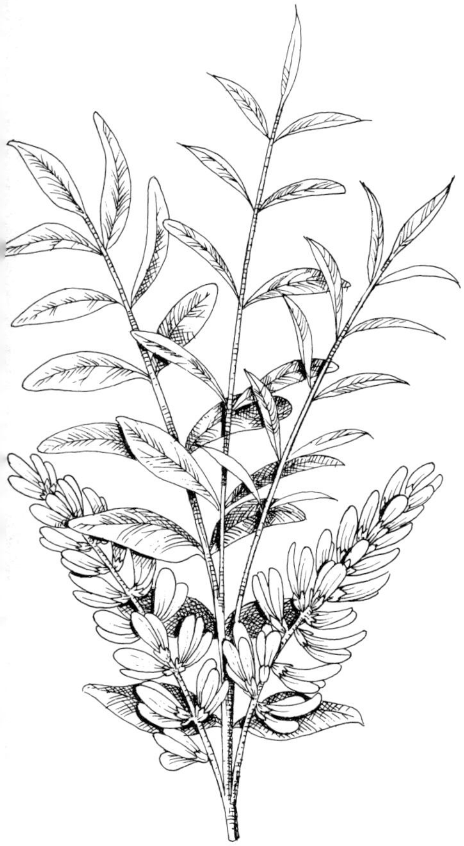

Today, licorice *(Glycyrrhiza glabra)*, one of the oldest of herbal remedies, has taken on a new lease of life as the provider of the most useful drug so far discovered in the treatment of gastric ulcer. Licorice is also now known to have a cortisone-like action.

To complete the basis of the major purpose of this chapter—an assessment of the future of healing plants—three further examples may be given of our indebtedness to Nature for herbs that heal.

For three millennia licorice has been used by mankind. One of the earliest records of this in on Assyrian tablets. It is also listed in the papyri of Ancient Egypt. Since then it has been used medicinally by civilization after civilization—Sumerians, Babylonians, Hindus, Chinese, Greeks, and Romans—right down to the present day. The Romans thought so highly of it that it was included in the rations of the Roman legions. Records of its use in Britain date back to the thirteenth century, and both Chaucer and Shakespeare refer to it.

Its uses have been multifarious, ranging from the Chinese, who valued it as a rejuvenator, to more plebeian uses as a soother of congested throats and lungs and overworked alimentary tracts. As one old herbal nicely expresses it, it is "a protection against the acrimony of food." In more recent times one of its main uses has been to disguise the taste of nauseating medicines. This it achieves by virtue of the fact that the important constituent of its root, glycyrrhizin, is fifty times sweeter than cane sugar. It is this constituent which also makes it popular as a confectionery, and explains its widespread use in the United States in tobacco and snuff.

The sequel to this history of ancient lineage, whereby licorice leapt to the fore as one of the most valuable of modern drugs, is one of the most intriguing who-done-its of modern times. During World War II a Dutch doctor, Dr. F. E. Revers, noticed that some of his patients with peptic ulcer were doing particularly well. The one thing these patients had in common was that they were taking a preparation supplied by a local pharmacy. This preparation, he found, contained the equivalent of 40 percent of powdered licorice extract.

Why licorice should be of value in the treatment of peptic ulcer he knew not, but he decided to find out. This he did and, to cut a long story short, the upshot was the synthesis from glycyrrhizin of a substance known as carbenoxolone. This has been described by an extremely knowledgeable doctor in this field as "one of the most significant contributions to the treatment of gastric ulcer for fifty years," while another expert has described it as "the first drug which convincingly has been shown to accelerate the healing of chronic gastric ulcer. To say that it melts away ulcers would be an exaggeration. To say that it considerably facilitates the healing process and enables patients to be treated as outpatients and not in hospital is a fair comment."

Among the 1800 species of plants with medicinal or toxic properties which, according to the Indian Council of Scientific and Industrial Research, are known to grow in India (and this, it is stressed, is a minimum figure) is one know as *Rauvolfia serpentina: Rauvolfia* in honor of Leonard Rauwolf, the distinguished sixteenth-century physician-botanist; *serpentina* because of the snake-like appearance of its root. (Incidentally on the principle of the Paracelsian Doctrine of Signatures, it was this snake-like appearance that dictated its use in the treatment of snakebite.)

Its major traditional use, however, dating back several thousand years was as a soother of the mind and an antidote to lunacy. So incorporated had it become into the folklore of the country that it was regularly chewed by the holy men of India seeking tranquillity for their meditations, and Mahatma Gandhi is said to have been a regular drinker of a tea made from it. Gradually, over the years, it became a common prescription for all sorts of mental diseases. When in the post-1918 era Indian chemists began to analyze it and isolate its active constituents, these were ever more widely used for their characteristic tranquillizing and relaxing effects. Over the course of time Indian doctors working with mentally disturbed patients noticed

Rauvolfia serpentina, India's major contribution to modern medicine. One of the traditional remedies for soothing the troubled mind; modern research has confirmed this age-old claim. With this tranquilizing action it combines a valuable action reducing high blood pressure.

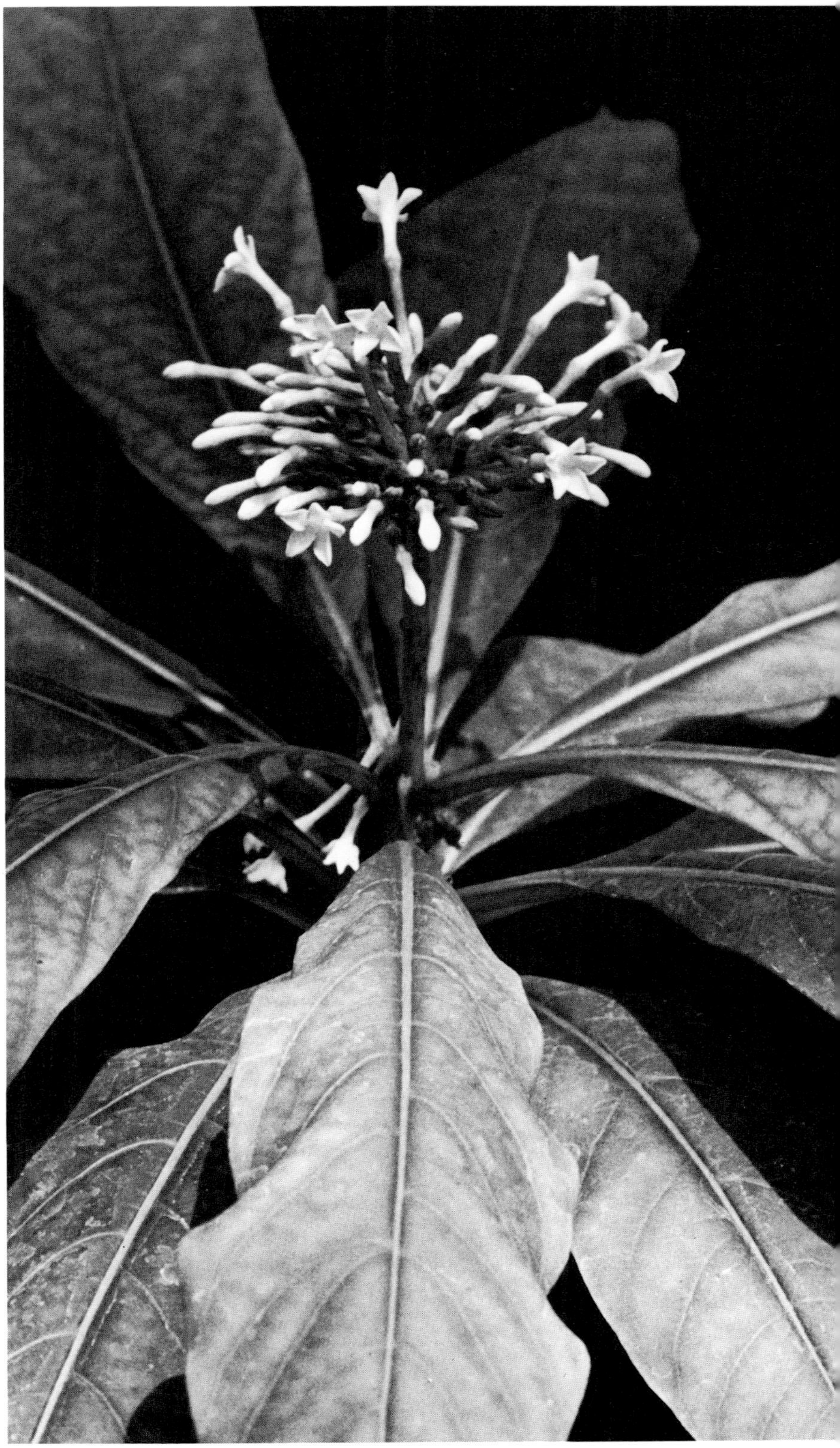

that *Rauvolfia* often produced a lowering of blood pressure, and by the 1940s, it has been estimated, at least a million Indians were being treated with *Rauvolfia* for high blood pressure.

None of this aroused any interest in western medical circles, but in 1949 the *British Heart Journal* published an article by Dr. Rustom Jal Vakil, the distinguished Indian cardiologist, in which he reported that 44 percent of his patients with high blood pressure showed a definite lowering of it when given *Rauvolfia.* This report was read by Dr. Robert W. Wilkins, Chief of the Hypertension Clinic of the Massachusetts General Hospital, Boston, who in due course commented that their "clinical experiences with *Rauvolfia* preparations have taught us that they are more than just further additions to the rapidly growing list of hypotensive agents.... Current indications are that these preparations may find their chief usefulness in many psychoneuroses and tension states, in addition to essential hypertension.... Its most beneficial effect is to decrease 'neurotic' symptoms in all patients and to lower the blood pressure, particulary in young labile hypertensive subjects with tachycardia" (a rapid pulse).

This unleashed the floodgates of the pharmaceutical industry, whose scouts started scouring the earth for *Rauvolfia.* So locust-like were they that they practically cleared every single plant out of India, thereby forcing the Indian government to ban its export. Fortunately it was soon found to be fairly widely scattered throughout the tropics, particularly *Rauvolfia serpentina* in India, Burma, Thailand, Malaysia, and Java, and *Rauvolfia vomitoria,* or African *Rauvolfia,* in tropical Africa.

It is not only in human medicine, however, that *Rauvolfia* is proving of value. The aging male turkey is liable to develop high blood pressure, which may prove fatal by rupturing the aorta, the main artery leading from the heart to the circulatory system. Whether this be the price he pays

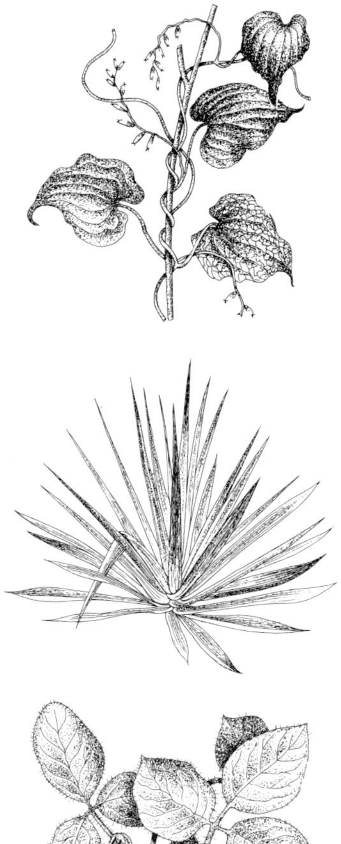

For the production of the steroid group of drugs, which include cortisone, and the constituents of the contraceptive pill, we are dependent on herbs. Without plants such as yams, sisal, soya bean, and fenugreeek, the production of the steroid drugs now playing such an important role in medicine and in helping to prevent a world population explosion would be impossible.

for the outbursts of temper to which he is subject, is an open question, but it can result in serious economic loss. An enterprising American veterinarian therefore had the bright idea of adding *Rauvolfia,* with its two-pronged action as a hypotensive drug and a tranquilizer, to the drinking water of turkeys. His idea worked. It lowered the blood pressure and reduced mortality, which was the main thing, but alas, it did not apparently moderate their outbursts of wild rage.

The publication from the Mayo Clinic, in 1949, of the report of the dramatic effects of cortisone in the alleviation of rheumatoid arthritis unleashed such a torrent of interest as has seldom been experienced in the history of medicine. The problem about cortisone from the point of view of the pharmaceutical industry was the difficulty in synthesizing it, and it soon became clear that the only solution to the problem was to try and find some source in Nature from which it could be made. The obvious source was the group of steroidal saponins, as they are known. These, incidentally, are the materials from which the sex hormones incorporated in the contraceptive pill are synthesized.

In due course, and after the pharmaceutical industry learned many a salutary lesson the hard way, a satisfactory source of this vital precursor was found in the yams, or *Dioscoreae,* of Mexico. For long a staple food on account of their high starch content, these Mexican yams, and many of the other six hundred species, are today the most important source of raw material for the world's steroidal industry. Thus, of the 1000 tons of raw steroid used in 1973, 77 percent came from plant sources (50 percent from Mexico, 15 percent from the United States, 6 percent from Africa, 5 percent from China, and 1 percent from India), 10 percent from animal sources, and the remainder from total synthesis.

Other herbal sources of steroids include fenugreek seed, sisal, and soya bean *(Glycine soja).* The most important of these is sisal *(Agave sisalana),* from which a sapogenin is obtained which is converted into sex hormones in Britain and Italy, and is providing a most helpful addition to the income of East Africa. Fenugreek *(Trigonella foenumgraecum)* is not such a lucrative source of sex hormone precursors, but it has an interesting history in this context. One of its many medicinal reputations is as a stimulant of lactation and for what has been described as the "encouragement of an alluring roundness of the breast." For this latter purpose it has long been used by the ladies of the harems of North Africa and the Middle East. Is it possible that there is an association between this reputed action on the breast and its current reputation as a source of the sex hormones? Truth is often stranger than fiction.

These are but a few examples of the many valuable drugs that we have obtained from herbs, but they are sufficient to indicate the wealth of potential healing riches that Nature can provide if only we shall mend our ways. Instead of playing what has been described as molecular roulette with synthetic substances in highly mechanized computerized research ivory towers in the hope that "something will turn up," the pharmaceutical industry must give much more attention to the study and development of herbs that heal. What is wanted is that the research worker should study herbs that are known to be effective in certain diseases, and with that information as a starting point, then proceed to synthesize modifications in the hope that they will be more effective, or have a wider range of action, than the original herb.

How this should be done must vary according to circumstances, but many a useful lesson could be learned from the Orient and from the other side of the Iron Curtain. In China, for instance, where an interesting merging of traditional and western medicine is taking place, as the country emerges from its long self-imposed quarantine of the Mao period, an intensive attack is being made on this problem of

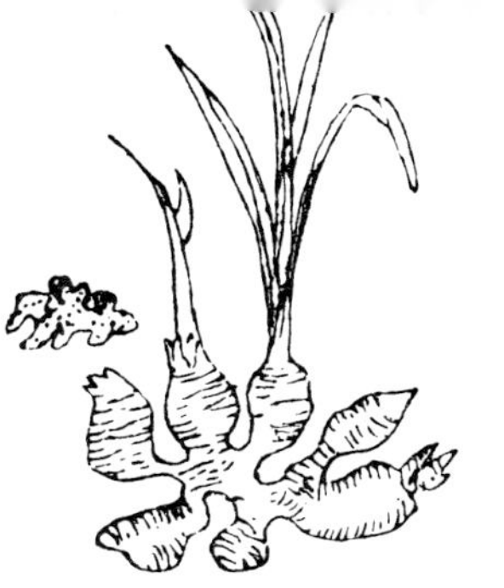

This lovely old drawing of *Zingiber officinale,* the plant from which we get ginger, typifies how old herbal remedies still play a useful part in alleviating at least some of the ills to which man is heir.

how best to utilize the therapeutic value of the country's vast herbal riches. In *China Medicine as We Saw It,* a publication of the John E. Fogarty International Center for Advanced Study in the Health Sciences, Dr. W. Stuart Maddin has commented: "Throughout China a very high priority has been accorded research efforts into the medical use of herbs. Teams of experts, using pharmaceutical assay equipment, are conducting tests in the search for new and better remedies." An interesting point he makes is that "there is little time for backtracking. Although some researchers are seeking specific answers to explain the curative qualities of certain plant substances, most, which have survived the test of centuries, are being left alone." The scope on which this research work is being made is illustrated by the fact that there are fifty research institutes on traditional herbal drugs in China.

That there is some "backtracking," and that this is turning up interesting facts is illustrated by an excerpt from a Chinese brochure quoted by Dr. Maddin: "Experimental workers, in the investigation of the pharmacological actions of Chinese herbs, have ascertained preliminarily that the herbs commonly used for treating acute abdominal diseases possess the properties of arresting the growth of bacteria, reducing inflammation, promoting bile secretion, regulating gastro-intestinal peristalsis, increasing blood flow and lowering capillary permeability of intestines. Pharmacologists have made a variety of new preparations of herb medicines with better therapeutic effect and greater convenience..."

Here then is the two-pronged attack that we in the occident should emulate: a careful, detailed, and systematic investigation of those herbal remedies already in use, and an equally systematic investigation of those herbs that have so far been ignored. In this research, cooperation is essential between orthodox medicine and herbal medicine.

For too long these two advocates of the healing art have been at daggers drawn. To apportion blame for this unfortunate state of affairs is irrelevant. There have been faults on both sides. Not the least of these have been the extravagant claims made by herbalists for their wares. There is an old tradition, dating back to the "quacks" of the middle ages vending their "wonder drugs" to goggle-eyed peasants on market days, of grossly over stated claims made for their medicaments—a tradition that was taken up enthusiastically by the proprietary-medicine manufacturers of the last century on both sides of the Atlantic. Today, however, herbalists are putting their house in order and, largely through the intermediary of pharmacognosists, are showing a welcome desire to cooperate with the medical profession.

This is a move that should be actively welcomed by the medical profession. For too long have the more academically minded among them pooh-poohed the claims of the herbalists—often with a superciliousness compounded of ignorance and rudeness. Granted that many of the vaunted herbal remedies are merely placebos, but this is no criticism of them. Placebos have an important part to play in the healing art—as every experienced clinician is the first to admit. Indeed, on not a few occasions they are more effective, and certainly safer, than their potent analogues. Where so many herbalists have gone astray is in not admitting—as the wise experienced doctor does—that the benefit following the use of the herb (or medicine) in question is a placebo effect.

Even when orthodox medicine has taken an interest in herbs, all too often they have gone about it in the wrong way. With their blinkered, orthodox approach to the problem they have overlooked the elementary facts of Nature. Two classical examples of this have been described in this chapter: the cases of digitalis and ergot. The intentions of the research pharmacologists were credible, but they forgot that unbalanced research work on herbs can lead to chaos.

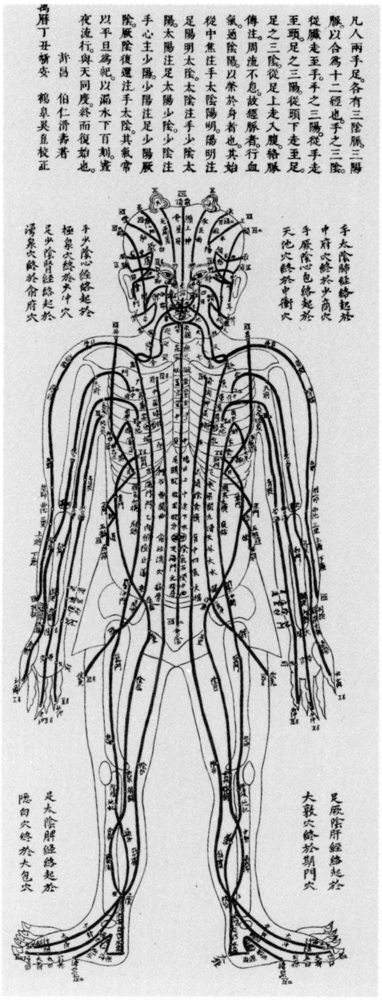

The herbal wisdom of China has done much to enrich the healing art. Today, in her wisdom, China is adapting this ancient learning to modern conditions and linking it with the best of western medicine. It is in the same tradition that western medicine is beginning to appreciate the value of acupuncture. Its rationale, as shown in this drawing, may be obscure, but it works.

His approach must be that of his counterparts in India and Russia, for example, as well as China, where a systematic approach is being made to a scientific study of the healing properties of the multiplicity of herbs and plants growing in their national domains. In both countries this has proved of value. In India, for instance, as already mentioned, it has produced *Rauvolfia,* one of our most valuable tranquilizers and hypotensive agents. In Russia it has produced a series of valuable drugs which have a digitalis-like action in coping with the failing heart, such as lily-of-the-valley, oleander, and Indian hemp.

Whether the attack should be on a wide front or a more narrow one is a question of tactics and priorities. If possible it should be a case of combined operations, with the emphasis on an investgation of all the more reasonable claims made for well-established herbal remedies. To attempt to put all herbs through a routine barrage of screening tests would obviously not be practicable. The start must be made with what qualified herbalists consider to be well-based claims. What is equally important is that the investigations must not be exclusively laboratory-oriented. Careful study in pharmacological laboratories will be necessary, but clinical trials must also be carried out to ensure that mistakes such as those made over ergot are not repeated. No matter what the research wallahs may say, the final and deciding test of a drug—whether herbal or synthetic—depends on what it does in the patient—not in a test tube, culture, or animal. Already much valuable information has been obtained in this way from a study of the effect of herbs in several diseases. For example, in the last decade some 75,000 different plant species have been systematically screened in the United States for anticancer activity. Commenting on this search, one prominent research worker in the field of the chemotherapy of cancer has said: "Recent studies in the isolation and structural elucidation of tumor inhibitors of plant origin are yielding a fascinating array of novel types of growth-inhibitory compounds. There appear to be reasons for confidence that this approach may point the way to useful templates (i.e., molds) for new synthetic approaches to cancer chemotherapy." Here at long last is an indication that the more thoughtful medical reseach workers in our midst are "seeing the light", appreciating that, as has been said, "we live in a natural world that promotes the process of healing, a world that contains herbs and medicinal salts beneficial to man," and beginning to realize the necessity for making a determined effort to discover what Nature has to provide in the way of herbs that heal.

As I have said elsewhere: "The fact that, according to Holy Script, we are made in the image of God is no excuse for ignoring Nature. We are part and parcel of her, and it is by co-operating with her, and exploring her mysteries that we are most likely to live the life we all desire, and to have it more abundantly. This is no idle philosophical fancy, with the slogan of 'back to Nature.' It is an integration of mind, body and spirit which is much more likely to fulfill our hopes and ambitions than the arid atmosphere in which the modern synthesist, whether chemist, pharmacologist, or biologist, spends his life, resembling in many ways the alchemist of old in his futile search for gold. The psalmist's 'riches of the earth' are ours. Why then do we not explore them for what they are producing in the way of herbs that heal?"

William A.R. Thomson, M.D.

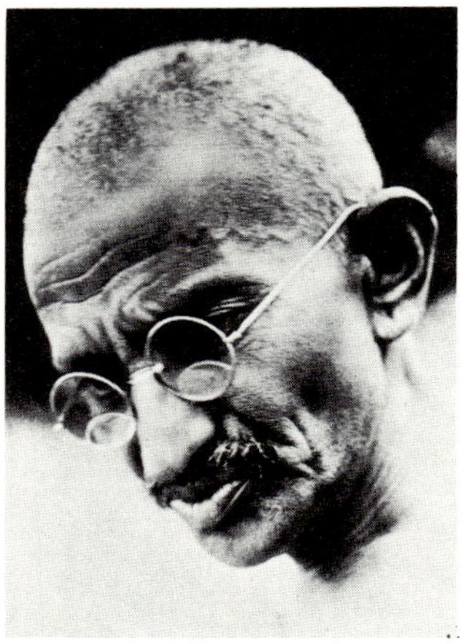

The herbal wisdom of the orient is gradually percolating through to the occident. Tranquillity, one of the main aims of so many of the religions of the East, might well be induced without the aid of herbs, but their use for this purpose was not overlooked. Mahatma Gandhi is said to have been a regular drinker of a tea made from *Rauvolfia serpentina,* the traditional tranquilizer of his country.

The great herbals of Europe from the Middle Ages onward have provided a fund of knowledge and aesthetic pleasure. The title page of John Parkinson's *Paradisi in Sole,* published in 1629, provides a fitting epilogue to this review of medicines from the earth. Here is epitomized, with a pleasing lightness of touch, the integration of man and nature in the provision of herbs that heal.

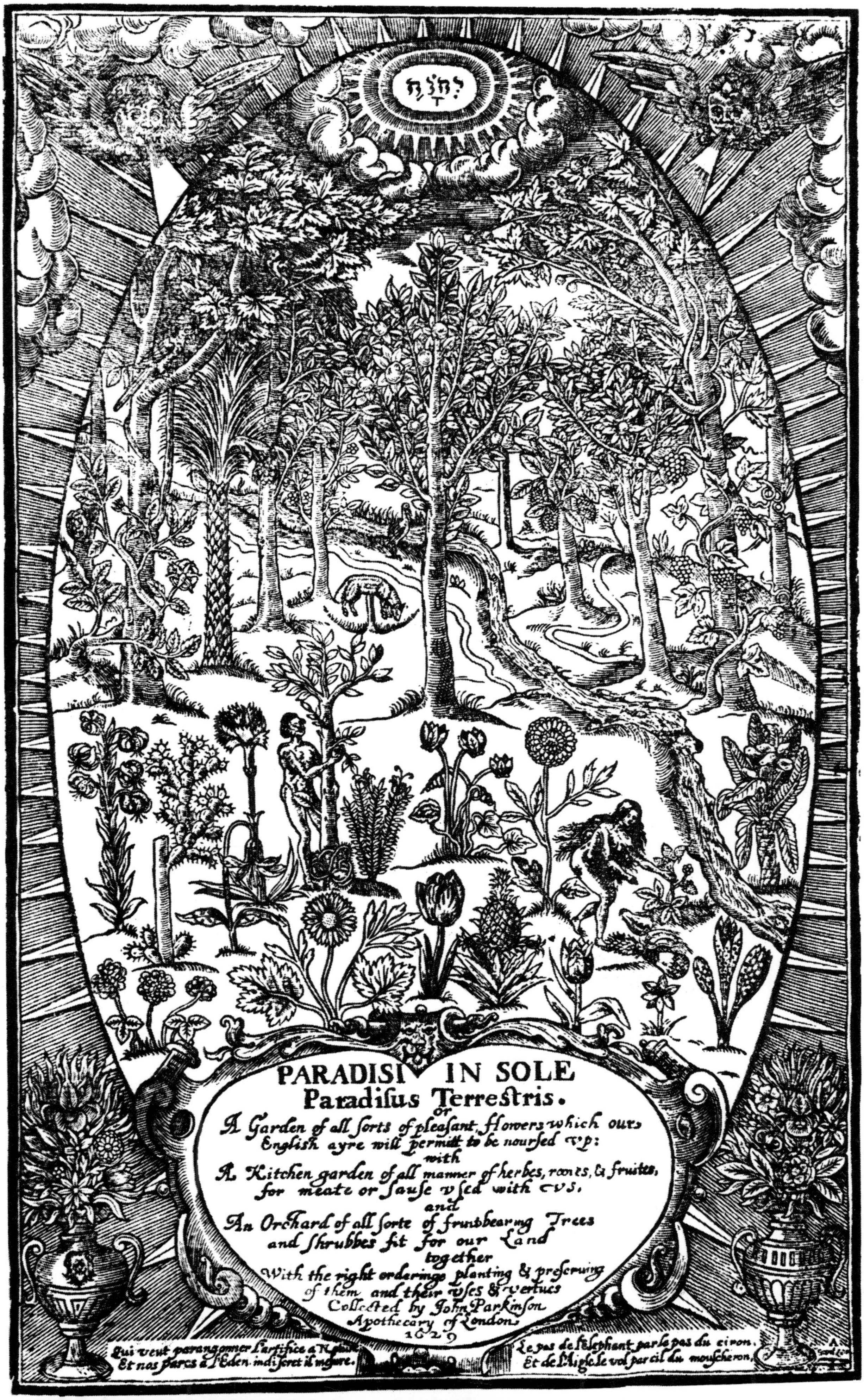
יְהֹוָה
PARADISI IN SOLE
Paradisus Terrestris.
or
A Garden of all sorts of pleasant flowers which our English ayre will permitt to be noursed vp:
with
A Kitchen garden of all manner of herbes, rootes, & fruites, for meate or sause vsed with vs,
and
An Orchard of all sorte of fruitbearing Trees and shrubbes fit for our Land
together
With the right orderinge planting & preseruing of them and their vses & vertues
Collected by John Parkinson
Apothecary of London.
1629
Qui veut parangonner l'artifice a
Et nos parcs a l'Eden indiscret il mesure.
Le pas de l'elephant par le pas du ciron.
Et de l'Aigle le vol par cil du mouscheron.

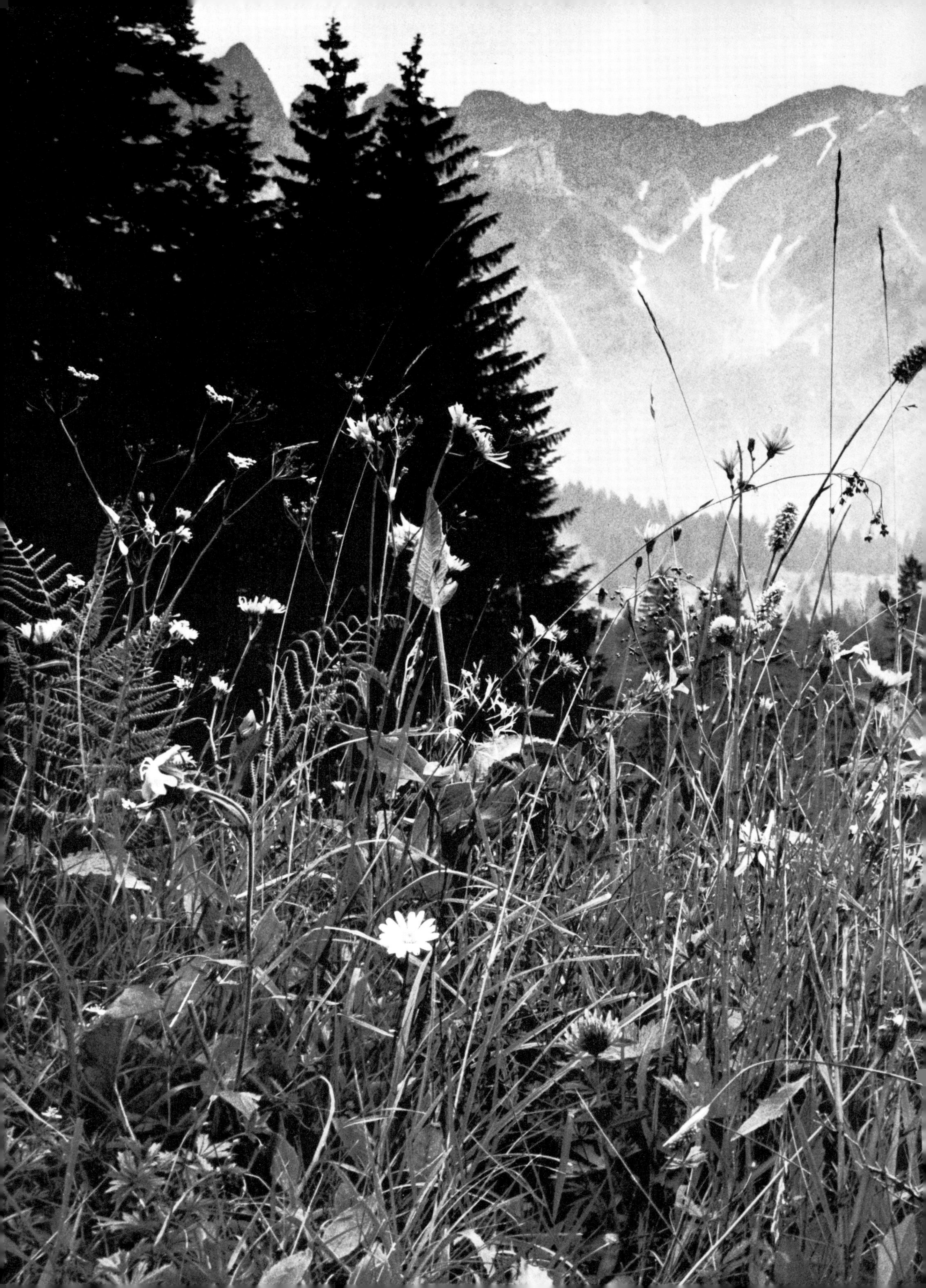

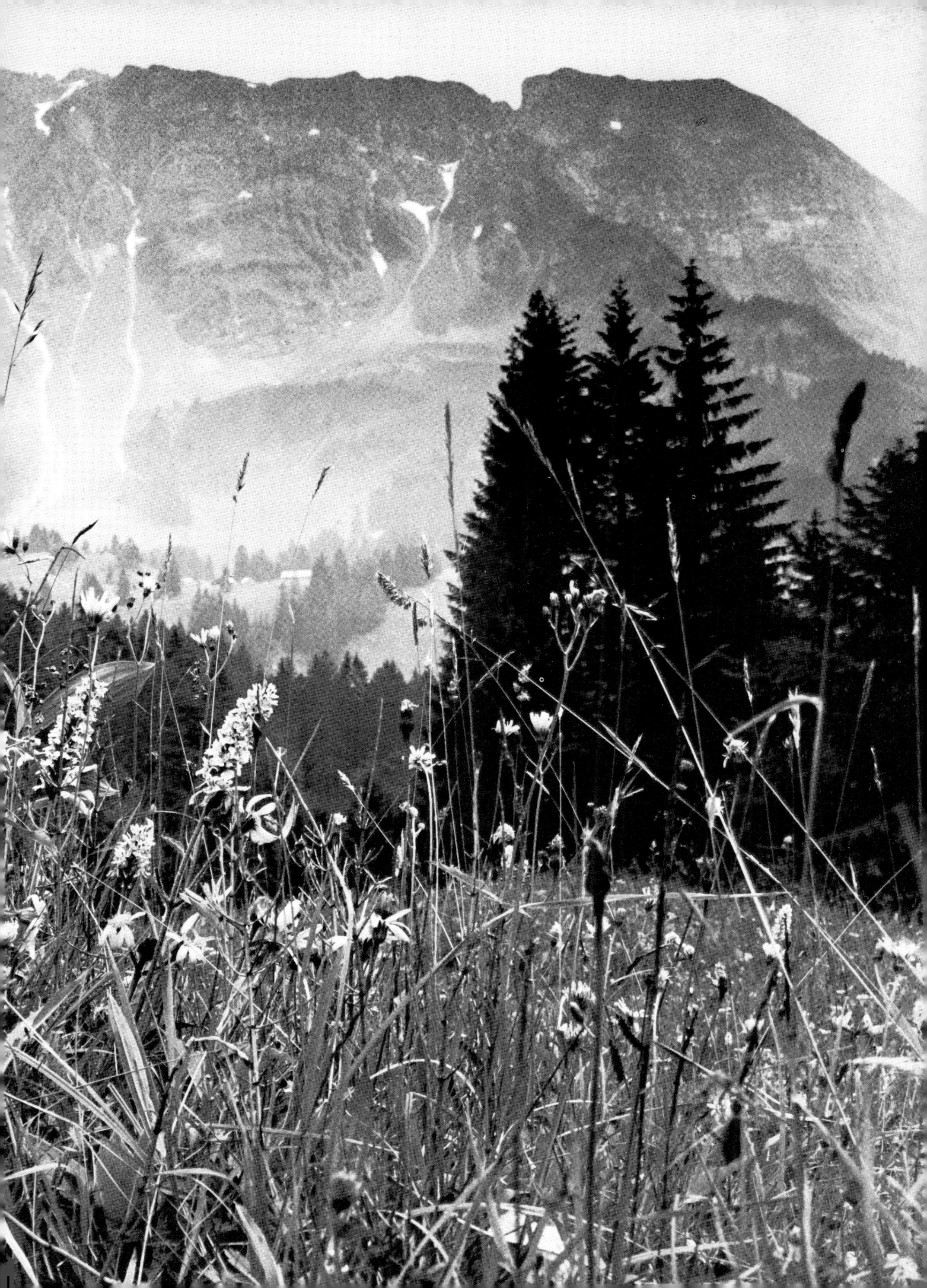

PLANT INDEX
Latin/English
English/Latin

Information given in this index:

• LEXICON REFERENCE NUMBER: Refers to the location of each major plant in the Lexicon on pp. 33–112, where botanical descriptions of the 247 principal plants are given.
• LATIN NAME: Standard botanical name of each plant discussed in this book.
• AUTHOR: Abbreviated name in italics of the botanists responsible for the Latin nomenclature of the plants. The abbreviations are explained in the key below.
• ENGLISH NAME(S): Common English names of the plants. Alternate English names may be found in the English/Latin Plant Index which follows.
• PAGE NUMBERS: Because the Plant Lexicon and Reference Sections I, II, III of this book are arranged in alphabetical sequence, no page references to those sections are given here. Page numbers in italics refer to chapters other than the Lexicon and Reference Sections.

Acharius	Erik Acharius
Ait.	William Aiton
Baill.	Henri Ernest Baillon
Bak.	Edmund G. Baker
Balf.	John H. Balfour
Bartl.	Friedrich Bartling
Bartr.	William Bartram
Beauvois	Ambroise de Beauvois
Benth.	George Bentham
Bernh.	Johann Jacob Bernhardi
Bertol.	Antonio Bertoloni
Blume	Carl Ludwig von Blume
R. Br.	Robert Brown
Britt.	Nathaniel Lord Britton
Brot.	Felix Brotello
Buch.-Ham.	C. Francis Buchanan (Lord Hamilton)
Cham.	Ludolf Adalbert von Chamisso
Choisy	Jacques Denis Choisy
J. Coult.	John Merle Coulter
DC.	Augustin de Candolle
J. F. Ehrh.	Friedrich Ehrhart
Endl.	Stephen Friedrich Endlicher
G. Forst.	Johann Georg Adam Forster
Gaertn.	Joseph Gaertner
P. Gaertn.	Philipp Gottfried Gaertner
Gilib.	Jean Emmanuel Gilibert
C. C. Gmel.	Carl Christian Gmelin
H. B. K.	Friedrich Wilhelm von Humboldt, Aimé Bonpland, and Carl Kunth
Hayne	Friedrich Gottlob Hayne
Hemsl.	William B. Hemsley
A. W. Hill	Arthur William Hill
J. Hill	John Hill
Hoffm.	Johann Joseph Hoffmann
Huds.	William Hudson
Jacq.	Nickolaus Joseph von Jacquin
King	George King
W. D. J. Koch	Wilhelm Daniel Joseph Koch
Körte	Franz Körte
L.	Carolus Linnaeus (Carl von Linné)
Labill.	Jacques de La Billardière
Lam.	Jean Baptiste de Lamarck
Lem.	Charles Antoine Lemaire
L'Hér.	Charles Louis L'Héritier de Brutelle
Liebl.	Franz Kaspar Lieblein
Link	Johann Heinrich Link
Mattuschka	Heinrich Gottfried von Mattuschka
Maxim.	Carl Johann Maximowicz
Medicus	Friedrich Casimir Medicus
Mill.	Philip Miller
Moench	Conrad Moench
Mol.	Juan Ignacio Molina
Nees	Christian Nees von Esenbeck
Nutt.	Thomas Nuttall
Nyman	Carl Fredrik Nyman
Oliv.	Daniel Oliver
Pall.	Peter Simon Pallas
Pav.	José Antonio Pavón
Perrine	Henry Perrine
Pers.	Christiaan Henrik Persoon
Raf.	Constantine Samuel Rafinesque
Räuschel	Ernst Adolf Räuschel
Rchb.f.	Heinrich Gustav Reichenbach
A. Rich	Achille Richard
Roscoe	Wilham Roscoe
Rose	Joseph Nelson Rose
Roth	Albrecht Wilhelm Roth
Ruiz	Hipólito Ruiz Lopez
Scherb.	Johannes Scherbius
Schott	Heinrich Wilhelm Schott
Schweigger	August Friedrich Schweigger
Scop.	Giovanni Antonio Scopoli
Small	John Kunkel Small
K. Spreng.	Kurt Polycarp Joachim Sprengel
Stapf	Otto Stapf
St.-Hil.	Augustin de Saint-Hilaire
Thunb.	Carl Pehr Thunberg
Tulasne	Edmond Louis René Tulasne
Vahl	Martin Hendriksen Vahl
Warb.	Otto Warburg
Wiggers	Friedrich Heinrich Wiggers
Willd.	Carl Ludwig Willdenow

Latin/English

35 Berberis vulgaris, *L.*	(European or common) Barberry, *152*
36 Betula pendula, *Roth*	Birch, *156*
B. pubescens, *J. F. Ehrh.*	Birch
Borago officinalis, *L.*	Borage, *151, 160*
37 Brassica nigra, *(L.) W. D. J. Koch*	Black mustard
38 Brassica oleracea var. capitata, *L.*	Winter cabbage, *156*
39 Bryonia dioica, *Jacq.*	Red bryony, Wild hop
40 Calendula officinalis, *L.*	Marigold, Pot marigold, *151, 156, 157, 158*
Cannabis sativa, *L.*	Hemp, Marijuana, *15, 139, 140, 141, 194*
41 Capsella bursa-pastoris, *(L.) Medicus*	Shepherd's purse
42 Capsicum annuum, *L.*	Green pepper, Chili pepper
43 Carex arenaria, *L.*	Sedges
44 Carica papaya, *L.*	Papaya
45 Carlina acaulis, *L.*	Carline thistle, *151*
46 Carum carvi, *L.*	Caraway
47 Cassia angustifolia, *Vahl*	(Alexandrian) Senna
48 Castanea sativa, *Mill.*	Spanish or European chestnut
49 Ceanothus americanus, *L.*	New Jersey tea, Redroot
Centaurea solstitialis, *L.*	St. Barnaby's thistle, *137*
50 Centaurium umbellataum, *Gilib.*	Centaury, *156*
51 Cephaelis ipecacuanha, *(Brot.) A. Rich.*	Ipecac, Ipecacuanha, *148*
52 Cetraria islandica, *(L.) Acharius*	Iceland moss
53 Chelidonium majus, *L.*	Celandine, Celandine poppy, *151*
54 Chionanthus virginicus, *L.*	Fringe tree, Old man's beard
Chondodendron tomentosum	Curare, *185*
55 Chondrus crispus, *(L.) Stackhouse*	Irish moss
56 Chrysanthemum vulgare, *(L.) Bernh.*	(Common) Tansy
57 Cichorium intybus, *L.*	Chicory, Succory
58 Cimicifuga racemosa, *(L.) Nutt.*	Black cohosh, Black snakeroot
59 Cinchona succirubra, *Pav.*	Yellowbark cinchona, *12, 15, 148, 187*
60 Cinnamomum zeylanicum, *Blume*	Cinnamon
61 Citrus aurantium, *L.*	Bitter orange, Sour orange, *151*
62 Claviceps purpurea, *Tulasne*	Ergot, *142, 143, 147, 186, 189*
63 Cnicus benedictus, *L.*	Blessed thistle
64 Cochlearia officinalis, *L.*	Scurvy grass, Spoonwort
65 Coffea arabica, *L.*	Coffee, *12*
66 Cola acuminata, *Schott et Endl.*	Cola, *147*
67 Colchicum autumnale, *L.*	Autumn crocus, Meadow saffron
68 Convallaria majalis, *L.*	Lily-of-the-valley, *194*
69 Corydalis cava, *(L.) Schweigger et Körte*	Cordyalis
70 Crataegus oxyacantha, *L.*	(English) Hawthorn, *156*
C. monogyna, *Jacq.*	(English) Hawthorn
71 Cucurbita pepo, *L.*	Pumpkin, Squash
72 Curcuma longa, *L.*	Turmeric
73 Cydonia oblonga, *Mill.*	Quince
74 Cynara scolymus, *L.*	(Globe) Artichoke
75 Cynoglossum officinale, *L.*	Hound's tongue
76 Cytisus scoparius, *(L.) Link*	(Scotch) Broom
77 Datura stramonium, *L.*	Thornapple, Jimsonweed, *148*
Dichroa febrifuga	*141*
78 Digitalis purpurea, *L.*	Foxglove, *11, 13, 14, 15, 142, 144, 186, 187, 188*
D. lanata, *J.F. Ehrh.*	Grecian foxglove, *13, 15*
79 Dioscorea villosa, *L.*	(Wild) Yam, *14, 15*
80 Drosera rotundifolia, *L.*	Sundew
81 Dryopteris filix-mas, *(L.) Schott*	Male fern
82 Echinacea angustifolia, *DC.*	Purple coneflower
83 Ephedra sinica, *Stapf*	Ephedra, Joint pine, *137*
E. distachya, *L.*	Ma-huang, *140–141, 185*
84 Equisetum arvense, *L.*	(Common) Horsetail, Scouring rush, *156, 159*
85 Erigeron canadensis, *L.*	Fleabane, Horseweed
86 Erythroxylum coca, *Lam.*	Coca, *138, 148*
87 Eschscholzia californica, *Cham.*	California poppy
88 Eucalyptus globulus, *Labill.*	Eucalpytus, Blue gum (tree)
89 Eupatorium cannabinum, *L.*	Hemp agrimony
90 Euphrasia rostkoviana, *Hayne*	(Drug) Eyebright
91 Ficus carica, *L.*	(Common) Fig
92 Filipendula ulmaria, *(L.) Maxim.*	Queen-of-the-meadow
93 Foeniculum vulgare, *Mill.*	Fennel, *151, 156, 157*
94 Fragaria vesca, *L.*	(Woodland) Strawberry
Frangula alnus, *Mill.*	Alder buckthorn
95 Fraxinus excelsior, *L.*	Ash
96 Fucus vesiculosus, *L.*	Rockweed
97 Fumaria officinalis, *L.*	Fumitory, Earth smoke

98	Galega officinalis, *L.*	(European) Goat's rue
99	Galeopsis ochroleuca, *Lam.*	Hempnettle
100	Galium odoratum, *(L.) Scop.*	Sweet woodruff
101	Galium verum, *L.*	Bedstraw, Our Lady's bedstraw, *152*
102	Gaultheria procumbens, *L.*	Wintergreen, Teaberry, Checkerberry
103	Gelidium amansii, *Lamoureux*	Agar agar
104	Gelsemium sempervirens, *(L.) Ait.*	Yellow jessamine
105	Gentiana lutea, *L.*	Yellow gentian, Drug gentian, *156*
106	Geranium robertianum, *L.*	Herb robert
107	Geum urbanum, *L.*	Avens, Cloveroot
108	Ginkgo biloba, *L.*	Ginkgo, Maidenhair
109	Glycyrrhiza glabra, *L.*	Licorice, *154, 155, 190*
110	Gossypium herbaceum, *L.*	Cotton
111	Gratiola officinalis, *L.*	Hedge hyssop
112	Guaiacum officinale, *L.*	Lignum vitae
113	Hamamelis virginiana, *L.*	Witch hazel
114	Haronga madagascariensis, *Choisy*	Haronga tree
115	Harpagophytum procumbens, *DC.*	Grapple plant
116	Hedeoma pulegioides, *(L.) Pers.*	American pennyroyal
117	Hedera helix, *L.*	English ivy, *152*
118	Helichrysum arenarium, *(L.) Moench*	Everlasting flower
119	Helleborus niger, *L.*	Black hellebore
120	Herniaria glabra, *L.*	Rupturewort
121	Hibiscus sabdariffa, *L.*	Roselle, Jamaica sorrel
122	Hippophaë rhamnoides, *L.*	Sea buckthorn, *154, 155*
123	Humulus lupulus, *L.*	(Common) Hop
124	Hydnocarpus kurzii, *(King) Warb.*	Chaulmoogra, *141*
125	Hydrastis canadensis, *L.*	Goldenseal
126	Hyoscyamus niger, *L.*	(Black) Henbane
127	Hypericum perforatum, *L.*	Saint John's wort, *156, 157, 158, 159*
128	Ilex aquifolium, *L.*	European holly
129	Ilex paraguariensis, *St.-Hil.*	Paraguay tea, Maté
130	Inula helenium, *L.*	Elecampane, Scabwort
	Ipomoea, *L.*	Morning glory genus, *146, 147*
	I. violaceae, *L.*	Ololiuqui, *147, 149*
131	Juglans regia, *L.*	English walnut
132	Juniperus communis, *L.*	(Common) Juniper, *159*
133	Krameria triandra, *Ruiz et Pav.*	Peruvian krameria
134	Lamium album, *L.*	White deadnettle, *156*
135	Laurus nobilis, *L.*	Bay
136	Lavandula angustifolia, *Mill.*	(English) Lavender, *151, 156*
137	Leonurus cardiaca, *L.*	(Common) Motherwort
138	Levisticum officinale, *W. D. J. Koch*	Lovage
	Lilium, *L.*	Lily genus, *14*
139	Linum usitatissimum, *L.*	Flax
12	Lippia citriodora, *H. B. K.*	Lemon verbena
140	Lobelia inflata, *L.*	Indian tobacco
	Logania, *R. Br.*	Logania genus, *14*
	Lophophora, *J. Coult.*	Peyote, Mescal button genus, *138, 147*
141	Lycopus virginicus, *L.*	Bugleweed
142	Lythrum salicaria, *L.*	Purple or Spiked loosestrife
143	Malva sylvestris, *L.*	High mallow, Common mallow, *154, 155*
	Mandragora officinalis, *L.*	Mandrake, *139, 141*
144	Marrubium vulgare, *L.*	Horehound
145	Marsdenia cundurango, *Rchb. f.*	Eagle or Condor vine
146	Matricaria chamomilla, *L.*	German or Wild chamomile, *151, 156, 157, 159*
147	Melilotus officinalis, *L. (Pall.)*	Yellow sweetclover
148	Melissa officinalis, *(L.)*	(Common) Balm, *151, 156, 159*
149	Mentha piperita, *L.*	Peppermint, *151, 156, 159*
150	Menyanthes trifoliata, *L.*	Buckbean, Marsh trefoil, *151*
151	Monarda didyma, *L.*	Oswego tea, *35*
	Morus	Mulberry genus, *14*
	Muscari, *Mill.*	Grape hyacinth genus, *137*
152	Nasturtium officinale, *R. Br.*	Watercress, *151, 152*
153	Nerium oleander, *L.*	Oleander, *194*
	Nicotiana, *L.*	Tobacco genus, *146*
154	Olea europaea, *L.*	Olive
155	Ononis spinosa, *L.*	Prickly restharrow
156	Origanum vulgare, *L.*	(Wild) Marjoram, Oregano, *151, 156*
157	Orthosiphon stamineus, *(Thunb.) Bak.*	Java tea
	Paeonia mascula *(L.) Mill.*	Peony, *32*
158	Panax quinquefolius, *L.*	American ginseng
	P. ginseng, *C. A. Mey*	Asiatic ginseng
159	Papaver somniferum, *L.*	Opium poppy, *14, 138, 187, 188, 189*
160	Passiflora incarnata, *L.*	Wild passionflower, Maypop
	Penicillium potatum	Penicillin, *185*

161	Petasites hybridus *(L.) P. Gaertn., B. Mey, & Scherb*	Butterbur, Sweet coltsfoot
162	Petroselinum crispum, *(Mill.) Nyman ex A. W. Hill*	Parsley
163	Peucedanum ostruthium, *(L.) W. D. J. Koch*	Masterwort, Hogfennel
164	Peumus boldus, *Mol.*	Boldo
165	Phaseolus vulgaris, *L.*	(Common) Bean
166	Physostigma venenosum, *Balf.*	Calabar bean, *144, 145*
167	Phytolacca americana, *L.*	Pke, Pokeweed
168	Pilocarpus pennatifolius, *Lem.*	Jaborandi
169	Pimpinella anisum, *L.*	(Common) Anise
170	Pimpinella saxifraga, *L.*	Black caraway
	P. major, *Hudson*	
171	Pinus sylvestris, *L.*	Scotch pine
172	Piper methysticum, *G. Forst.*	Kava, Kava-kava
	Pisum, *L.*	Pea genus, *14*
173	Plantago psyllium, *L.*	Psyllium
174	Plantago lanceolata, *L.*	English plantain, Rib grass, *154, 155, 156*
175	Podophyllum peltatum, *L.*	Mayapple, *144, 145*
176	Polygala senega, *L.*	Seneca snakeroot
177	Polygonum hydropiper, *L.*	Smartweed
178	Polypodium vulgare, *L.*	European polypody, Sweet fern
179	Populus nigra, *L.*	Balsam poplar
180	Potentilla anserina, *L.*	Silverweed, *156*
181	Potentilla erecta, *(L.) Räuschel*	Tormentil
182	Primula veris, *L.*	Cowslip, *154, 155, 156*
	P. elatior, *(L.) J. Hill*	Cowslip
183	Prunus dulcis var. amara, *W. A. Webb*	Bitter almond
184	Prunus serotina, *J. F. Ehrh.*	(Wild) Black cherry
185	Prunus spionsa, *L.*	Blackthorn, Sloe
186	Pulmonaria officinalis, *L.*	Blue lungwort
187	Pulsatilla vulgaris, *Mill.*	Pasque flower
188	Quercus robur, *L.*	Oak
	Q. petraea, *(Mattuschka) Liebl.*	Oak
	Ranunculus, *L.*	Buttercup genus, *14*
189	Rauvolfia serpentina, *(L.) Benth.*	Indian snakeroot, *14, 16, 139, 140, 144, 185, 186, 190–192, 194*
190	Rhamnus frangula, *L.*	Alder buckthorn
191	Rhamnus purshiana, *DC.*	Cascara sagrada, *145*
192	Rheum palmatum, *L.*	(Medicinal) Rhubarb, *141*
	R. officinale, *Baill.*	(Medicinal) Rhubarb
193	Ribes nigrum, *L.*	(European) Black currant
194	Ricinus communis, *L.*	Castor bean
195	Rosa canina, *L.*	Dog rose, *152, 156, 159*
196	Rosmarinus officinalis, *L.*	Rosemary, *156, 159*
197	Rubia tinctorum, *L.*	(Common) Madder, *14, 15*
198	Rubus fruticosus, *L.*	European blackberry, Bramble
199	Rumex crispus, *L.*	Curled dock, Yellow dock
	R. acetosa, *L.*	Common sorrel
	R. alpinus, *L.*	Monk's rhubarb
200	Ruta graveolens, *L.*	(Common) Rue
201	Salix alba, *L.*	White willow
202	Salvia officinalis, *L.*	Garden sage, *156*
203	Sambucus ebulus, *L.*	Dwarf elder
204	Sambucus nigra, *L.*	European elder, *152, 156*
205	Sanguinaria canadensis, *L.*	Bloodroot
206	Sanicula europaea, *L.*	Snakeroot, Sanicle, *156*
207	Saponaria officinalis, *L.*	Soapwort, Bouncing bet
76	Sarothamnus scoparius, *L.*	(Scotch) Broom
208	Sassafras albidum *(Nutt.) Nees*	(Common) Sassafras
	Schefflera, *L.*	Rubber tree genus, *12*
209	Scopolia carniolica, *Jacq.*	Scopolia
210	Scrophularia nodosa, *L.*	Figwort, *14*
211	Sedum acre, *L.*	Mossy stonecrop
212	Selenicereus grandiflorus, *(L.) Britt. et Rose*	Night-blooming cereus
	Senecio, *L.*	Groundsel genus, *137*
213	Senecio fuchsii, *C. C. Gmel.*	Alpine ragwort
214	Serenoa repens, *(Bartr.) Small*	Saw palmetto
215	Silybum marianum, *(L.) Gaertn.*	Milk thistle
216	Smilax utilis, *Hemsl.*	Sarsaparilla, *146*
217	Solanum dulcamara, *L.*	European bittersweet, Bitter nightshade
218	Solidago virgaurea, *L.*	Goldenrod
219	Sophora japonica, *L.*	Chinese pagoda tree
220	Strophanthus kombé, *Oliv.*	Strophanthus, *144, 145*
	Strychnos, *L.*	Strychnos genus, *147*
221	Strychnos nux-vomica, *L.*	Nux-vomica
222	Swertia chirata, *Buch.-Ham.*	Chirata
223	Symphytum officinale, *L.*	(Common) Comfrey
224	Taraxacum officinale, *Wiggers*	Dandelion, *151, 152, 159*
225	Teucrium chamaedrys, *L.*	Germander

English/Latin

This list includes common and alternate English names of the 247 principal healing plants treated in this book. For each plant the Lexicon plant number and the Latin name are also given. For page references, see the Latin/English Plant Index preceding.

SELECT BIBLIOGRAPHY: FURTHER READING

Bailey, Liberty, and Bailey, Ethel: *Hortus Third: A Concise Dictionary of Plants Cultivated in the United States and Canada.* New York: Macmillan, 1976. London: Collier Macmillan, 1976.

Debuigne, Gérard: *Larousse des Plantes qui Guérissent.* New ed. Paris and New York: Larousse, 1974.

Flück, Hans: *Medicinal Plants and Their Uses.* Translated by J. M. Rowson. London: W. Foulsham and Co., 1976.

Grieve, M.: *A Modern Herbal,* 2 vols. Reprint. New York: Hafner Press, 1974.

Loewenfeld, Claire, and Back, Phillipa: *The Complete Book of Herbs and Spices.* Newton Abbott, England: David and Charles, 1974. Boston: Little, Brown, 1976.

Mességué, Maurice: *Of Men and Plants.* London: Weidenfeld and Nicolson, 1972. New York: Macmillan, 1973.

Mez-Mangold, Lydia: *A History of Drugs.* Basel, Switzerland: F. Hoffman-La Roche, 1971.

Morton, Julia F.: *Major Medicinal Plants.* Springfield, Ill.: Charles C. Thomas Publishers, 1977.

Quinn, Joseph R., ed.: *China's Medicine as We Saw It.* Washington, D.C.: U.S. Department of Health, Education and Welfare, Public Health Service, National Institute of Health, 1975. DHEW Publication No. (NIH) 75-684.

Sanecki, Kay N.: *The Complete Book of Herbs.* London: Macdonald, 1974.

Swain, Tony, ed.: *Plants in the Development of Modern Medicine.* Cambridge, Mass.: Harvard University Press, 1972.

Thomson, William A. R.: *Herbs That Heal.* London: A. & C. Black, 1976. New York: Charles Scribner's Sons, 1977.

Usher, George: *A Dictionary of Plants Used by Man.* London: Constable, 1974. New York: Hafner Press, 1974.

PICTURE CREDITS

Academisch Historisch Museum, Leiden: 13 (bottom)
Ägyptisches Museum Staatliche Museen Preuss. Kulturbesitz, Berlin. Photo: Jürgen Liepe: 139 (top, left)
Bayerische Staatsbibliothek, Munich: 137 (top)
Bodleian Library, Oxford: 7
Eugen Bossard, Zurich: 46 No. 29, 51 No. 48, 60 No. 76, 68 No. 105, 100 No. 215, 104 No. 225
Botanical Museum, Harvard University, Ware Collection of Plaschka Glass Models of Plants: 15 (top)
Lisbeth Bührer, Lucerne: 9 (bottom), 45 No. 26, 111 No. 246, 150, 151 (right), 153, 154, 155, 158 (top), 160
Franz Coray, Lucerne. Artwork in Plant Lexicon: Nos. 4, 10, 12, 14, 20, 21, 27, 36, 49, 54, 58, 66, 72, 79, 83, 85, 88, 89, 114, 115, 116, 118, 122, 124, 141, 145, 151, 157, 158, 172, 177, 184, 185, 189, 208, 213, 214, 219, 220, 222, 229, 231, 233, 239, 241
Fritz-Martin Engel, Ansbach: 189 (top)
Richard Erdoes, New York: 146 (top center)
Peter T. Furst: 146 (top right), 147 (right)
Giraudon, Paris: 140 (top), 143 (top)
Dr. Albert Hofmann, Burg i. Leimental: 149, 190 (top)
Hans Leuenberger, Yerdon: 144 (top)
Louvre, Antiquité Orientale, Paris. Photo: Service photographique de la Réunion des Musées nationaux: 138 (bottom)
Magnum Photo Library Print, New York. Photo: John Nance: 145 (top)
Mansell Collection, London: 12, 141 (top), 188 (left).
National Archaelogical Museum, Athens. Photo: TAP Service: 141 (center, left)
National Library of Medicine, Bethesda: 140 (bottom, left)
Dr. Allen Paterson, Curator of the Chelsea Physic Garden: 13 (top)
Peter, Teufen: 196/197
Popperfoto, London: 186 (top), 194
Prof. Dr. W. Rauh, Institut für Systematische Botanik und Pflanzengeographie der Universität Heidelberg: 6, 39 No. 5, 48 No. 38, 53 No. 55, 58 No. 71, 59 No. 74, 61 No. 81, 63 No. 87, 67 Nos. 102, 103, 69 No. 108, 72 No. 119, 75 No. 129, 82/83 No. 153, 91 No. 183, 96 No. 199, 98 No. 205, 99 No. 209, 111 No. 245, 142 (top), 144 (left), 191
Publishers Archives: 10/11, 151 (left)
Ringier Bilderdienst, Zurich: 147 (top, right)
Städelsches Kunstinstitut, Frankfurt am Main: 186 (left).
Traugott Steger, Emmenbrücke: 85 No. 160
Thames and Hudson, London: 140
Bruno Vonarburg, Lustmühle: 34, 50 No. 45, 112

PUBLISHED WORKS

Arber, Agnes: *Herbals, Their Origin and Evolution,* Cambridge University Press, 1953: 17
Artseny-Gewassen, Vols. I, V, C. J. Sepp en Zoon, Amsterdam, MDCCXCVI, MDCCC: Plant Lexicon: Nos. 106, 120, 161
Artus, *Hand-Atlas,* Vols. I+II: Plant Lexicon: Nos. 3, 7, 9, 11, 15, 18, 32, 33, 42, 46, 51, 52, 67, 68, 73, 86, 91, 93, 99, 110, 131, 148, 149, 162, 165, 197, 202, 204, 232, 243
Biedermann, Hans: *Altmexikos Heilige Bücher,* Akademische Druck- und Verlagsanstalt, Graz, 1971: 146 (bottom)
Brandon, S. G. F.: *Man and God in Art and Ritual,* Charles Scribner's Sons, New York, 1975: 8
Fuchs, Leonard: *New Kreuterbuch,* 1543, Reprint 1964 by Verlag Konrad Kölbl, Munich: 5, 11, 14
Hayne, Dr. Friedrich Gottlob: *Getreue Darstellung und Beschreibung der in der Arzneykunde gebräuchlichen Gewächse,* Vols. V, VI, Berlin, 1817: Plant Lexicon: Nos. 173, 174
Heilmann, Karl Eugen: *Kräuterbücher in Bild und Geschichte,* Verlag Konrad Kölbl, Munich, 1966: 113
Lehner, Ernst and Johanna: *Folklore & Odysseys of Food and Medicinal Plants,* Tudor Publishing Company, 1962: 145 (bottom), 195
Losch, F.: *Les Plantes Médicinales,* Biel: 35. Plant Lexicon: Nos. 2, 6, 8, 22, 30, 39, 57, 61, 62, 63, 80, 90, 92, 97, 105, 107, 111, 123, 130, 132, 142, 147, 156, 159, 163, 169, 171, 178, 180, 182, 186, 193, 194, 203, 206, 217, 218, 227, 228, 234, 235, 237, 242
Medicina Antiqua, *Codex Vindobonensis* 93, Österreichische Nationalbibliothek, Vienna, Vollständige Faksimileausgabe Akademische Druck- und Verlagsanstalt, Graz, 1971: 141 (center, right)
Mez-Mangold, Lydia: *Aus der Geschichte des Medikamentes,* 1971: 139 (top right), 152
Naturgeschichte des Pflanzenreichs nach Prof. Dr. G. H. von Schuberts: Lehrbuch der Pflanzengeschichte, Verlag von J. F. Schreiber, Esslingen bei Stuttgart, 1887: Plant Lexicon Nos. 1, 13, 19, 25, 28, 31, 35, 37, 40, 41, 43, 50, 56, 64, 65, 69, 70, 75, 78, 84, 94, 95, 96, 100, 101, 117, 126, 127, 128, 134, 137, 144, 150, 152, 154, 155, 167, 187, 195, 198, 201, 207, 210, 211, 230, 236, 240
G. Pabst: *Köhler's Medizinal-Pflanzen,* Vols. I, II, III, Verlag von Fr. Eugen Köhler, 1887: 187. Plant Lexicon: Nos. 16, 23, 24, 34, 44, 47, 53, 59, 60, 77, 104, 109, 112, 113, 125, 133, 135, 136, 138, 139, 140, 143, 146, 164, 166, 168, 170, 175, 176, 179, 181, 188, 190, 191, 192, 196, 200, 216, 221, 223, 224, 226, 238, 244, 247
Porta, J. B.: *Phytognomica octo libris contenta,* Naples, 1558: 9 (top), 143 (bottom)
Ronan, Colin: *The Forgotten Science of the Ancient World: Lost Discoveries,* McGraw-Hill, New York, 1973: 141 (center, second from right)
Schöffer, Peter: *Der Gart,* Mainz, 1485: 142 (left)
Severin, Timothy: *Vanishing Primitive Man,* American Heritage Publishing, New York, 1973: 147 (top left)
Strabo, Walahfrid: *"Hortulus." Vom Gartenbau,* first published by Joachim von Watt (Vadianus): 161
Wallnöfer, Dr. Heinrich, and Anna von Rattauscher: *Der goldene Schatz der chinesischen Medizin,* Schuler Verlagsgesellschaft, Stuttgart, 1959: 193
Zornn, Bartholomaeum: *Herbarium,* Thomae Panco VII, D, Cologne, 1673: 32